PERIPHERAL VASCULAR SONOGRAPHY

A Practical Guide

PERIPHERAL VASCULAR SONOGRAPHY

A Practical Guide

JOSEPH F. POLAK, M.D.

Associate Professor
Department of Radiology
Harvard Medical School
Brigham and Women's Hospital
Boston, Massachusetts

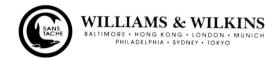

WILLIAMS & WILKINS
BALTIMORE · HONG KONG · LONDON · MUNICH
PHILADELPHIA · SYDNEY · TOKYO

Editor: Timothy H. Grayson
Managing Editor: Marjorie Kidd Keating
Copy Editor: Thomas Lehr
Designer: Norman W. Och
Illustration Planner: Ray Lowman
Production Coordinator: Kathleen C. Millet

Copyright © 1992
Williams & Wilkins
428 East Preston Street
Baltimore, Maryland 21202, USA

Printed in the United States of America

Library of Congress Cataloging-in-Publication Data

Polak, Joseph F.
    Peripheral vascular sonography : a practical guide / Joseph F.
Polak.
      p.   cm.
    Includes bibliographical references and index.
    ISBN 0-683-06914-4
    1. Blood-vessels—Ultrasonic imaging. I. Title.
    [DNLM: 1. Vascular Diseases—ultrasonography—handbooks.   WG 39
P762p]
RC691.6.U47P65 1992
616.1'307'543
DNLM/DLC
for Library of Congress
                                  91-19081
                                  CIP

92 93 94 95
2 3 4 5 6 7 8 9 10

To my wife,

Jo-Anne,

for her continued help and support

PREFACE

The chapters that constitute this handbook describe some of the various uses of peripheral vascular sonography for the diagnosis of venous and arterial diseases of the upper and lower extremities. The increasing role of ultrasound in the diagnosis of vascular disease has evolved concurrently with the increased dissemination of other noninvasive technologies, such as x-ray computed tomography and magnetic resonance imaging.

Although sonographic imaging of the aorta, vena cava, and varied vascular structures of the abdomen and pelvis can be performed, this handbook concentrates on the applications to which sonography is best suited, i.e., imaging of the vessels of the arms, legs, and neck. Magnetic resonance imaging, already an effective means of evaluating the major vessels of the body, is gaining importance for the evaluation of the peripheral vessels. Its effectiveness, as well as that of computed tomography, will ultimately need to be compared to that of sonography, using the more traditional venographic and arteriographic studies as the "gold standard" examination.

What are the advantages of sonography, especially duplex and more recently color flow imaging, compared to other noninvasive imaging modalities? The sonographic approach is portable, relatively inexpensive, capable of imaging structure and determining blood flow, and easily adapted to the performance of serial examinations in a given patient. This enables the physician to serially monitor patients for evidence of disease progression, to better decide on the timing of an intervention, and to monitor the effects of the intervention. These advantages apply to the evaluation of patients with both thromboembolic disease of the veins and obstructive atherosclerotic lesions of the arteries.

Sonography has been shown to be an effective and accurate screening modality for the diagnosis of venous thrombosis. This role is broadening to include monitoring of patients undergoing different therapeutic regimens. An example of a question that can be answered by sonography is whether the chronic morbidity noted following the successful treatment of acute deep vein thrombosis can be decreased by earlier and more aggressive treatment. Early thrombus resorption using thrombolytic agents such as urokinase, streptokinase, or t-PA may limit damage to the endothelial lining and the valves of the veins and decrease the incidence of chronic venous insufficiency. It is only by serially monitoring changes in the extent and character of the thrombosis that such a question will be answered.

Sonography is also used to help select among the specific therapeutic options available to treat peripheral and carotid artery disease. It can also noninvasively monitor the effects of fibrointimal hyperplasia, a process affecting arteries that have been subjected to endarterectomy, atherectomy, or angioplasty, as well as the veins that are used for arterial bypass surgery. This pathologic entity, which is distinct from atherosclerosis, causes progressive stenosis that ultimately leads to occlusion of the affected vessel. The effectiveness of new interventional techniques is judged by the ability of the techniques to reestablish and maintain normal blood flow to the extremity. The Doppler component of the sonographic examination offers the capability of measuring blood flow velocity changes at sites of developing stenosis. The effectiveness of the intervention and of any adjunctive pharmaceutical therapy aimed at reducing the myointimal proliferative process can then be quantitated and objectively evaluated by serial measurements.

More recently, high-resolution sonographic imaging has shown itself to be capable of visualizing early plaque deposition and thickening of the intima-media layer of the arterial wall. These changes are considered by many to represent the earliest forms of atherosclerosis. This not only may help in evaluating the extent of early artherosclerosis but also could open a whole new horizon for monitoring the effects of early medical interventions.

Sonography is considered to be heavily operator-dependent. The technical skill of the sonographer affects the quality of the study and the ability to detect pathological changes. The hard copy or videotape images reflect this inherent bias since they are selected by the sonographer. Computed tomography and magnetic resonance angiography are somewhat less operator dependent. Image acquisition and display are not dependent on operator skills. In peripheral sonography, therefore, appropriate training of the sonographer is of the utmost importance. The overall accuracy of the examinations described in this guide depends heavily on the skill of the sonographer.

This handbook has been developed from the author's experience in training sonographers to perform vascular ultrasound as well as teaching a broader audience composed of technologists, physicians specializing in peripheral vascular diseases, and general practitioners. The issues addressed in this manual are a reflection of the questions commonly asked by this varied audience. A great deal of care has been taken to describe these techniques with a "hands-on" approach. This guide also includes more basic data that are increasingly needed for the application of clinical decision making. For example, the clinical care of patients presenting with suspected thromboembolic disease remains an important challenge. An understanding of both the pathophysiological mechanisms at play and the capabilities of sonographic imaging is often necessary to deliver optimal care to the patient. The information contained in the following chapters should help the clinician in deciding when sonography is best used to help diagnose and monitor patients with peripheral vascular disease.

Joseph F. Polak, M.D.

CONTENTS

Color Plate I

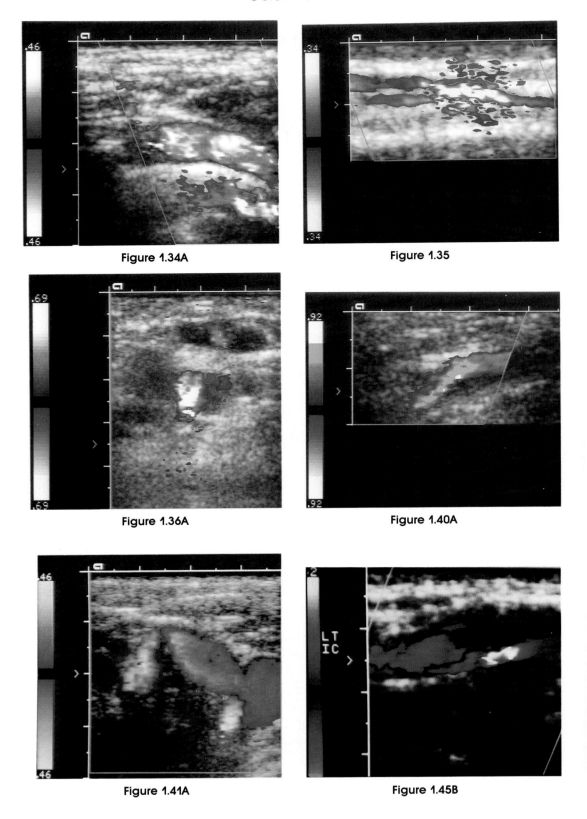

Figure 1.34A

Figure 1.35

Figure 1.36A

Figure 1.40A

Figure 1.41A

Figure 1.45B

Color Plate II

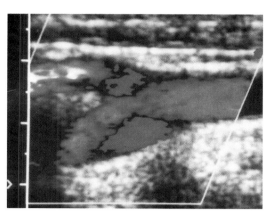

Figure 4.5D

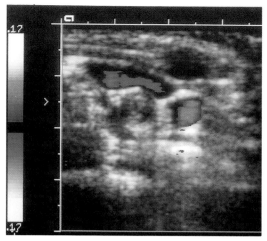

Figure 4.30A

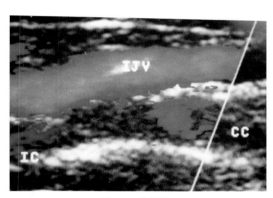

Figure 4.30E

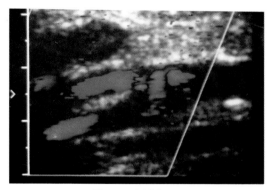

Figure 4.32A

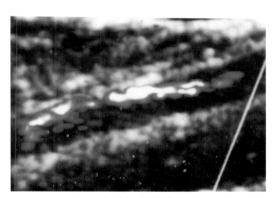

Figure 4.33D

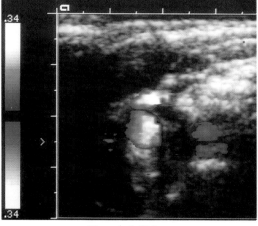

Figure 4.46A

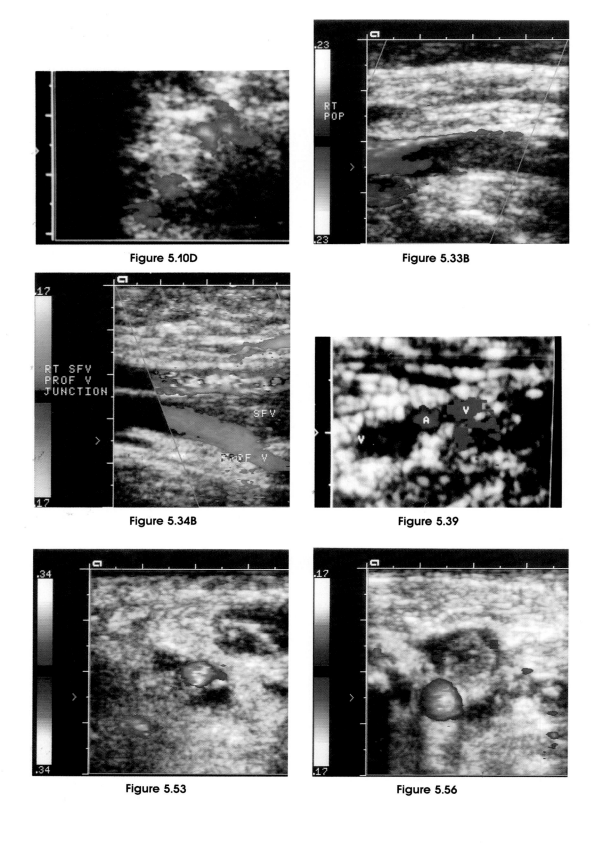

Color Plate III

Figure 5.10D

Figure 5.33B

Figure 5.34B

Figure 5.39

Figure 5.53

Figure 5.56

Color Plate IV

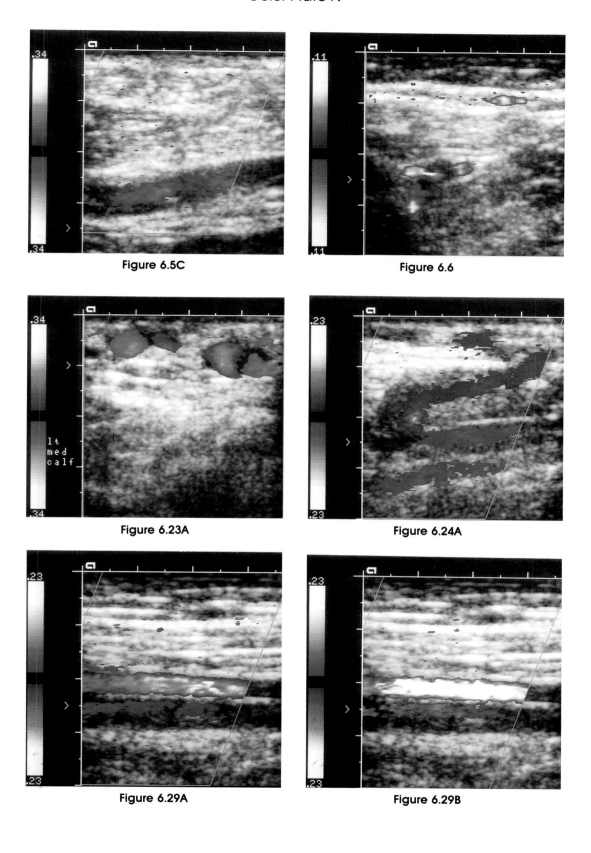

Figure 6.5C

Figure 6.6

Figure 6.23A

Figure 6.24A

Figure 6.29A

Figure 6.29B

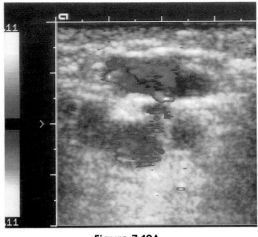

Figure 7.12A

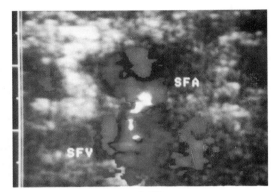

Figure 7.17E

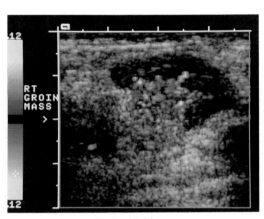

Figure 7.20A

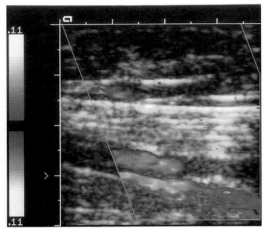

Figure 7.27A

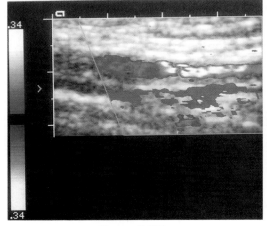

Figure 7.29A

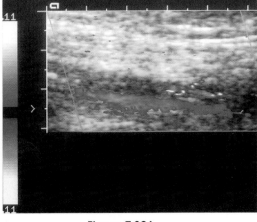

Figure 7.30A

Color Plate VI

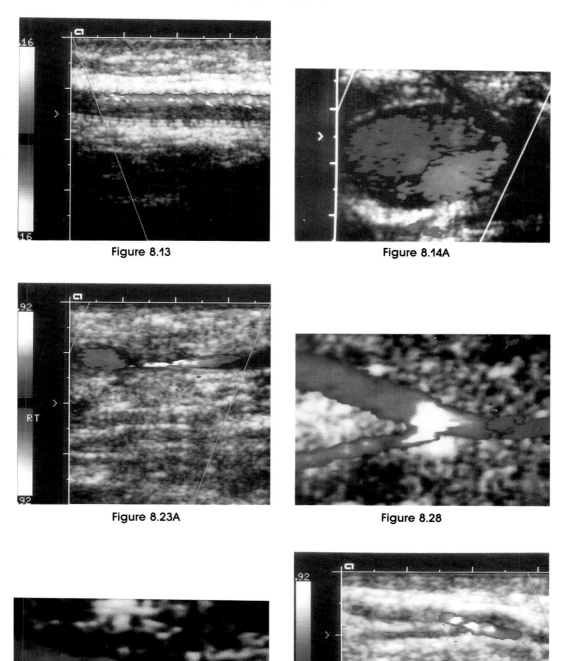

Figure 8.13

Figure 8.14A

Figure 8.23A

Figure 8.28

Figure 8.29

Figure 8.30A

CHAPTER ONE

Doppler Sonography: An Overview

Gray-Scale Imaging

Gray-scale imaging is accomplished by detecting and displaying the echoes returning when a short pulse of radiofrequency (RF) energy is applied to either one or a group of piezoelectric crystals in contact with the skin. We are dealing with sound waves of a high frequency—3 million to 10 million cycles per second (Hz)—as compared to the human hearing threshold of 20,000 Hz. These sound waves travel poorly in air compared to their transmission in water and in the soft tissues of the body. To ensure proper transmission between the crystals used in sonography and the soft tissues of the body, an interface with acoustic properties similar to water is applied on the skin to act as an acoustic interface. This is done with a water-soluble gel. The piezoelectric crystal absorbs electrical energy in the form of an RF signal and then emits this energy as a sound wave. This penetrates the soft tissues and is reflected back toward the transducer whenever interfaces of different acoustic properties are encountered. Position encoding of the returning echoes is reflected by the time between the transmitted sound pulse and the detection of the returning signal. These returning sound waves interact with the crystal(s), this time with the opposite effect, transforming sound energy into electrical energy. Since the speed of sound in soft tissues is relatively constant at 1540 cm/sec, time delays can be translated into physical displacement relative to the crystals. The ultrasound beam also loses energy as the depth of the tissue increases (Fig. 1.1). This attenuation causes the echoes returning from the deeper-lying structures not to have as much energy and hence less intensity. A time-gain compensation (TGC) is normally applied to the returning echoes to equalize the intensity of the signals as they are displayed on the television monitor—this is called the TGC curve (Fig. 1.2).

The intensity of the returning echoes is also a function of the type of biologic tissue encountered by the sound beam. The muscles and the different soft tissues within the extremity interact with the ultrasound beam by a scattering interaction. This interaction is the source of strong returning echoes, since the size of most of the physical structures within the soft tissues is roughly the same as the wavelength of the ultrasound beam. In contrast, the red blood cells within vessels appear dark because they are much smaller than the ultrasound wavelength and do not send off

Figure 1.1. The effects of transducer frequency and imaging depth on the signal intensity of returning ultrasound echoes is summarized in this graph. There is a significant loss of sound beam penetration as the frequency increases. In addition, at a given frequency, there is also rapid loss of strength of the returning echoes as the depth of the structure being imaged increases.

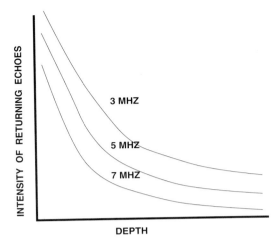

Figure 1.2. The time-gain compensation (TGC) curve is used to normalize the appearance of the returning echoes into a more even and acceptable image. Because of the effects of attenuation, the intensity of returning echoes normally decreases dramatically with depth from the transducer face (*top*). The *black dots* correspond to the location of a vessel of interest. The time-delay compensation or TDC performs amplification of the returning echoes as a function of the delay between transmission and receipt of the sound waves (*middle*). The deeper the structure, the longer the delay and the more amplification is given to the signal containing the returning echoes. The final result of this operation is shown in the lower figure. There is now a more even distribution of the returning echoes. This makes it easier to compare the echogenic structure of a venous thrombus or a carotid plaque to the surrounding soft tissues.

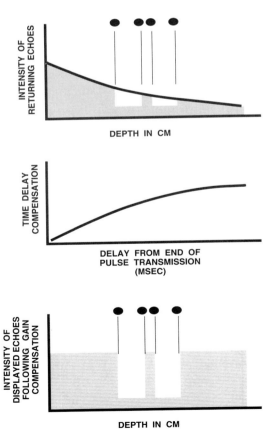

strong returning echoes (Fig. 1.3). This type of physical interaction is called Rayleigh scattering. The sharp contrast between structures of different acoustic properties can also be accentuated whenever the structure—often the artery wall—is perpendicular to the ultrasound beam. This type of interaction is called specular reflection (Fig. 1.4). The appearance of the gray-scale image is due to the combination of these effects (Fig. 1.5). The interaction or scattering of the ultrasound beam is related to the structural components within the tissue of interest. The term used to describe the density of the signal that returns is echogenicity. The echogenicity of a tissue or region of interest is the sonographic appearance of this region relative to the surrounding tissues. A material that is poorly echogenic or hypoechoic appears black on the ultrasound image. A material that contains more structure and returning echoes is normally termed isoechoic. Finally, if the echoes within the structure of interest have increased intensity with respect to the surrounding soft tissues and muscles, the structure is termed hyperechoic.

Ultrasound transducers consisting of a single crystal have come into disfavor for imaging of the peripheral vascular system. These transducers were used to create two-dimensional sonographic images in one of two ways. The first was in conjunction with an articulated mechanical arm device through which the position of the echoes returning from structures of interest was mapped on a display screen. This device was large, difficult to master, did not have the capability to do Doppler imaging, and did not permit rapid interactive positioning and mapping of structures of interest. The static scanner has been, to all practical extent, replaced by the real-time ultrasound device.

The real-time mechanical scanners consist of a crystal mounted in such a way that either it moves or sound issuing from it is

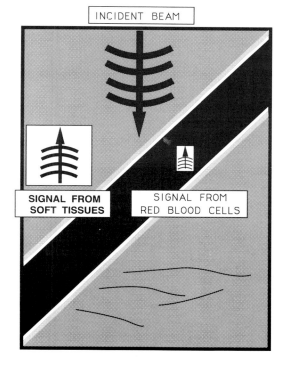

Figure 1.3. The echoes used to create an ultrasound image are created through the physical process called scattering. The signal intensities returning from different tissues are a function of the density of these scatterers, the size of the scatterers, and the distribution of the scatterers within these tissues. In general, the wavelength of the ultrasound beam is approximately the size of the structures responsible for the scattering process in muscles and other nonvascular structures. This is responsible for most of the background signals seen on a sonogram. Red blood cells also interact with the ultrasound beam through a form of scattering called Rayleigh scattering. The wavelength of the ultrasound beam is larger than the red blood cells. This type of interaction is not angle dependent. The strength of the returning echoes increases as the fourth power of the ultrasound frequency. The echoes from red blood cells have a signal intensity 10,000 to 1 million times less than those from contiguous soft tissues.

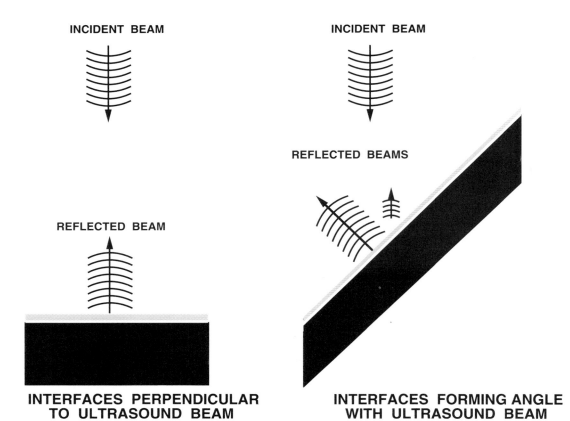

INCIDENT BEAM

INCIDENT BEAM

REFLECTED BEAMS

REFLECTED BEAM

INTERFACES PERPENDICULAR TO ULTRASOUND BEAM

INTERFACES FORMING ANGLE WITH ULTRASOUND BEAM

Figure 1.4. Specular reflection is the interaction between tissue and ultrasound beam at the interface between materials of different acoustic properties (impedance). It is mostly responsible for the ability to identify arterial wall interfaces and to clearly distinguish their boundaries. This type of interaction is highly angle dependent as shown in this figure. Arterial wall interfaces perpendicular to the beam are clearly seen. As the angle between the beam and the interface increases, most of the reflected echoes are directed away from the location of the transducer and do not contribute to the signal intensity.

reflected from a mirror that moves very rapidly, back and forth, over a short area. The angle defined by the motion of the assembly defines a field of view in the shape of a sector—hence the name sector scanner (Fig. 1.6). These devices are capable of resolving most vascular structures of interest. The transducers are unfortunately subject to mechanical wear and tear. They have imaging frame rates limited by the mechanical components of the transducers. Simultaneous real-time two-dimensional imaging and Doppler sonography is not possible. Either a second ul-trasound crystal has to be used (Fig. 1.7) or the motion within the transducer has to be suspended (Fig. 1.8) in order to acquire signals that can be further processed to give Doppler spectral waveforms.

The use of multiple small piezoelectric crystals arranged in arrays of different shapes and forms has come to replace the more traditional mechanical sector scanner (Fig. 1.9). This type of imaging technology has developed concurrently with the increased use of dedicated microprocessors capable of coordinating the tasks necessary for image formation. Three basic shapes are available for peripheral vascular imaging: sector, linear array, and curvilinear array transducers. All three share the property that they do not have any moving parts. Focusing of the ultrasound beam is normally done by introducing a delay in the time at which a given crystal in the array is emitting its pulse of ultrasound energy. This is accomplished by introducing a delay of variable length in the delivery of a small pulse of RF energy to the crystal. By varying the sequence and location of the RF pulse, it is possible either to focus more ultrasound signal at a given depth from the crystal face (thereby improving resolution) or to steer the angle

of interrogation of the array as a whole (Fig. 1.10). This latter capability is useful when imaging a vascular channel that takes a sharp turn with respect to the transducer-skin interface. The ability to focus ultrasound energy at a given depth also improves detail discrimination at that depth (Fig. 1.11). This can be accomplished either by changing the way the sound beam is emitted or by using special algorithms to process the returning echoes—so-called dynamic focusing.

We have found the linear array transducer to be well suited for vascular imaging. There is no geometric distortion, so straight arterial segments do not appear

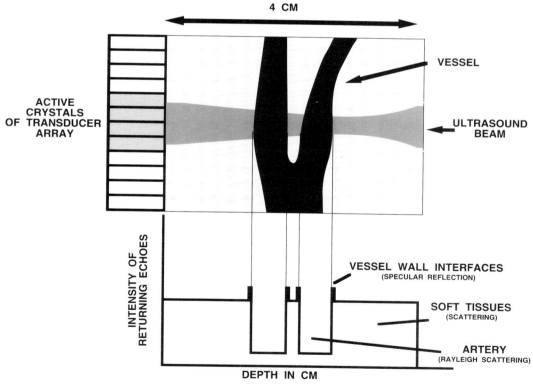

Figure 1.5. This figure summarizes the source of the signals on a sonographic image. The arterial wall interfaces, when imaged perfectly perpendicularly, act as specular reflectors. This causes the relative intensity of the returning echoes to be slightly brighter at these interfaces. The echoes from the soft tissues are due to scattering. Small specular reflectors oriented in different directions contribute to the background signal. Signals from the red blood cells are due to Rayleigh scattering. Their intensity is several orders of magnitude less than that of signals from surrounding soft tissues.

Figure 1.6. The mechanical sector scanner was the first type of transducer built to be capable of generating ultrasound images in real time. A crystal vibrates to generate a sound wave. This sound wave travels through a liquid milieu until it reaches a mirror. The beam is then reflected in a direction defined by the position of the mirror with respect to the crystal. The mirror is in continual motion. The lower illustration shows that this has the effect of redirecting the sound beam. The range of motion of the mirror defines a sector, hence the name sector scanner. The mirror will normally move back and forth over this sector from 5 to 30 times per second, depending on the depth of the structure being imaged. The frame rate decreases as the depth and the size of the sector increase.

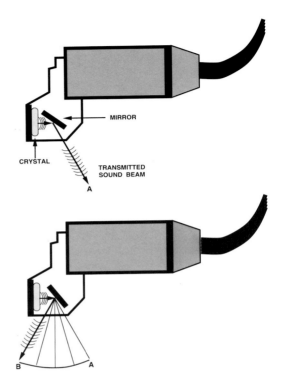

curved at the edges of the imaging field. This phenomenon is shared by both the sector and curvilinear transducers and becomes worse with depth. An imaging field of view of 4 to 6 cm permits consecutive sampling of long arterial segments in a reasonable amount of time (Fig. 1.12). This geometric configuration is easily used to cover the length of the upper- and lower-extremity vessels.

The sector and smaller curvilinear transducers have certain advantages whenever the vessels are tortuous or lie underneath structures that block sound wave transmission. They are more easily placed against the anterior iliac spine for imaging of the iliac arteries. Visualization of the subclavian artery and vein as they wind underneath the clavicle is also facilitated. In general, they perform best whenever the acoustic window is small and the vascular segments that need to be imaged lie quite deeply. Because of the shape of the emitted sound waves, the sector and cur-

vilinear scanners will show longer segments of artery and vein as depth increases.

The shape of the linear array transducer also has an effect on the operator's ability to perform certain diagnostic tasks. For example, a slight taper to the shape of the transducer will decrease the surface area put in contact with the skin. This facilitates transmission of pressure from the transducer face to the more deeply located veins when compression sonography is being performed.

The vascular structures of interest in the upper and lower extremities range in size between 1 mm and 1 cm in diameter. A high-resolution ultrasound device is normally needed to accurately visualize structures of this size range. Since resolution in an ultrasound transducer is directly linked to the operating frequency of the transducer (in fact proportional to it), increasing the transducer frequency improves visualization of both arteries and veins. An unfortunate side effect of increasing the transducer frequency is reduced penetration depth of the ultrasound beam. This also has a more pervasive effect on the distribution of frequencies that return to the transducer. Although an ideal instrument could potentially transmit at only one frequency, there is in fact a distribution or spectrum of frequencies emitted by the transducer and reaching the soft tissues at different depths. Similarly, a spectrum of frequencies is reflected and returns to the transducer. The effect of the

soft tissues in the path of the ultrasound beam is to more greatly attenuate the higher-frequency components within the spectrum, thereby causing more of the lower-frequency components to return to the transducer. This degrades the ability to discriminate finer detail or resolution (Fig. 1.13). This effect is more pronounced the deeper the structure of interest lies in the soft tissues. Contrast resolution also changes as a function of frequency. The internal structure of forming thrombus may not be seen when imaging at 3 MHz

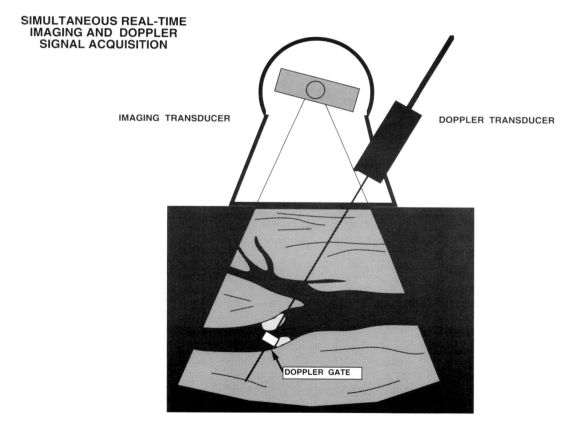

Figure 1.7. Duplex imaging is also possible when an additional crystal is added to a mechanical sector scanner. The real-time image is used to locate the site where the Doppler gate is to be positioned. A separate Doppler transducer then processes Doppler shift information from this location. A simultaneous display of a real-time gray-scale image and of a Doppler waveform is achieved. The coupling between the Doppler transducer must be perfectly aligned to the imaging transducer to prevent inconsistencies in the placement of the Doppler gate. This is often the source of problems and requires careful maintenance of the transducer assembly. The additional transducer is often placed to the side of the imaging transducer and is often a hindrance.

**FROZEN REAL-TIME
IMAGE DURING DOPPLER SIGNAL ACQUISITION**

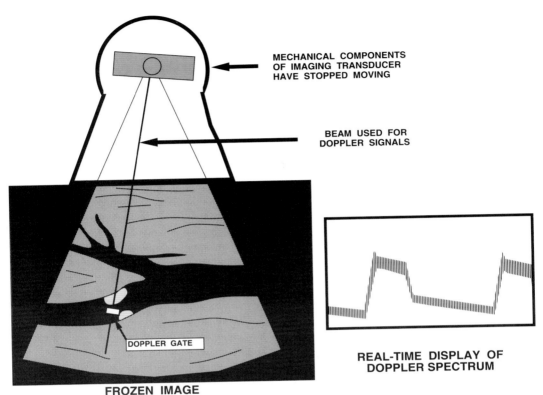

MECHANICAL COMPONENTS
OF IMAGING TRANSDUCER
HAVE STOPPED MOVING

BEAM USED FOR
DOPPLER SIGNALS

DOPPLER GATE

REAL-TIME DISPLAY OF
DOPPLER SPECTRUM

FROZEN IMAGE

Figure 1.8. The mechanical transducers that use the same transducer crystal to obtain Doppler frequency shift information require that the transducer stop moving during Doppler imaging. The Doppler gate is interactively positioned at the site of interest during real-time imaging. However, real-time imaging must stop while the Doppler frequency shift information is acquired and processed to create a Doppler waveform. Inconsistencies in placement of the Doppler gate can occur due to inadvertent operator movement when switching between modes. The other limitations of these mechanical devices include wear and tear of the mechanical components and the need to introduce coupling fluid in the transducer assembly.

but can often be perceived at frequencies of 5 to 7 MHz.

A transducer with a carrier frequency of approximately 5 MHz is the most useful for most clinical applications in peripheral vascular imaging. On occasion, greater resolution may be required. This is the case when imaging a more superficial vascular structure such as the carotid artery and characterizing early atherosclerotic plaque. Higher frequencies of 7 to 10 MHz

are then used. For imaging of the lower extremity veins, specifically the deeper-lying femoral vein and artery, the 5-MHz transducer performs well in most subjects. On occasion, patients with very large thighs and deeply lying vessels may require the use of a lower-frequency transducer, such as 3.5 MHz. Conversely, detection of early thrombus in the muscular veins of the calf is often facilitated by operating at a higher frequency such as 7 MHz.

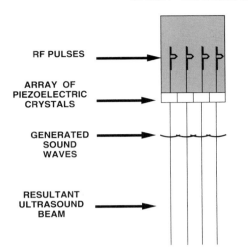

LINEAR PHASED ARRAY TRANSDUCER

RF PULSES

ARRAY OF PIEZOELECTRIC CRYSTALS

GENERATED SOUND WAVES

RESULTANT ULTRASOUND BEAM

Figure 1.9. The linear array transducer consists of an array of 96 to 128 crystals arranged in series. Radiofrequency signals applied to the individual crystals make them vibrate and generate sound waves. These then travel in the soft tissues. The crystals are excited for only a small amount of time (microseconds). Most of the remaining time is taken up by a listening period when the echoes returning from the soft tissues underneath the transducer can interact with the crystals. These in turn generate small radiofrequency signals in response to the sound waves hitting them. The signals are then processed to create the ultrasound image.

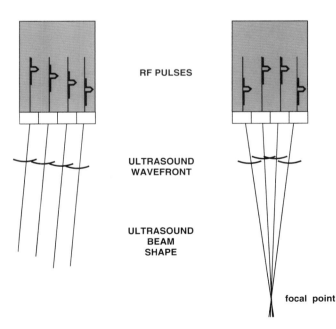

BEAM STEERING

BEAM FOCUSING

RF PULSES

ULTRASOUND WAVEFRONT

ULTRASOUND BEAM SHAPE

focal point

Figure 1.10. Adjacent crystals in the linear array transducer are exciting at different times to achieve beam steering or beam focusing. These same effects can also be achieved by introducing variable time delays in the signals received by the crystal elements of the transducer. On the *left,* a group of four crystals are excited with increasing delays, causing the beam to steer toward the left. On the *right,* the center crystals are excited later to achieve a more focused beam. These effects are achieved by operating on a small number of crystals at a time—often four, as in the example—rather than on the whole array.

Doppler Imaging

There are three forms of Doppler imaging currently in use: continuous-wave Doppler, pulsed Doppler, and color Doppler sonography.

CONTINUOUS-WAVE DOPPLER: PRINCIPLES

Continuous-wave (CW) Doppler was first developed in the early 1950s. In essence, a piezoelectric crystal is used to send out signals continuously while the re-

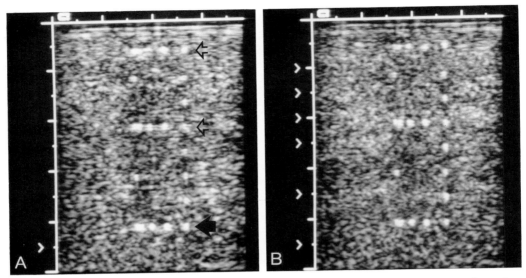

Figure 1.11. **A,** The effect of selectively focusing different components of the linear array transducer is shown. Selective focusing at a depth of 4½ cm clearly shows a separation between the farther pins (*solid arrow*), while the nearest pins are not as clearly seen (*open arrows*). This focusing is achieved either by introducing varying time delays to the radiofrequency signals being applied to the transducer crystals or by processing the signals being received by these crystals. **B,** Focusing at all the different levels makes all the pins clearly discernible. The imaging frame rate is severely reduced by this type of focusing.

turning echoes are continuously detected by a second crystal (Fig. 1.14). The returning signals lie in line of sight of the probe containing the piezoelectric crystals.

The underlying physical principle used is that of the Doppler shift. Specifically, red cells, or in fact any soft tissues, moving relative to the ultrasound probe will cause a frequency shift in the returning ultrasound signal (Fig. 1.15). This frequency shift is proportional to the velocity at which the structure moves with respect to the transducer. It is also affected by the relative angle between the direction of the ultrasound beam and the direction of the moving structure. In summary, the frequency shift increases as the structure moves toward the transducer and decreases as the structure moves away from the transducer. This relationship is summarized by the Doppler equation first pro-

posed by Christian Doppler in 1889 (Fig. 1.16).

When first used clinically in the early 1960s, this information was encoded in the form of an audio signal or displayed as an average value of the Doppler shift detected by the probe. The frequency shifts caused by moving blood are in the range of human hearing. For example, using a Doppler probe with a carrier frequency of 5 MHz forming an angle of 60° with a blood vessel, a velocity of 20 cm/sec in a vein causes a frequency shift of 640 Hz. The peak velocities in a normal carotid artery (i.e., 80 cm/sec) cause a shift four times as great, or 2560 Hz. If the ultrasound beam intersected both the artery and the vein, the frequency of the signals returning from the vein would be 4,999,360 Hz while the signals returning from the artery would be 5,002,560 Hz. If the ultrasound probe were pointing in the opposite direction and the venous flow directed toward the probe and the arterial flow away, the returning frequencies would be 5,000,640 Hz and 4,997,440 Hz, respectively. This frequency shift is affected by the carrier frequency of the ultrasound beam. For the same velocity of blood flow (proportional to degree of stenosis and inversely to vessel diameter), the measured frequency shift will increase as the carrier frequency increases (Fig. 1.17). In earlier applications, the instantaneous average of the frequency shifts was detected and displayed. The device used

to do this is called a zero-crossing detector. It permits a rough quantitation of the average velocity of blood flow but also gives qualitative information on the pattern of blood flow.

All moving structures in the line of sight of the beam emanating from the ultrasound probe cause returning signals that contain frequency shift information. It is therefore not possible to locate the source of the returning echoes and relate them to a given anatomic structure. To gain the ability to localize the source of the returning echoes, a focusing characteristic is of-

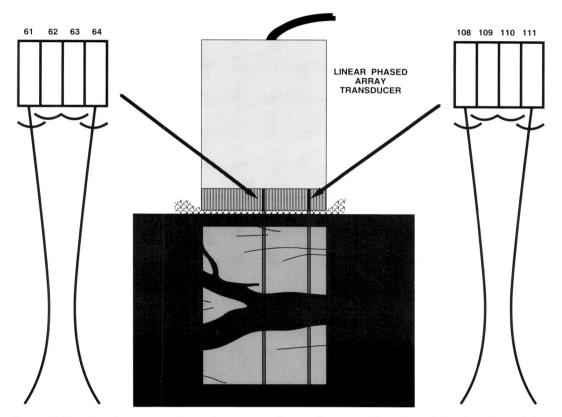

Figure 1.12. The linear array transducer encodes position as a function of the location of the different crystals. To the *left,* four crystals in the middle of the array are being used. Crystals are often fired in groups of four as shown here. The second group of crystals is located 47 crystals away. The interval of time taken for an image line to be acquired is a function of imaging depth, with each centimeter of depth corresponding to roughly 13 microseconds. It will therefore take 2.5 msec for imaging to progress to the second set of crystals when a 4-cm imaging depth is used.

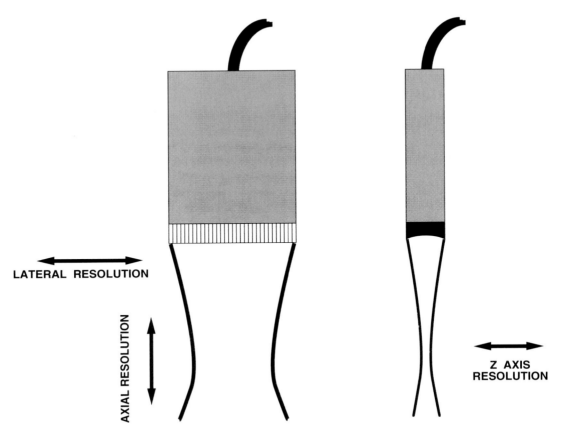

LATERAL RESOLUTION

AXIAL RESOLUTION

Z AXIS RESOLUTION

Figure 1.13. There are three ways of evaluating resolution. The first is rarely mentioned. It refers to the z-axis resolution. It is determined by the shape of the crystal array when looked at from the edge of the transducer. It cannot be modified during imaging unless a standoff is used. Lateral resolution refers to the ability of discriminating two objects located side by side on the image. It is achieved by the active focusing of the transducer crystals. Axial resolution can be slightly modified by changing the way returning echoes are processed. It is mostly dependent on the duration and shape of the radiofrequency pulse used to excite the crystal element of a transducer.

ten built into the piezoelectric crystals. The ultrasound beam is then capable of interrogating signals arising at varied depths, for example 2 to 3 cm, from the tip of the transducer. Penetration of the ultrasound beam is also improved when the carrier frequency is decreased (Fig. 1.18).

A limitation of the zero-crossing detector is the ambiguity caused by the processing of average frequency shifts (Fig. 1.19). Blood flowing in contiguous vessels but moving in opposite directions can cancel each other out on the Doppler frequency

shift display. A major step forward in the practical application of Doppler sonography was the development of the spectrum analyzer, which made it possible to display the distribution of frequency shifts caused by moving blood.

A spectrum analyzer consists of a special electronic device capable of performing a mathematical transformation called the Fourier transform (Fig. 1.20). In essence, returning signals holding frequency shift information are detected by the transducer and then decoded into their compo-

C-W DOPPLER PROBE

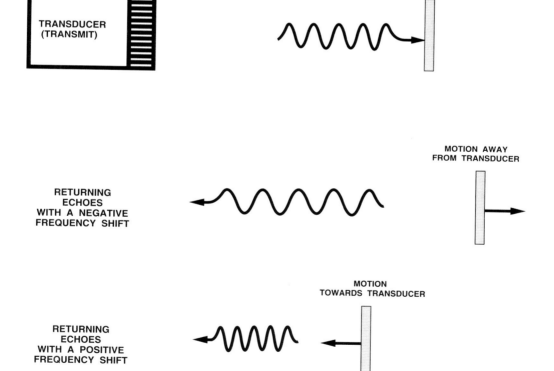

RECEIVE CRYSTAL

TRANSMIT CRYSTAL

FOCAL ZONE

INSONATED VESSEL

Figure 1.14. The traditional non-imaging Doppler device is the CW (continuous-wave) probe. It is so named because it sends off sound signals continuously from one crystal while the other is in a constant receive mode. These probes will sample signals from every structure in the line of sight. However, most devices have crystals shaped so that they have an effective focal zone varying from 1 to a few centimeters.

TRANSDUCER (TRANSMIT)

RETURNING ECHOES WITH A NEGATIVE FREQUENCY SHIFT

MOTION AWAY FROM TRANSDUCER

RETURNING ECHOES WITH A POSITIVE FREQUENCY SHIFT

MOTION TOWARDS TRANSDUCER

Figure 1.15. The Doppler effect can be simplified as follows: The returning echoes from a nonmoving object do not cause any change in the frequency of the ultrasound beam. Echoes returning from an object moving away from the transducer have a lower frequency. The difference between the received and the emitted frequencies corresponds to a negative Doppler frequency shift. Echoes returning from an object moving toward the transducer have a higher frequency than the emitted frequency. The difference is a positive Doppler frequency shift.

DOPPLER RELATIONSHIP

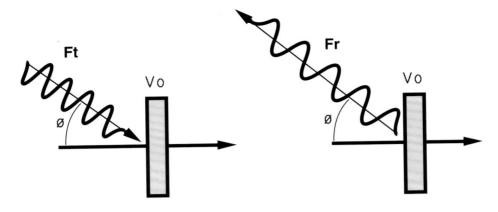

$$FD = Fr - Ft = 2\ \frac{Ft\ Vo\ cos\emptyset}{c}$$

Figure 1.16. The Doppler equation is the essential key to the use of sound to measure the velocity of flowing blood. The essential terms are as follows: The frequency of the transmitted ultrasound beam (*Ft*) is also called the Doppler carrier frequency. The frequency of the returning or reflected echoes is called *Fr*. The Doppler frequency shift caused by motion of the object is termed *FD*. It is equal to the difference between *Ft* and *Fr*. The Doppler shift, for example, rarely reaches 20,000 Hz, whereas *Fr* and *Ft* are normally between 3 million and 5 million Hz. The velocity *Vo* of the moving object is proportional to *FD,* the measured Doppler shift. Measurement of the actual velocity requires knowledge of the velocity of sound ($c = 1540$ cm/sec) and of the angle formed between the direction of motion of the object and the ultrasound beam (ϕ). The term θ is often used to describe this angle.

Figure 1.17. The curve describing the relationship between frequency shift and lumen narrowing of an artery is similar in shape for different Doppler carrier frequencies. The values corresponding to the presence of a critical stenosis are different, however. In the three cases shown, a 50% stenosis will cause a 3,000, 4,000, or 5,000 Hz frequency shift at the carrier frequencies of 3, 4, and 5 MHz, respectively. Knowledge of the angle—assumed to be 60° if it was not measured—and of the velocity of sound are all that are needed to determine the velocity of blood flow according to the Doppler equation. This effectively cancels out the effect of the carrier frequency.

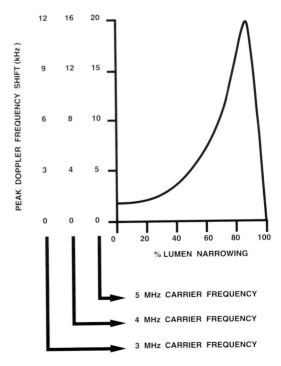

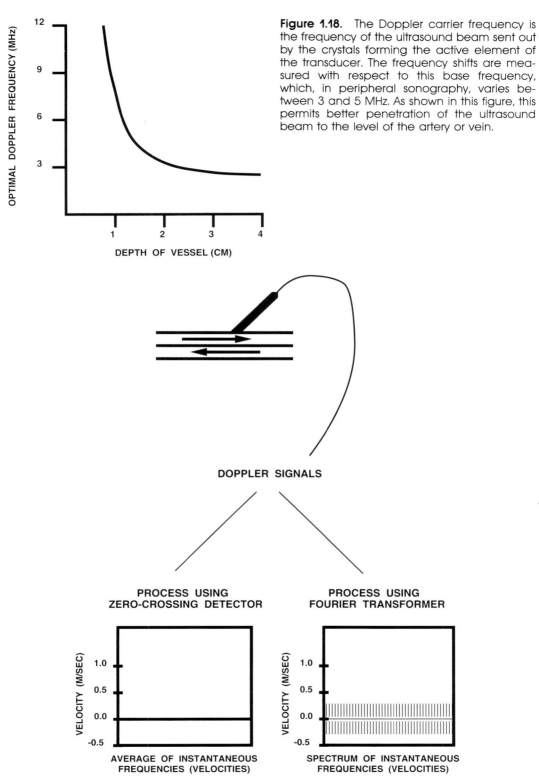

Figure 1.18. The Doppler carrier frequency is the frequency of the ultrasound beam sent out by the crystals forming the active element of the transducer. The frequency shifts are measured with respect to this base frequency, which, in peripheral sonography, varies between 3 and 5 MHz. As shown in this figure, this permits better penetration of the ultrasound beam to the level of the artery or vein.

DOPPLER SIGNALS

PROCESS USING
ZERO-CROSSING DETECTOR

PROCESS USING
FOURIER TRANSFORMER

AVERAGE OF INSTANTANEOUS
FREQUENCIES (VELOCITIES)

SPECTRUM OF INSTANTANEOUS
FREQUENCIES (VELOCITIES)

Figure 1.19. The older-generation Doppler devices give an output signal that is proportional to *the average or mean velocity of moving red blood cells.* As such, motions of equal amplitude but in opposite directions tended to cancel out as shown here. The modern Doppler spectrum analyzer actively displays *the velocity distribution of moving red blood cells.*

FOURIER ANALYSIS

AUDIO SIGNAL (DOPPLER SHIFT)

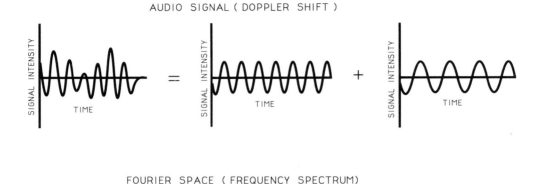

FOURIER SPACE (FREQUENCY SPECTRUM)

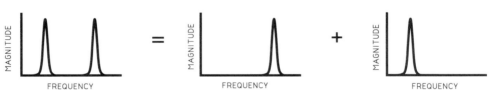

Figure 1.20. The basic method used to extract and process the Doppler frequency shift contained in the returning echoes of an ultrasound beam is the Fast Fourier Transform. This algorithm is used to decompose the audio signal of the Doppler shift into spectra showing the actual distributions of the frequencies in the returning echoes. On the top line, the complex audio signal on the left corresponds to a combination of the two Doppler frequency shifts shown on the right. These signals processed following the Fast Fourier Transform are shown on the bottom line. The frequency shifts are now shown as spectra. On the left, the complex audio signal is shown to contain both a low- and a high-frequency component equivalent to adding the two spectra on the right.

nent frequency values (Fig. 1.21). This process results in the creation of a spectrum or display of the distribution of velocities for a given time interval. In most devices, this sampling takes place every 1 to 5 msec. During this small time interval, the full distribution of frequency shifts in the signal returning to the ultrasound probe is sampled, processed, and displayed. The continued refreshment of these spectra throughout the cardiac cycle creates what is commonly referred to as the Doppler spectral waveform. The intensity of the returning signal at a given frequency corresponds roughly to the actual number of moving blood cells with the same velocity. The intensity of the Doppler spectral waveform is encoded to be proportional to

the number of the returning echoes and is therefore roughly proportional to the number of red cells traveling at the corresponding velocity.

DUPLEX SONOGRAPHY

The two major limitations of the CW Doppler devices are the inability to accurately localize the sites where the signals holding Doppler frequency shift information are sampled and the difficulty in determining the actual velocity of moving blood. Late in the 1970s emerged the concept of spatially localizing the site where the Doppler frequency shifts were originating: duplex sonography. Rather than using a continuous-wave probe, a small

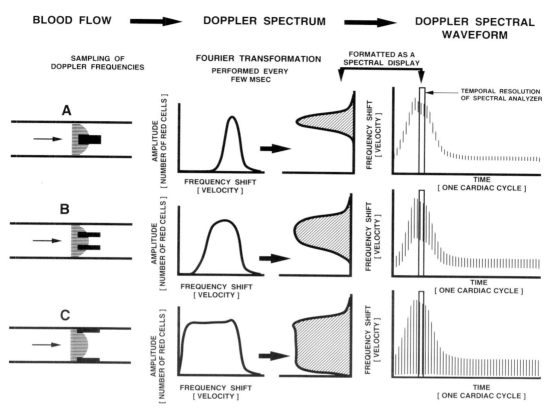

BLOOD FLOW ➡ **DOPPLER SPECTRUM** ➡ **DOPPLER SPECTRAL WAVEFORM**

Figure 1.21. The Doppler spectral waveform is created from the frequency shift information contained in the echoes returning from a physical location defined by the Doppler gate. Important factors influencing the appearance of the waveform are the location and size of the gate as well as the vessel and the type of flow within it. On the top row, a narrow Doppler gate has been positioned in the center of an artery with laminar (parabolic) flow. A Fast Fourier Transform is used to create a spectrum or distribution of the number of red cells (scatterers) with a given frequency shift. This spectrum is normally acquired every 1 to 10 msec, depending on the manufacturer of the device and the depth of the Doppler gate. The spectrum is then formatted into a part of the final Doppler waveform shown on the right. This takes place by first displaying the spectrum in the vertical direction and then encoding the amplitude of the spectrum as the intensity of the Doppler waveform tracing. In the second row, the same steps have been taken with a wider Doppler gate. This forces the transducer to receive a broader distribution of red cell velocities. The effect is to widen the Doppler waveform on the right and to narrow the window below the tracing—the spectral tracing. In the last row, the width of the Doppler gate has been magnified to demonstrate the source of artificial "spectral broadening" of the Doppler waveform. The Doppler gate now includes all the velocities of red cell movement in the vessel, including the slower, near-zero velocities near both walls. The spectrum is broader than the two above. The spectral window or vertical expanse of the Doppler waveform is almost completely filled in. The persistent narrow band of absent signals at the base of the spectrum is due to the wall filter. This filter is so named because it excludes low-frequency (low-velocity) signals normally caused by the motion of the arterial wall during the cardiac cycle.

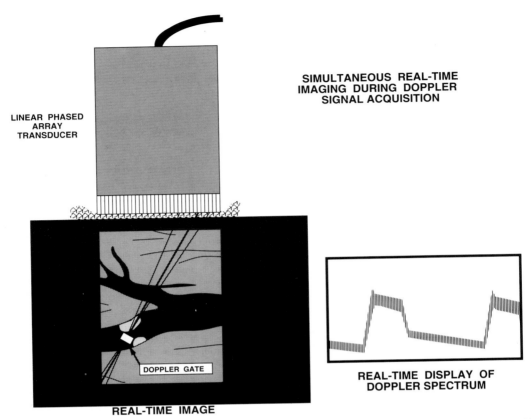

Figure 1.22. Duplex sonography refers to the combined use of real-time imaging and the acquisition of Doppler spectral information. It is increasingly implemented on the type of linear array transducer shown here. There are no moving components. The returning echoes reach the transducer and are processed to generate both the real-time image and the Doppler waveform. The Doppler gate is more accurately positioned since the examiner can interactively use the real-time image. The same electronic timing circuits used to create the image also help localize the Doppler gate. The ultrasound pulses sent to measure Doppler shifts to create the Doppler waveform are longer in duration than those used for imaging. The processing is also markedly different. The Doppler analyzer and the gray-scale image are competing against each other for imaging time. The maximal rate at which pulses used to measure Doppler shifts are sent is called the pulse repetition frequency (PRF). The maximal PRF is dependent on the depth of field of the image, which sets the time taken to reach the more distant object in the image and to return. The PRF can also be increased by decreasing the real-time image frame rate. The maximal velocity that can be measured by pulse Doppler analysis is directly proportional to the PRF.

pulse of radiofrequency signals was delivered to the transducer crystal. This small pulse is capable of encoding spatial information by the fact that the time delay between transmission and receipt of the signal is twice that taken for the pulse to reach the structure of interest. Since the speed of sound is constant, this delay corresponds to the distance covered by the ultrasound pulse. The relative location of the returning echo pulse can therefore be determined. Frequency shift information carried by this pulse and caused by the interaction with a moving object also returns to the transducer. By performing the Fourier transform operation on this returning signal, a Doppler spectrum is obtained from a given location in the imaging field

(Fig. 1.22). Knowledge of the angle formed between flow in the vessel lumen and the ultrasound beam (Fig. 1.23) permits a calculation of the velocity of moving blood (Fig. 1.24).

The major limitation of this approach is that each pulse can be transmitted only after the returning echoes from the preceding pulse train have been received. Therefore, time delays equal to the length of time taken for an ultrasound pulse to return from the farthest structure in the imaging field must elapse before another pulse can be transmitted. This pulse repetition rate sets an upper limit to the frequency content of the signals that are accurately displayed following the Fourier transform operation (Fig. 1.25). This limit is commonly referred to as the sampling theorem or Nyquist limit. In essence, the electronics of the sonographic device behave as a stroboscope. The relative frequency of the signals returning are processed similarly to the way we perceive the visual information transmitted when a stroboscope is used on a moving object. A stroboscope can create the impression that a rotating bicycle wheel is turning at a slower rate than is the case. This is due to the limited spatial sampling caused by the stroboscope. A similar phenomenon can be noted on the Doppler spectrum. The information contained by the higher frequency shifts is displayed at a lower frequency (Fig. 1.26). This phenomenon is called aliasing. The electronics of the sonographic device can process the information from the ultrasound echoes at a maximal rate defined by the peak repetition frequency (PRF). If the PRF increases, higher frequency shifts can be displayed and aliasing is less likely. This is more likely at shallow depths. If the PRF decreases, the likelihood is greater that aliasing will occur.

COLOR DOPPLER SONOGRAPHY

Color Doppler imaging is a variation in the technology of pulse Doppler processing. The frequency shift information contained in the radiofrequency pulses returning to the transducer is decoded at multiple points on the gray-scale image. Color Doppler images are created by superimposing this frequency shift information on the spatial information of the gray-scale image (Fig. 1.27). The gray-scale image is formed by calculating the strength of echoes as they return with different delays between transmission and receipt of the pulses sent by the transducer. The relative frequency shifts experienced at these different points is further extracted. Rather than going through the full process of Fourier transformation at every point on the image, more efficient techniques are used. These processing algorithms, currently kept relatively simple due to cost constraints, create a display of the mean frequency shifts (velocity) very similar to the zero-crossing detector used with the older CW Doppler probes. In addition, the information on more than one frame of the image is needed to create the color Doppler display. At least three separate frames are needed. Because of this, the peak repetition frequency is slower with color Doppler imaging. This causes color Doppler to alias earlier—at lower frequency shifts—than pulsed Doppler.

PRACTICAL CONSIDERATIONS

The implementation of pulsed Doppler or color Doppler varies between the different manufacturers of sonographic scanners.

Pulsed Doppler is normally performed at a lower frequency than the imaging frequency. It therefore penetrates the soft tissues more deeply and can return echoes containing velocity information even when the gray-scale image, created at a higher carrier frequency, cannot resolve structures of interest.

Since the pulsed Doppler and gray-scale imaging functions share processing in the sonographic device, the PRF can be in-

Figure 1.23. This diagram summarizes the effect of small errors made in estimating the angle between the ultrasound beam and the direction of moving blood when performing Doppler measurements. The angle determination is normally made by twisting a small knob or depressing a toggle switch, which moves a mobile cursor in increments of 1°, 2°, or 5°. Small errors in the determination of this angle have less of an effect at lower Doppler angles in zone A. The effect is worse as the angle between the ultrasound beam and the vessel increases above 70° (zone C).

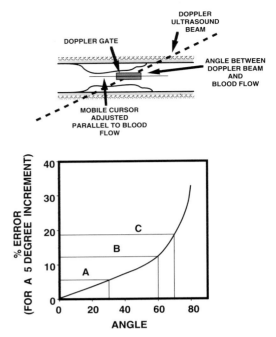

Figure 1.24. Although the carrier frequencies (here 3 and 5 MHz) of two Doppler devices may be different, the Doppler equation factors in this value as the "carrier" frequency. Application of the equation will therefore give the same velocity values irrespective of the carrier frequency.

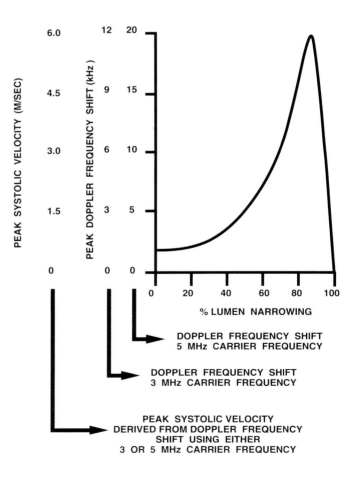

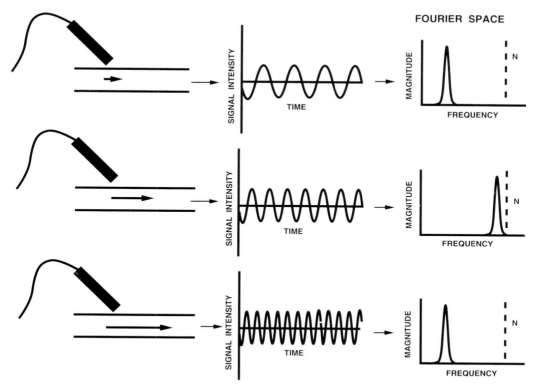

Figure 1.25. This diagram demonstrates the effect of aliasing on the display of the Doppler shift information. It shows the Doppler frequency shift information in Fourier space, at the next to last step in the creation of the Doppler frequency spectral display. The *dashed vertical line* corresponds to the Nyquist frequency. This frequency is equal to one-half the rate at which ultrasound pulses used for pulsed Doppler analysis are transmitted. The PRF or pulse repetition frequency is therefore twice the Nyquist frequency. On the top, the constant velocity within an idealized vessel corresponds to a small Doppler frequency shift. This frequency shift is displayed in Fourier space as a signal peak of low frequency. In the middle, the velocity is now twice that shown above. The resultant frequency shift is higher and so is the location of the signal peak in the Fourier space display. In the lower row, the frequency shift is thrice that of the first row. It is, however, higher than the Nyquist frequency. Therefore it cannot be accurately processed by the electronics within the Doppler signal processor. The final result is an ambiguity in the actual measurement of the frequency shift. The output of the signal processor is a signal peak in the low-frequency portion of the spectrum.

creased in certain devices by "freezing" or at least lowering the frame rate of the gray-scale image. This reduces the likelihood that aliasing will occur.

More than one crystal in the array of the multi-crystal linear array transducer is often used to acquire the Doppler spectra. This increases the sensitivity of the pulsed Doppler signal. The sensitivity of the Doppler component is slightly less than that of gray-scale imaging, despite the lower op-

erating frequency of the pulsed Doppler signals.

An important asset to the use of duplex sonography devices is the capability of performing separate steering of the Doppler beam and of the gray-scale image. In general, for vascular applications, the arterial or venous interfaces are best detected when the ultrasound beam is perpendicular to them. Unfortunately, this imaging configuration is unacceptable for Doppler

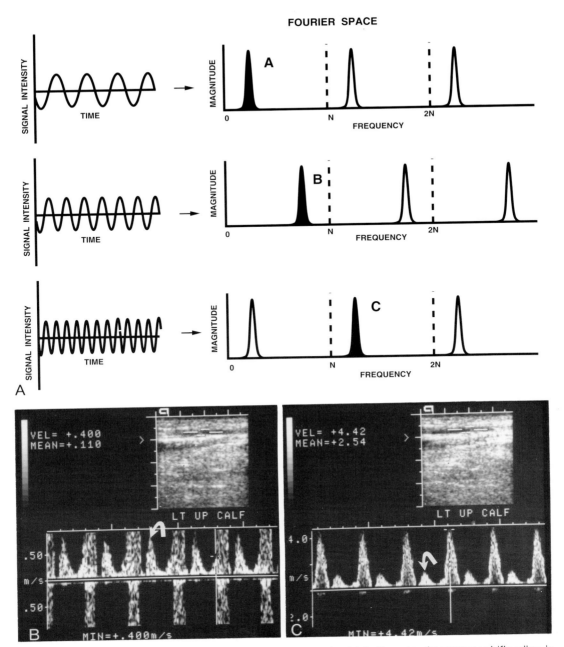

Figure 1.26. A, A complete explanation of the reason why high Doppler frequency shifts alias is beyond the scope of this book. The mathematical process that transforms frequency shift information into values in Fourier space does not do so by establishing a one-to-one correspondence. Instead, a series of repeating windows that contain the same information are created. The size of each of these windows is defined by the value of the Nyquist frequency. Under normal circumstances, the information collected is below the Nyquist frequency. It is therefore displayed within the first window (*shadowed peaks*). The two top rows show this effect. Notice that there are appropriately placed signal peaks (not shadowed) in the other "windows." An even higher frequency shift would normally be placed in the second window (*shadowed peak*). However, because of the sampling process, the peak is read as being present in the first window. A simple example of this effect is the science laboratory experiment using a stroboscopic light. The motion of a spinning bicycle wheel appears slowed by the appropriate frequency of the stroboscopic flashing light,

GRAY SCALE IMAGE

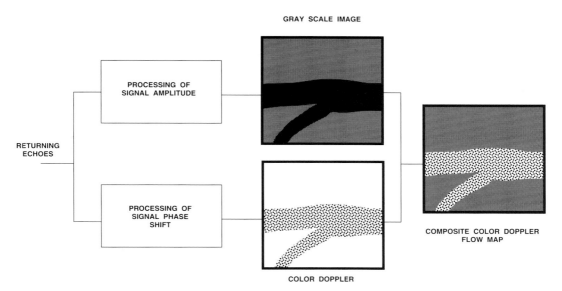

RETURNING ECHOES

PROCESSING OF SIGNAL AMPLITUDE

PROCESSING OF SIGNAL PHASE SHIFT

COLOR DOPPLER

COMPOSITE COLOR DOPPLER FLOW MAP

Figure 1.27. The color Doppler image is a combination of two types of information. It is composed of the normal gray-scale image which, in essence, is created by processing the amplitude of returning echoes. The color Doppler component is normally created at a lower frequency than the gray-scale image. It arises from a special processing of the returning echoes to extract the direction and phase shifts of the returning echoes. The mathematical process used is called autocorrelation. This requires a minimum of three echoes, but the results are improved as the number of echoes utilized increases—typically to 8 or up to 16. The image is processed as if it were composed of a series of Doppler gates distributed evenly throughout the image. The color Doppler image therefore possesses a PRF. The color Doppler image frame rate can increase as the PRF increases. This also increases the maximal frequency shift (velocity) that can be displayed. Unfortunately, this will decrease the real-time image frame rate since both are competing for a larger fraction of the imaging time. Both types of information are combined into a final color flow image with the aid of special algorithms. Care is taken, for example, to suppress color signals from strongly echogenic structures, since they are unlikely to represent blood.

imaging. The best Doppler signals arise when the beam forms an angle of 30° to 60° to the vessel. Both functions are therefore best dissociated by permitting separate steering.

It is recommended that the angle between the ultrasound beam and the vessel where velocities are sampled be less than 60° (Fig. 1.28). This is not to say that spectra obtained at 70° or 80° should be ignored. The phenomenon that limits the use of more obtuse angles is a rapid progression in the magnitude of the error caused by determining the angle between

despite its rapid motion. A similar effect is seen in the old western movies. The motion of the spinning wagon wheel is artifactually slowed and even reversed by the frame rate of the film in the movie projector. In both cases, the physical device used has a limited rate at which information is displayed. A similar process occurs because of the electronics of the Doppler analyzer. The result is a limited and "aliased" view of reality. **B,** Aliasing of the Doppler spectrum can cause confusion and inability to accurately quantitate the presence of high-grade stenosis. The peak systolic velocity cannot be accurately measured. The early diastolic velocity (*curved arrow*) has a value of 0.8 m/sec. **C,** A peak systolic velocity of 4.4 msec corresponds to a high-grade stenosis. The early antegrade diastolic flow (*curved arrow*) measures 0.8 m/sec, the same value as above. This resizing of the spectral display was achieved by increasing the PRF.

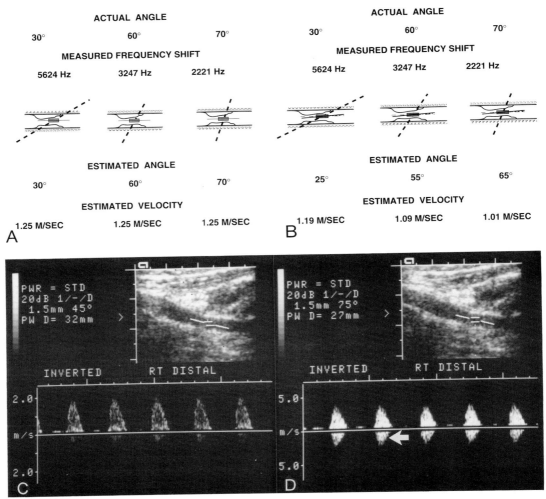

Figure 1.28. **A,** The frequency shifts caused by moving blood are shown here as a function of the angle made between the vessel and the direction of the ultrasound beam used to acquire the Doppler signals. Application of the Doppler equation with accurately measured angles will give the same velocity—1.25 m/sec—in all three cases. **B,** The same frequency shifts are then used to calculate the velocity with the addition of the same 5° error purposely made in each case. The error causes the velocity to be severely underestimated when the Doppler angle is greatest at 70°. It is almost negligible at an angle of 30°. **C,** The effect of proper angle correction is shown. A 45° angle is used to measure frequency shifts at a distinct stenosis at the level of this popliteal artery. Peak systolic velocities are measured near 2.0 m/sec. A small amount of spectral broadening suggests that the sampling is done slightly beyond the actual physical neck of the stenosis. **D,** A corresponding image taken with a steeper angle of interrogation (75°) shows significant changes in the velocity spectra. The measured peak systolic velocity is higher, close to 2.5 msec, corresponding to a 25% difference in the estimate. Artifactual retrograde blood flow is now apparent (*arrow*).

the ultrasound beam and the vessel of interest. At 30°, an error of 5° in setting the angle causes a 5% error in the velocity estimate. At 60°, this causes a 12% error, at 70° a 19% error, and at 80° a 33% error (Fig. 1.28). Counteracting this effect is the reduced sensitivity of the Doppler device at shallow angles, especially when linear-array probes are used. A shallow (<30°) angle of intersection of the returning echoes with the transducer decreases the strength of the echoes reaching the crystal elements.

The limitations for color Doppler imaging are similar to those of pulsed Doppler sonography. Images of flowing blood are often seen on the color Doppler image despite the absence of any resolvable structure on the gray-scale image. The lower frequency of the color Doppler mapping can then be used to detect deeper-lying vessels and serve as a guide for the placement of the Doppler gate for further Doppler spectral analysis.

On certain devices, the gray-scale image can be frozen or slowed down to lower

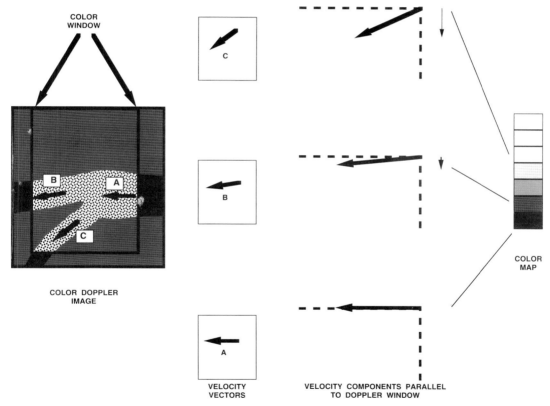

Figure 1.29. The relative angle between the color window and the motion of flowing blood affects the signal intensity displayed on the color map. In this case, the color window is pointing straight down on the vessel. Motion can be decomposed into components parallel to the color window (maximal signal) and those perpendicular to the window (absent signal). On the right side, case *A* shows that there are no components parallel to the window and therefore no signal on the color map. For case *B*, the sampling angle between the vessel and the color window is very mild and corresponds to a low velocity on the color map. Case *C* shows the effect of a steeper angle with higher velocity values on the color velocity map.

frame rates to give more signal and a faster frame rate for the color Doppler display. Such a strategy is rarely useful, since the gray-scale image remains the most important component of the sonographic evaluation of the peripheral vessels and is heavily relied on for the hand-eye coordination needed during the sonographic examination. However, it is possible to increase the frame rate during color Doppler imaging and therefore diminish the aliasing frequency by limiting the size of the color window. Instead of tying up the computer processing information outside this region of interest, more computer power is de-

voted to this small portion of the image. Similarly, the processor need not wait for signals arising outside the sample volume, thereby reducing ambiguity in the returning signals.

Although signals from all the crystals are normally used to create the color flow images, the efficacy of collecting signals containing frequency shift information varies with the angle made to the transducer face. Maximal amplitude of the returning echoes is always obtained for a beam perpendicular to the transducer. The sensitivity of the returning echoes decreases as the angle made with the trans-

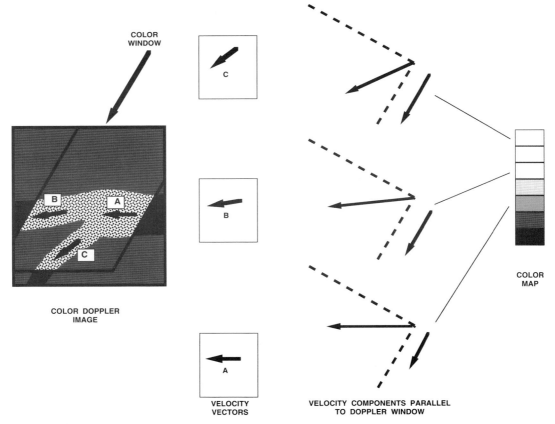

Figure 1.30. Changing the direction of the color window will mostly emphasize the different velocities of blood moving parallel to the transducer. The greatest change is seen for case A. The previously barely perceptible motion of blood is now encoded with a much larger component of blood flow parallel to the Doppler window. The changes for case B are similarly quite significant. In case C, the differences are not as substantial.

ducer face decreases. A shallow angle diminishes the magnitude of the signal available for processing the frequency shift information. This effect tends to decrease the magnitude of the signals used to create the color flow image.

Separate steering of the color Doppler and gray-scale images is of utmost importance in peripheral vascular imaging. The flow information obtained with angulations of 60° or 70° is much superior to that obtained perpendicular to the vessel (Figs. 1.29 and 1.30). However, the images are likely to suffer from a loss of intensity as the angle decreases further. The ability to steer the beam separately may also help circumvent obstructions such as calcified plaque.

Pulsed and color Doppler imaging both require faster frame rates to minimize aliasing. The effect of increasing the frequency of the ultrasound signals used for Doppler imaging is to increase the sensitivity to slower flow while decreasing beam penetration. One might believe that a higher carrier frequency might increase the maximal velocity that can be displayed before aliasing occurs. This is not the case. In fact, the higher the carrier frequency, the lower the velocity at which aliasing occurs.

Gray-Scale versus Doppler Imaging

The importance given to the different components of the sonographic examination is a reflection of the clinical question being asked. Under many circumstances, high-quality gray-scale or real-time imaging is essential since it accurately displays soft tissue interfaces, specifically the interface between the lumen of the vessel and its wall as well as that of the wall with respect to the surrounding soft tissues. This type of imaging task requires higher ultrasound frequencies. Structural details

used for plaque characterization are better perceived at 7 MHz than at 5 MHz.

The type of Doppler device used depends on the type of blood flow analysis desired. A simple non-imaging probe can often suffice for measuring arterial waveforms in the dorsalis pedis or posterior tibial artery at the ankle (Fig. 1.31). For simple spectral analysis of short arterial segments such as the carotid, a CW probe with a spectral analyzer can perform quite efficiently. High accuracies, in the 90% range, have been reported for detecting significant internal carotid artery stenoses. For deeper-lying structures, and for more accurate identification of the source of blood flow signals, the pulsed Doppler device—duplex sonography—is more practical. For example, for stenosis grading within peripheral arteries, bypass grafts, or even the carotid arteries, velocities must be obtained both at the site of suspected stenosis and at more proximal locations so that velocity ratios can be calculated.

The color Doppler map offers a simple two-dimensional display of both anatomic information and blood flow dynamics. It is therefore possible to quickly survey large volumes for the presence and pattern of blood flow. Specific areas that show patterns outside of the normal range can be interrogated with the use of a pulsed Doppler analyzer.

Artifacts

Artifacts can plague both gray-scale and Doppler ultrasound imaging. They can be quite disconcerting to the beginning vascular sonographer.

One of the most common artifacts is generated by the presence of calcification or gas—such as air—in the soft tissues. The ultrasound beam is incapable of penetrating these areas. In addition, transmission of the ultrasound beam cannot cross behind these zones of acoustic shadowing

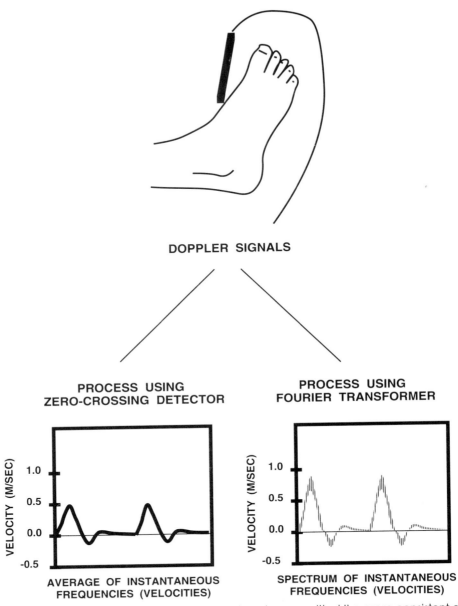

DOPPLER SIGNALS

PROCESS USING
ZERO-CROSSING DETECTOR

PROCESS USING
FOURIER TRANSFORMER

AVERAGE OF INSTANTANEOUS
FREQUENCIES (VELOCITIES)

SPECTRUM OF INSTANTANEOUS
FREQUENCIES (VELOCITIES)

Figure 1.31. The modern use of the spectrum analyzer has permitted the more consistent determination of the distribution of moving blood cells in arteries. It is the method currently used with duplex imaging. Previously published measurements of blood velocities were made using the non–spectral analyzer approach. These values are estimates of the mean velocity of moving blood. Varied parameters of blood flow dynamics, such as the pulsatility index, are determined from these mean velocity contours. The values derived from a Doppler spectral display should not be expected to be the same.

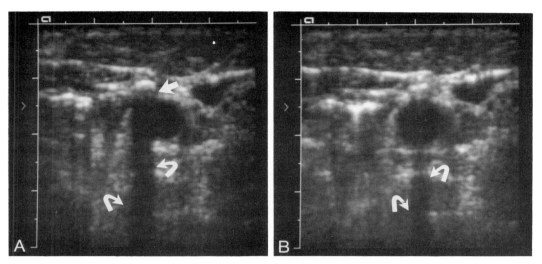

Figure 1.32. **A,** On this first transverse image, a zone of signal loss (*curved arrows*) projects from the wall of the carotid artery (*arrow*). **B,** The second image was taken when the patient was swallowing. The zone of signal loss (*curved arrows*) has moved, suggesting that it is extrinsic to the carotid wall. At first appearance, the finding shown here is typical of a calcified carotid plaque. Signal loss distal to the plaque is due to the fact that almost no energy from the ultrasound beam can travel through calcium. This loss of signal also occurs when the ultrasound beam encounters a gas such as air. The entity responsible for the artifact is in fact a small air-containing diverticulum arising from the larynx—a laryngocele. Its location changes with swallowing.

(Fig. 1.32). This affects both the gray-scale image and the Doppler component.

Reverberation artifacts can artificially project distant structures onto other structures in the image. The reverberation of the sound beam from the interface of the jugular vein can be projected into the lumen of the carotid artery and mimic a carotid dissection (Fig. 1.33). The mirror image is created by the reflection of the sound beam against an interface between zones of high and low acoustic impedance. This can happen at the lung interface and create a mirror artifact of the subclavian artery (Fig. 1.34).

Turbulence caused by the dissipation of the kinetic energy stored in high-velocity jets of blood flow can set up vibrations in the adjacent soft tissues (Fig. 1.35). This is commonly seen distal to high-grade stenoses or at AV fistulous communications.

Other, more benign artifacts can be confusing. The color Doppler signals will often overflow the physical confines of a blood vessel. This color "overflow" can obscure smaller lesions such as plaques or small non-obstructing venous thrombi. Color "flash" can be elicited by rapid motion of the transducer on a structure that is hypoechoic. This artifact arises from the basic premise of many color Doppler processing algorithms, which give a high likelihood for assigning color signals to "black structures" such as the blood vessel lumen. Other areas, such as cysts or zones of acoustic shadowing, can then also have color Doppler signals inappropriately assigned to them.

A basic limitation of color Doppler imaging is the fact that only the mean frequency shift (velocity) is displayed. Zones containing large numbers of red cells rapidly moving in opposite directions will of-

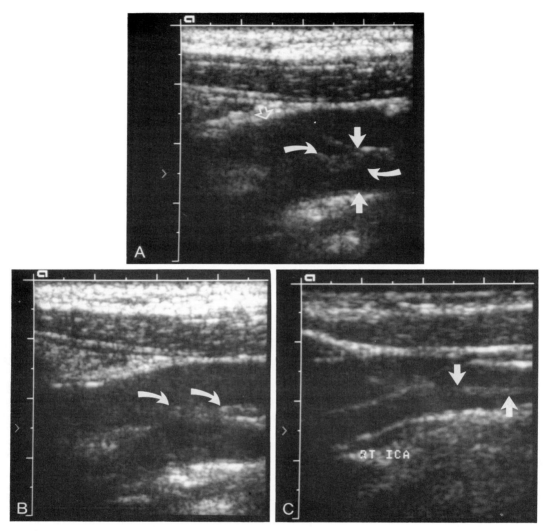

Figure 1.33. **A,** This first longitudinal image shows a line of increased echogenicity (*curved arrows*) in the common carotid artery (*straight arrows*), just inferior to the jugular vein (*open arrow*). The appearance is suggestive of a long plaque. **B,** The second longitudinal image was taken in a different phase of respiration. The suspicious line (*curved arrows*) has moved outside of the carotid artery and is now appreciated in the jugular vein. This is a reverberation artifact. **C,** This linear artifact can also mimic an arterial wall dissection (*arrows*).

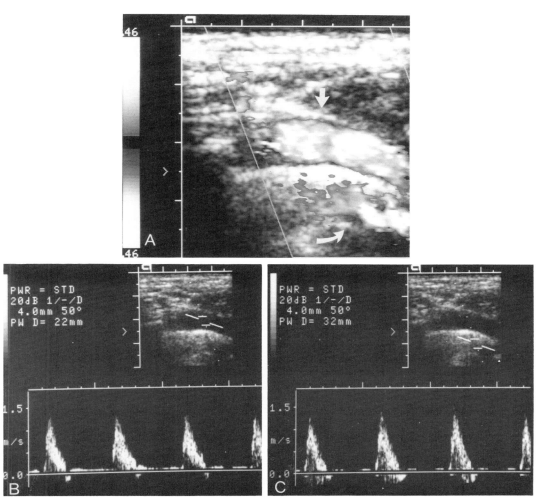

Figure 1.34. **A** (see color plate I), This color Doppler image of the subclavian artery shows apparent duplication of the vessel. The more proximally located vessel (*arrow*) is the true subclavian artery. The more distally located color lumen (*curved arrow*) corresponds to an artifact. The artifact is due to a misregistration in the location of the Doppler signal secondary to reflection of the sound beam at the high acoustic interface with the lung. This is termed the "mirror" artifact. **B,** The true lumen of the subclavian artery shows a typical triphasic pattern of blood flow. **C,** The mirror image of the artery also contains flow signals with a similar spectral distribution.

Figure 1.35. (See color plate I). The soft tissue vibrations induced by either a stenosis or an AV fistula can be visualized on the color Doppler image. In this instance, a high-grade stenosis at the distal anastomosis of a femoral-tibial bypass graft has caused soft tissue vibrations distal to the stenotic jet (*arrows*). This phenomenon, considered an artifact by many authors, corresponds to the physical effect of the high-velocity jet as it hits the vessel wall and disperses energy. It is better perceived at the higher-sensitivity settings and at the lower-velocity range of the color Doppler display.

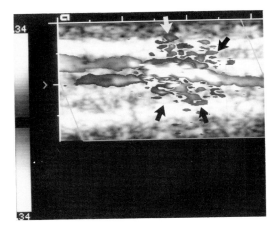

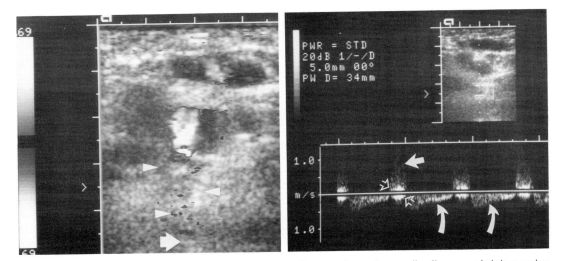

Figure 1.36. **A** (see color plate I). This color Doppler image shows two collections containing color signals. This corresponds to a complex pseudoaneurysm arising from a femoral artery puncture. The femoral artery lies deep in the soft tissues (*arrow*). The actual physical communication with the collection is outlined by the *arrowheads*. No color signals are seen within the channel due to turbulence. **B,** Flow into this pseudoaneurysm consists mostly of a component of high-velocity antegrade flow (*arrow*) and marked turbulence (*open arrows*) affecting a much greater number of red blood cells. The latter is caused by the tortuosity and small size of the communicating channel. Low-intensity, high-amplitude velocities (*arrow*) are superimposed on strong-intensity components of antegrade and retrograde flow due to the turbulence (*open arrows*). These signals, arising during systole, mostly cancel each other out. This explains the net low-amplitude signal on the color Doppler image. The pressure difference between the collection and the artery causes a more typical retrograde diastolic flow into the artery (*curved arrows*).

ten show up as having low velocities. The color image will display the net motion of these red cells, which mostly cancels out, and only a net vector of small magnitude will be registered on the color image (Fig. 1.36).

Flow Patterns of Interest (Synopsis)

NORMAL ARTERIES

The pattern of flow within the peripheral or more central arteries is principally that of antegrade flow during most of the cardiac cycle. In the carotid system, antegrade flow is present throughout the length of systole and diastole. Only rarely will a reversal in the direction of blood flow occur. The circumstances include the presence of severe aortic valve insufficiency with actual retrograde flow back toward the heart during a cardiac cycle and, on occasion, flow within the different lumina of an arterial dissection.

In the peripheral arteries, flow tends to be triphasic with a strong antegrade component of flow during systole followed by end-systolic flow reversal of short duration. A return to forward flow during late diastole is quite variable in its presence or extent and shows dramatic changes in response to both normal and abnormal physiologies. In normals, the typical response to exercise in the lower limb arteries is intense peripheral vasodilation and an overall decrease in peripheral resistance. This decrease in peripheral resistance is reflected by a marked change in the Doppler spectral waveform. There is loss of the high-resistance pulsatile waveform, which is replaced by a pattern very similar to what is seen within the internal carotid—a low-resistance flow profile showing antegrade flow during both systole and diastole.

A similar pattern can be seen in severe peripheral arterial disease distal to a steno-sis. Under these circumstances, the vasodilation is caused by a physiologic response recruiting and dilating arteries within the muscles. This peripheral vasodilation and the presence of collateral branches decrease the overall resistance seen by the vessel distal to a stenosis and lead to a low-resistance profile with antegrade flow during both systole and diastole.

The distribution of blood flow across the lumen of an artery follows a laminar pattern (Fig. 1.37). The highest velocities are seen near the center of the arterial lumen. The velocity of blood decreases as a function of the square of the distance from the wall, where velocity is nearly stagnant at the interface of blood with the endothelial lining of the intima.

This normal pattern is perturbed at the sites of bifurcations or in tortuous segments. At bifurcations, such as the carotid, a zone of flow separation and even reversal of the direction of blood flow is measurable by Doppler sonography both in vivo and in vitro (Fig. 1.38). This zone of relative stagnation is also the preferential site of atherosclerotic plaque formation. The pathophysiologic importance of the interaction between the endothelial lining of the artery and the slowly moving blood constituents is still a matter of conjecture.

Tortuous vessels will show zones of increased velocity at the outer curve of the vessel (Fig. 1.39). These differences in velocity are seen on both duplex sonography and color Doppler flow mapping (Figs. 1.40 and 1.41).

Stenotic Arteries

Progressive narrowing of arterial segments perturbs the normal laminar pattern of blood flow. The distribution of velocities across the lumen shows a more heterogeneous appearance. This is measured on the Doppler spectral waveform as the phe-

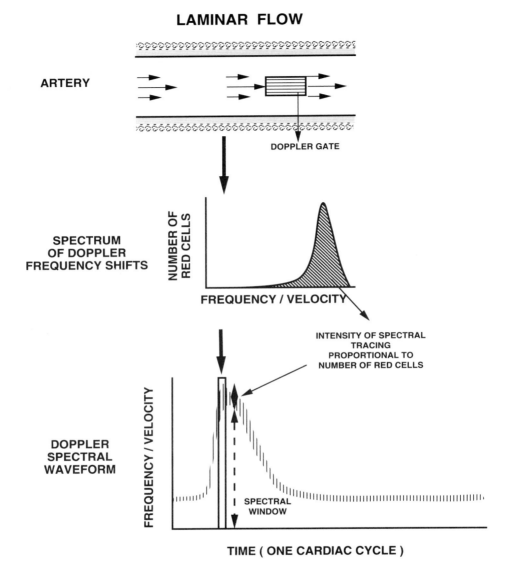

Figure 1.37.   The spectral display seen on the screen of the ultrasound device is created by sampling and calculating the frequency shifts of returning echoes. In this case, the echoes from the center of an artery with normal laminar flow have been sampled. A spectrum is calculated from the frequency shifts of the returning echoes. The result is a display of the distribution of the different frequency shifts seen over a time interval of 1 to 10 msec. This then becomes a component of the Doppler spectral waveform (in the interval indicated by the *arrow*). The intensity of the waveform is proportional to the amplitude of the signals on the spectral display. In this case, the velocities are sampled in the center of the vessel and therefore have a sharp spectrum representing red blood cells with essentially the same velocity. This translates as a Doppler waveform with a clean window.

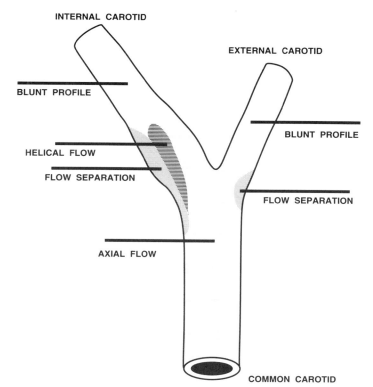

INTERNAL CAROTID

EXTERNAL CAROTID

BLUNT PROFILE

BLUNT PROFILE

HELICAL FLOW

FLOW SEPARATION

FLOW SEPARATION

AXIAL FLOW

COMMON CAROTID

Figure 1.38. The flow patterns in the normal carotid bifurcation are quite complex. The common carotid normally has a laminar pattern of blood flow (axial), which diverges from the midline at 1 to 2 cm from the carotid bulb. Two zones of flow separation—a zone where blood flow is stagnant and often reverses—are normally present. The larger is in the lateral wall of the internal carotid opposite the flow divider and the smaller is at the origin of the external carotid. A region of complex helical flow is believed to exist in vivo. It cannot be measured using Doppler techniques. The flow pattern downstream from the bifurcation may take some distance to return to a laminar pattern. In the interim, the velocity distribution across the artery is more blunt, with moving red cells grouped at the same velocity.

nomenon of spectral broadening (Fig. 1.42). There is a filling in of the Doppler spectrum, reflecting the more heterogeneous distribution in the velocities of flowing blood (Fig. 1.43). These effects are quite variable and difficult to quantitate, since even the size of the Doppler sample gate can mimic spectral broadening in the absence of a stenosis (Fig. 1.21).

As the severity of a stenosis increases, the most consistent measurable change is an increase in the peak systolic velocity (Fig. 1.44). The measured mean velocity yields similar information to the peak systolic velocity but shows more variability. The relative narrowing of the artery causes the blood to accelerate and reach a maximal velocity at the stenosis (Fig. 1.45). At this point, the stenosis "throat," all blood cells tend to travel at the same velocity and the Doppler spectrum is narrow. Distal to the stenosis, the velocity patterns are per-

turbed as energy is dissipated into a larger-diameter conduit. A flow jet is seen for stenoses above 50% in severity (Fig. 1.46). Just downstream of the stenosis, a vortex of reversed blood flow direction occurs. It lies to the side of the flow jet and is more apparent during systole. The heterogeneity in direction of flow is more notable at higher velocity values and tends to be maximal just distal to the zone of flow reversal.

Grading of the severity of stenosis can also be made by the use of the velocity ratio or using an absolute cutoff of velocity values. The maximal measured peak systolic velocity is compared to that obtained at a point located proximal to the suspected beginning of the stenosis. The derived ratio has been shown to be a good noninvasive correlate of the severity of the stenosis. The waveform seen at stenoses of the internal carotid shows a loss of the

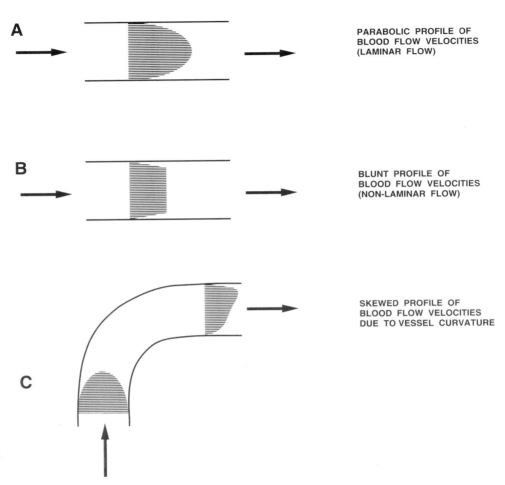

Figure 1.39. **A,** Laminar flow is present in most peripheral arteries. It consists of a parabolic shape in the distribution of the velocities of flowing blood across the lumen of the vessel. The slower velocities are located near the vessel wall, while the fastest component is located at the center. **B,** Plug or blunt flow refers to a relatively even grouping of the red cells, all having approximately the same velocity across the lumen of the vessel. It is seen at the site of a hemodynamically significant stenosis. **C,** The velocity profile at a vessel bend shows a skewed distribution of red blood cell velocities. There is a loss of the laminar pattern, with the fastest-moving red cells migrating to the outer aspect of the vessel as they exit the bend.

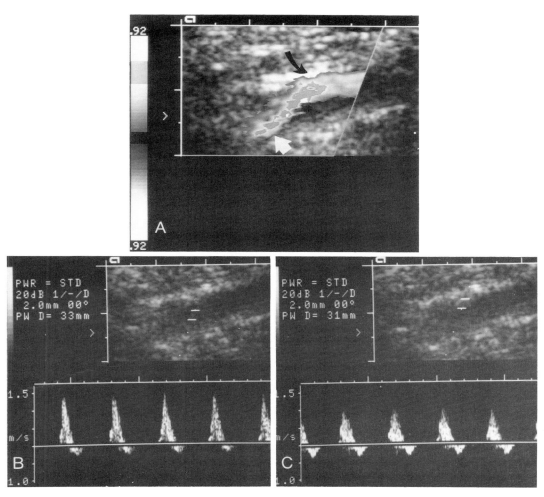

Figure 1.40. **A** (see color plate I), This color Doppler image of a femoropopliteal bypass graft shows the effect of a bend on the flow dynamics within a vessel. A green tag was used to select red blood cells whose velocity fell within a given velocity range. Red cells with the greater velocities are situated on the outside of the conduit (*arrow*), just proximal to the bend. Distal to the bend, there is redirection of blood flow toward the outer aspect of the vessel (*curved arrows*). **B,** The first Doppler spectrum is acquired in the region of the higher-velocity red blood cells as identified by the green tag. Peak systolic velocities are close to 1.5 m/sec. **C,** The second Doppler spectrum was acquired in the zone of slightly lowered red cell velocities at the bend proper. Peak systolic velocities are measured at 1.0 m/sec.

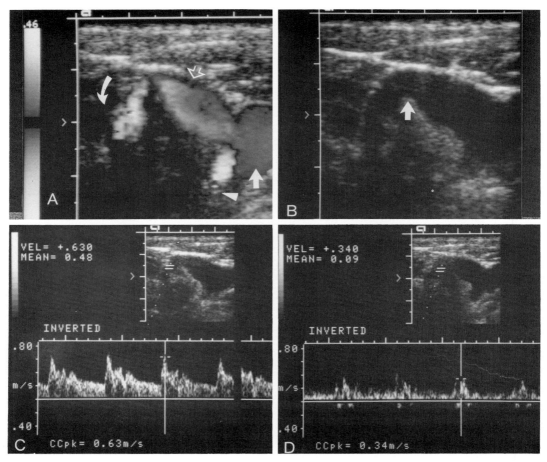

Figure 1.41. A (see color plate I), The flow dynamics at a sharp bend in the internal carotid artery can be confusing. The red encoding corresponds to flow directed toward the transducer in the carotid bulb (*arrow*) and in the proximal carotid artery (*open arrow*). Flow away from the transducer is encoded in blue. It is seen in the proximal internal carotid (*curved arrow*) and the proximal external carotid (*arrowhead*). **B,** The corresponding gray-scale image of this sharply angulated carotid can mimic the appearance of a stenosis (*arrow*). **C,** Beyond the actual physical bend, the highest velocities tend to be located on the far wall on the outside of the bend. Measurements obtained at this point show a peak velocity of 0.63 m/sec. **D,** Sampling of the velocity on the inside or near wall of the curve shows lower-amplitude velocities at 0.34 m/sec. The dynamics set up at the actual bend may vary under different hemodynamic situations. It is our habit to angle correct based on the direction of flow when a jet is seen on the color Doppler image or to angle correct parallel to the wall on the inside of the curve.

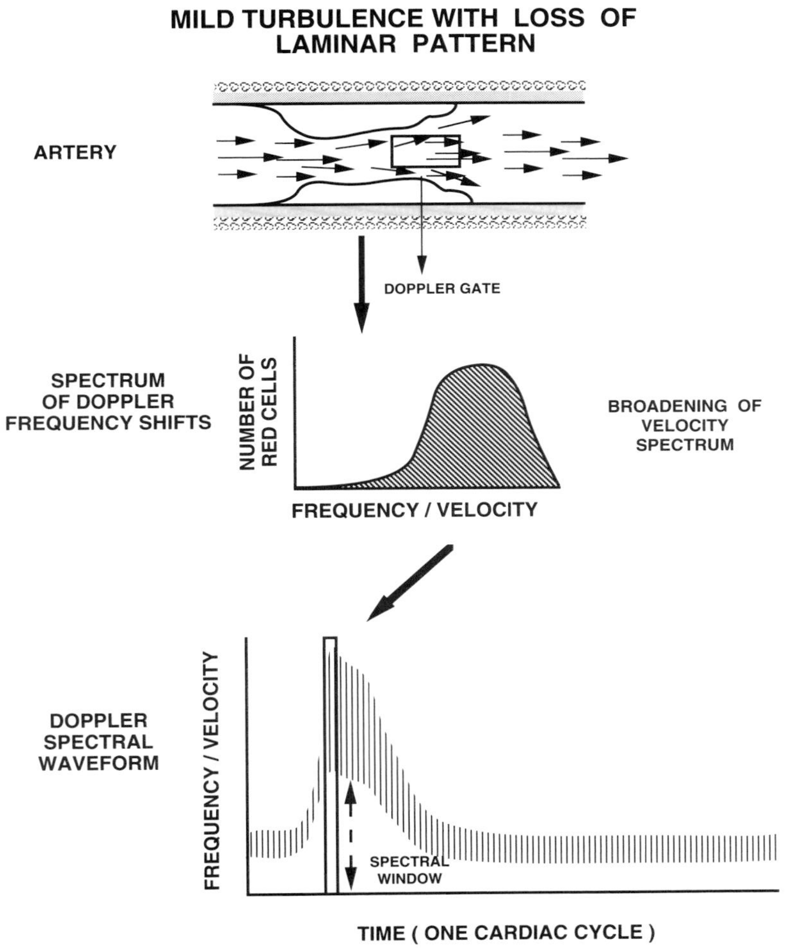

MILD TURBULENCE WITH LOSS OF LAMINAR PATTERN

ARTERY

DOPPLER GATE

SPECTRUM OF DOPPLER FREQUENCY SHIFTS

NUMBER OF RED CELLS

FREQUENCY / VELOCITY

BROADENING OF VELOCITY SPECTRUM

DOPPLER SPECTRAL WAVEFORM

FREQUENCY / VELOCITY

SPECTRAL WINDOW

TIME (ONE CARDIAC CYCLE)

Figure 1.42. A mild to moderate narrowing of an artery causes a loss in the normal laminar pattern of blood flow (*top*). This effect is more pronounced at the exit point of the narrowing. Sampling of the velocities at this point will show a broader frequency shift (velocity) distribution (*center*). This will then translate as a filling in of the Doppler spectral waveform (*bottom*).

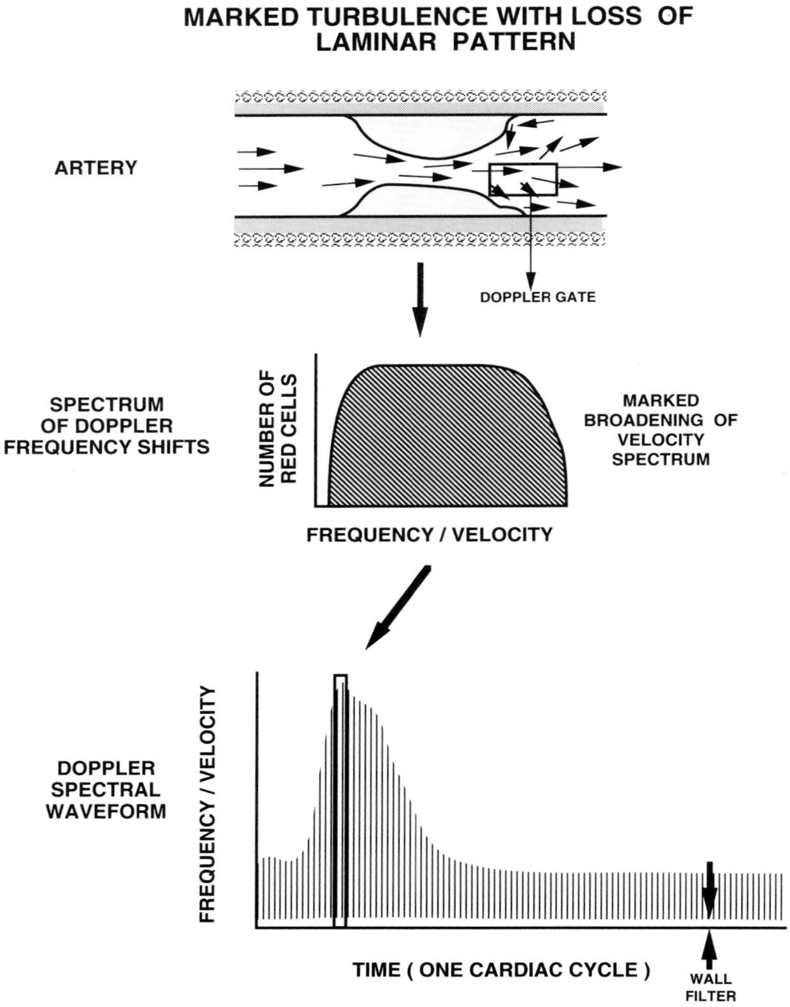

**MARKED TURBULENCE WITH LOSS OF
LAMINAR PATTERN**

ARTERY

DOPPLER GATE

SPECTRUM
OF DOPPLER
FREQUENCY SHIFTS

NUMBER OF
RED CELLS

MARKED
BROADENING OF
VELOCITY
SPECTRUM

FREQUENCY / VELOCITY

DOPPLER
SPECTRAL
WAVEFORM

FREQUENCY / VELOCITY

TIME (ONE CARDIAC CYCLE)

WALL
FILTER

Figure 1.43.   A more pronounced loss in the laminar distribution of blood flow will develop distal to a higher-grade stenosis. Sampling of the Doppler frequency shifts in this region will show a marked broadening of the spectrum of velocities.

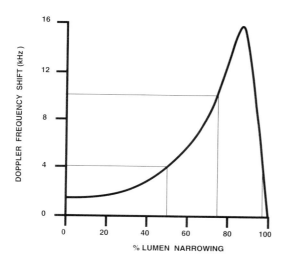

Figure 1.44. The relationship between peak systolic frequency shift and lumen narrowing of an artery is the basic principle that permits the use of Doppler sonography to detect and grade significant stenoses of the carotid and peripheral arteries. This curve has different components, which are well worth examining. The first is the low-frequency shift region below 50% narrowing. Although frequency shifts slowly increase as a function of non-critical narrowings, measurement error normally limits the use of peak-systolic frequency shifts for this range of stenosis severity. A narrowing of 50% of the lumen diameter is considered to be hemodynamically significant. The Doppler frequency shift increases more or less linearly with stenosis severity for stenoses ranging between 50 and 75%. Above 75% stenosis, frequency shifts will continue to increase until stenoses of 90% are reached. They will then start to fall. This portion of the Doppler curve is a possible source of error in estimating stenosis severity. Very high-grade stenoses might potentially be missed. One mechanism available to protect against this type of error is the use of the periorbital Doppler signals. These will likely be abnormal for stenoses more severe than 90%. The recent use of color Doppler mapping and the ability to see very narrowed flow lumina may also help clarify this type of situation.

pulsatile component. Increased diastolic as well as increased systolic flow velocities can be used to grade stenosis severity. In the peripheral arteries, the diastolic component of flow is quite variable and is in fact often absent. Because of this variability, the peak systolic velocity is favored as a better indicator of the presence of a significant stenosis.

Normal Venous Channels

The normal flow pattern within the veins of the upper and lower extremities tends to be constant antegrade flow returning toward the heart with superimposed oscillations due to normal respiration (Fig. 1.47) and transmitted atrial pulsations. The amplitude of these superimposed oscillations depends on the loca-

tion of the vein, the state of hydration, and the presence of proximal obstruction and right-sided heart failure. A simple physiologic maneuver can be used to accentuate venous return. Squeezing of the peripheral veins within the calf with a hand causes a relative increase of venous blood flow. This can be measured by sampling the Doppler spectrum in a vein proximal to the calf. This venous flow accentuation or augmentation can be used to exclude obstruction of a venous channel. An added advantage of this maneuver is that it increases blood flow velocity, thereby making it possible to detect Doppler frequency shifts in the vein lumen. These may not have been detectable due to a low resting velocity of blood flow. The maneuver can be used to great advantage to localize vessels and to confirm patency of the segment being imaged.

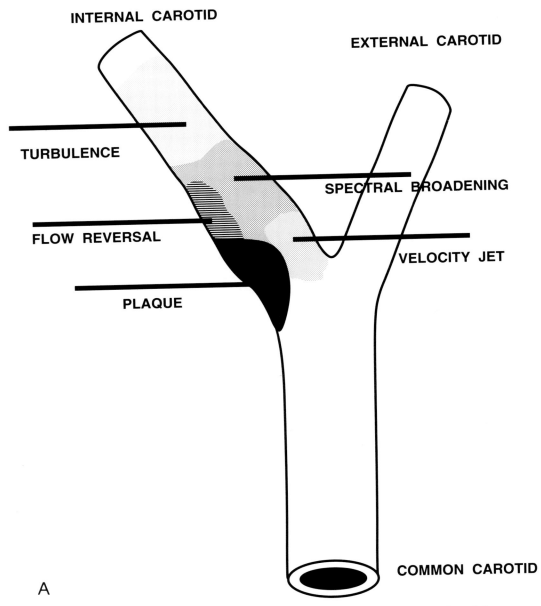

INTERNAL CAROTID

EXTERNAL CAROTID

TURBULENCE

SPECTRAL BROADENING

FLOW REVERSAL

VELOCITY JET

PLAQUE

COMMON CAROTID

A

Figure 1.45. A, A significant stenosis caused by a large carotid plaque will disrupt the normal pattern of blood flow. A zone of flow separation will develop downstream of the plaque. The velocity jet will extend from the throat (narrowest point) of the stenosis for a variable distance. Turbulence is expected slightly farther downstream, where the energy of the red cells is rapidly dissipated. **B** (see color plate I), The typical color Doppler appearance of a high-grade stenosis is shown here. The color Doppler signals change according to the color Doppler map from a red low-intensity saturation in color to white (*open arrow*) and finally alias into the higher-velocity range now identified by blue (*curved arrow*). This change in signal intensities corresponds to the physical phenomenon of aliasing. The higher-velocity signals cannot be accurately processed by the algorithms used to create the color Doppler flow image. The transitions from red, to white, and then to blue correspond to increasing blood flow velocities. These have gone above the maximal dynamic range of the

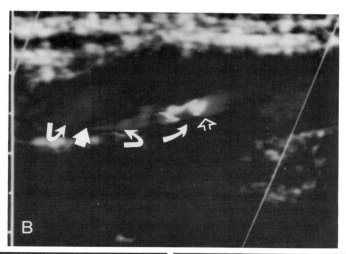

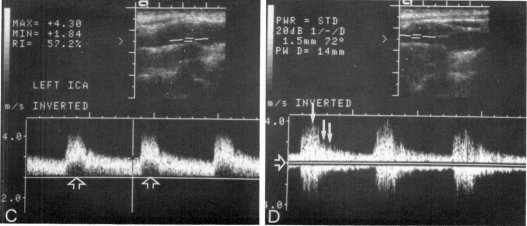

device. The presence of flow reversal can be distinguished from a stenosis, since the transition between the red and blue color signals goes through low-frequency shifts (low velocities) indicated by the black zone (*large arrow*) between the zones of forward and reverse flow (*curved arrows*). **C,** The typical appearance of the Doppler waveform in the actual throat or narrowest part of the stenosis is that of a high-velocity signal with increased peak systolic velocities. The spectral window shows some clearing (*open arrows*) consistent with the fact that the cohort of red cells across the stenosis is moving at roughly the same velocity. The smaller dark line at the base of the spectra corresponds to the wall filter. This filter eliminates low-velocity signals that are caused by physical motion of the arterial wall during the cardiac cycle. **D,** Beyond the actual stenosis is a region where turbulence and flow reversal coexist. In this image, the irregular-appearing envelope of the Doppler waveform corresponds to the presence of random motion (turbulence; *arrows*). A component of flow reversal suggests that the Doppler gate was positioned near a boundary layer between the antegrade (which shows the highest forward velocities) and retrograde motion outside the actual jet of fluid motion. The wall filter is well appreciated (*open arrow*) in this image.

Figure 1.46. Blood flow proximal to a high-grade stenosis is laminar **(A)**. At the stenosis proper, all the red cells tend to travel at the same velocity **(B)**. The spectrum is therefore more narrow than that sampled in the artery proximal to the stenosis, and it has a larger amplitude since all of the red cells must pass through the orifice. *Fmax* is the maximal systolic frequency shift (velocity). Distal to the stenosis, a more distinct jet of increased velocities develops **(C)**, surrounded by a zone of flow reversal **(D)**. The jet is often asymmetrical, hitting one or the other of the arterial walls rather than being directed toward the center of the artery. The amplitude (number of red cells in the spectrum) is smaller than that at the stenosis. The zone of flow reversal is seen as a site where eddy currents cause the blood to flow back on itself as the energy accumulated at the stenosis is dissipated. Negative velocity and frequency shifts are due to flow reversal.

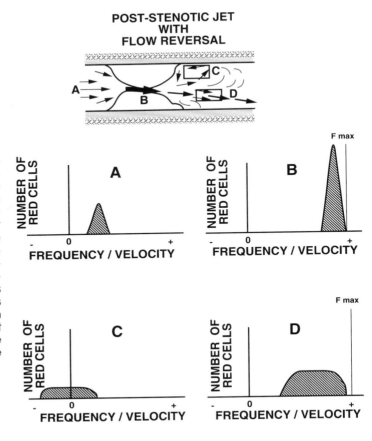

POST-STENOTIC JET WITH FLOW REVERSAL

Figure 1.47. Common femoral venous flow is mostly constant with a superimposed cyclical variation caused by breathing. The small amount of retrograde flow (*curved arrow*) represents a change in the direction of blood flow, which is physiological. This retrograde flow is due to a combination of reflux of the blood necessary to aid the closing of more proximally located valves in the superficial femoral and deep femoral veins. There is also a slight increase in the capacity of these large-diameter vessels in response to the increased venous pressure.

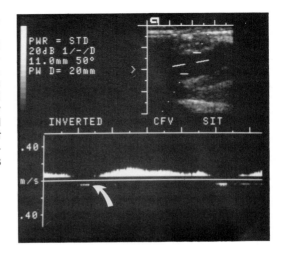

Obstructed Veins

With venous obstruction, there is loss of the normal respiratory variation secondary to the obstructive process. Similarly, there is loss of the normal response to venous augmentation. Indirect evidence of obstruction can also be obtained by the loss of the normal response to forced respiratory maneuvers. For example, in the lower extremity, a Valsalva maneuver increases intra-abdominal pressure and causes distention of the leg veins. In the upper extremity, a deep inspiration commonly results in collapse of the vein lumen through the transmission of a negative pressure wave. The presence of this normal vein wall apposition excludes the presence of obstructing thrombosis.

An indirect sign of venous obstruction is the development of venous collaterals: multiple smaller veins are often seen in the soft tissues at the level of the suspected obstruction.

Venous Incompetence

There is increasing interest in detecting and grading the extent of venous insufficiency as well as localizing its site in either the superficial or deep veins of the leg. The normal response to a Valsalva maneuver is cessation of flow without retrograde flow. With venous incompetence, there is frank retrograde flow down the incompetent veins. Similarly, proximal compression should not cause any distal augmentation or retrograde venous flow. Incompetent veins will show an abnormal response and retrograde flow. Finally, in the upright position, incompetent veins can easily be identified by squeezing the calf veins. Following antegrade flow in response to the squeeze, incompetent venous segments will show reflux and retrograde flow.

Arteriovenous Communications

The use of duplex sonography for the diagnosis of congenital arteriovenous malformations of the lower extremities is possibly a redundant function. Most congenital AV malformations are easily detectable close to the skin and manifest themselves by cutaneous changes. Color Doppler sonography may, on occasion, help identify the feeding arterial channel. In general, these distended vascular channels contain strong flow signals. Deeper-lying AV malformations can be detected by Doppler sonography. More recently, color Doppler sonography has increased the ease with which feeding arteries can be identified and mapped. Serial sonographic studies are currently being investigated as a means of evaluating the success of interventions aimed at eliminating these malformations.

Iatrogenic arteriovenous fistulas secondary to either catheterization, trauma, or surgery can also be readily detected. The presence of high velocity turbulent signals within the vein, more commonly the femoral, are suggestive. Other signs include low-resistance signals in the artery proximal to the communication and high-resistance signals distal to it. The recent use of color Doppler mapping now permits the actual localization of the site of fistulous communication.

Masses

The utility of Doppler sonography for evaluating peripheral masses consists mostly in excluding the presence of blood flow in a clinically felt mass. It is mostly the absence of blood flow in a peripheral mass that suggests that a biopsy or aspiration can be safely performed.

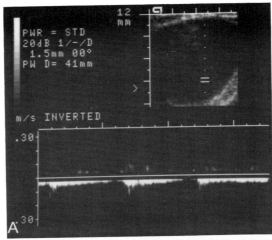

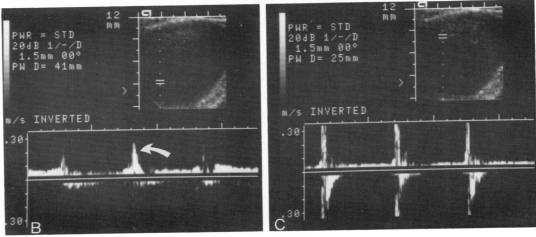

Figure 1.48. The blood flow pattern within pseudoaneurysms can be quickly and efficiently documented by color Doppler imaging. Duplex imaging will show quite different patterns, depending on where the Doppler gate has been placed. **A,** Mostly retrograde flow is seen in this lower portion of a pseudoaneurysm. **B,** Closer to the entry site of the jet feeding the pseudoaneurysm, a strong antegrade component of flow (*curved arrow*) is seen. **C,** The jet of blood entering the collection remains directed toward the wall farthest from the entry site.

Figure 1.49. The flow pattern within the communication between artery and pseudoaneurysm shows a combination of both antegrade (*arrow*) and retrograde (*open arrow*) flow. Antegrade flow into the collection occurs during systole, when arterial pressures are greater than the pressures within the soft tissues. The longer-duration, lower-amplitude diastolic flow occurs while systemic arterial pressures are higher than the pressure within the pseudoaneurysm.

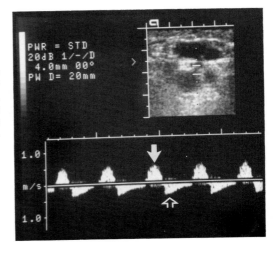

A typical pattern of swirling motion is almost pathognomonic for the presence of a pseudoaneurysm, a localized tear in the arterial wall. The Doppler spectral waveforms are much more variable (Fig. 1.48). The communication to the originating artery can often be visualized on color Doppler mapping. It will show a typical to-and-fro motion on Doppler spectral analysis (Fig. 1.49).

Aneurysmal dilatation in native arteries or at sites of surgical anastomoses can show a disruption in the normal flow pattern with reversal during systole.

SUGGESTED READINGS

Abu-Yousef MM, Wiese JA, Shamma AR. The "to-and-fro" sign: duplex Doppler evidence of femoral artery pseudoaneurysm. AJR 1988;150:632–634.

Banjavic RA. Design and maintenance of a quality assurance program for diagnostic ultrasound equipment. Semin Ultrasound 1983;4:10–26.

Barber FE, Baker DW, Nation AW, Strandness DE Jr, Reid JM. Ultrasonic duplex echo-Doppler scanner. IEEE Trans Biomed Eng 1974;21:109–113.

Kasai C, Namekawa K, Koyano A, Omoto R. Real-time two dimensional blood flow imaging using an autocorrelation technique. IEEE Trans Sonics Ultrason 1985;SU-32:458–463.

Kremkau FW. Diagnostic ultrasound. Principles, instruments, and exercises. 3rd ed. Philadelphia: WB Saunders, 1989.

Middleton WD, Erickson S, Melson GL. Perivascular color artifact: pathologic significance and appearance on color Doppler US images. Radiology 1989;171:647–652.

Mitchell DG, Needleman L, Bezzi M, et al. Femoral artery pseudoaneurysm: diagnosis with conventional duplex and color Doppler US. Radiology 1987;65:687–690.

Musto R, Roach MR. Flow studies in glass models of aortic aneurysms. Can J Surg 1980;23:452–455.

Ojha M, Johnston KW, Cobbold RS, Hummel RL. Potential limitations of center-line pulsed Doppler recordings: an in vitro flow visualization study. J Vasc Surg 1989;9:515–520.

Reneman RS, Spencer MP. Local Doppler audio spectra in normal and stenosed carotid arteries in man. Ultrasound Med Biol 1979;5:1–11.

Robinson DE, Wilson LS, Kossoff G. Shadowing and enhancement in ultrasonic echograms by reflection and refraction. JCU 1981;9:181–188.

Spencer MP, Reid JM. Quantitation of carotid stenosis with continuous-wave (C-W) Doppler ultrasound. Stroke 1979;10:326–330.

Wilkinson DL, Polak JF, Grassi CJ, Whittemore AD, O'Leary DH. Pseudoaneurysm of the vertebral artery: appearance on color-flow Doppler sonography. AJR 1988;151:1051–1052.

CHAPTER TWO

Pathophysiology

Venous Thrombosis
INCIDENCE AND PREVALENCE

Determination of the incidence or prevalence of venous thrombosis arising in the upper and lower extremities is a difficult epidemiologic task.

An estimate can be arrived at by using the reported rate of fatal pulmonary emboli. The annual death rate due to pulmonary emboli peaked at 8 cases per 100,000 persons per year in the mid-1970s. By the early 1980s, this had decreased to 6 cases per 100,000 per year. Since cases of fatal pulmonary emboli probably account for less than 10% of the total number of episodes of pulmonary emboli occurring each year, this would give a yearly rate of *60 to 80 cases per 100,000 persons per year* or approximately 120,000 to 160,000 episodes in the United States each year. This number is a lower-range estimate, since pulmonary embolism is most likely underdiagnosed as a cause of death. The difficulty lies in extrapolating from this number the incidence of lower-extremity, pelvic, or upper-extremity venous thrombosis.

Acute pulmonary embolism is associated with a lower-extremity vein thrombus more than 80% of the time. This has been estimated by looking at the number of times phlebography is positive in patients who have pulmonary embolism (Fig. 2.1). The incidence of venous thrombosis would therefore, at the very least, range between 48 and 160 episodes per 100,000 persons per year. Additional factors related to race and diet most likely account for a 50% greater incidence in blacks and a lower incidence in orientals. This estimate combines both symptomatic and asymptomatic deep vein thrombosis.

Objective evidence of the incidence of symptomatic lower-extremity deep venous thrombosis (DVT) comes from a Swedish study in which phlebography was used on symptomatic patients. The incidence observed was *90 episodes per 100,000 persons per year*. This distribution of vein thrombosis in symptomatic individuals favors the popliteal and femoral veins, where it is obstructive in nature. Conversely, evidence of pulmonary embolism is seen in up to 50% of patients with a venous thrombosis. This estimate applies to a mostly white population.

Asymptomatic venous thrombosis is more commonly associated with surgical procedures and immobilization in hospitalized patients. For example, an incidence

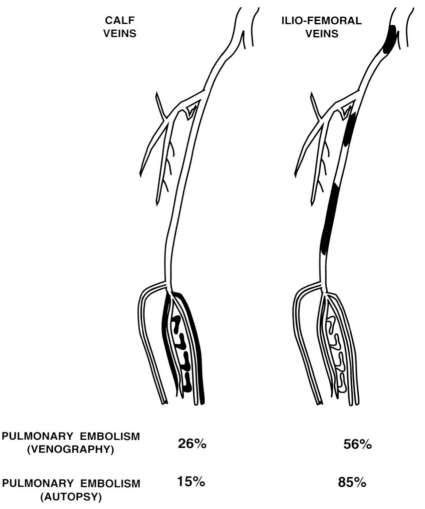

Figure 2.1. Our understanding of the relationship between peripheral venous thromboses and the presence of pulmonary embolism is somewhat skewed. The distribution of peripheral thromboses examined by peripheral venography following an acute episode of pulmonary embolism shows that the majority originate from the femoropopliteal veins. Cases with involvement limited to the calf veins may represent instances in which the more proximal portion of the blood clot has broken free. Finally, a likely source of the embolism is not found in up to 20% of cases. Again, some of these may represent instances in which all of the thrombus has embolized. Autopsy studies have shown that all instances of pulmonary emboli were associated with a peripheral thrombosis. The vast majority originate in the femoropopliteal veins, although a significant proportion may have come from the calf veins. The incidence of pulmonary embolism in cases with peripheral thromboses is 20 to 30%, with four of five being asymptomatic.

of DVT between 20 and 50% has been reported in certain high-risk postsurgical groups (patients who have had neurosurgical, orthopedic, and urologic procedures). Under these circumstances, there is a high prevalence of asymptomatic venous thrombosis involving the calf veins and less commonly, the popliteal and femoral veins (Fig. 2.2). The incidence of asymptomatic pulmonary embolism in this patient group has probably been underestimated. It is likely to occur in more than half of patients with lower-extremity venous thrombosis. In general, these non-obstructing thrombi tend to be self-limited and spontaneously lyse later in the postoperative course. They may spread in approximately 20% of cases and become a more serious threat for significant pulmonary embolism. Close to 80% of these thrombi are apparent within the first 5 to 7 postoperative days.

Rare causes of lower-extremity DVT include the spread of entities such as pelvic vein thrombosis following extensive pelvic surgery and ovarian vein thrombophlebitis. The Budd-Chiari syndrome can cause relative obstruction and thrombosis spreading to the inferior vena cava. Spread of thrombosis from the renal vein in renal cell carcinoma, or from tumor-related thrombosis of the inferior vena cava in pancreatic tumors are rare causes of proximal deep vein thrombus spreading downward to the femoral veins.

In pregnancy, the incidence of prepartum DVT is 0.7 per 1000. There is preferential spread of thrombus from the iliac vein

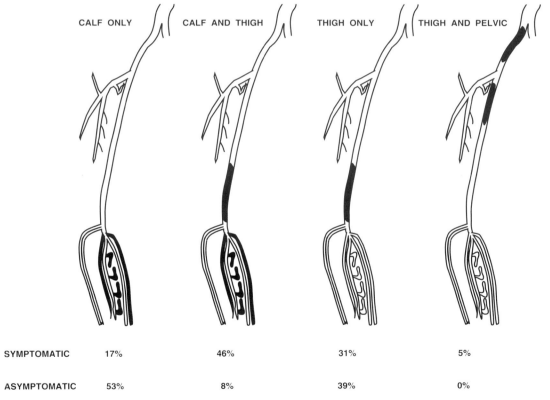

	CALF ONLY	CALF AND THIGH	THIGH ONLY	THIGH AND PELVIC
SYMPTOMATIC	17%	46%	31%	5%
ASYMPTOMATIC	53%	8%	39%	0%

Figure 2.2. There are two clinical patterns of deep vein thrombosis. The first type is seen mostly in symptomatic patients. These are typically outpatients presenting with localized symptoms in an extremity. They tend to have mostly obstructive thrombosis. The second type predominates in asymptomatic patients who have had recent surgical intervention. They tend to form nonobstructing thromboses of their deep veins. At presentation, almost three-fourths of the symptomatic patients have thromboses of the femoral veins. The pattern of thrombosis also suggests contiguous spread from the calf veins in more than half. The small incidence of proximal (iliofemoral vein) thromboses is due to patients who tend to form thrombus in the iliac vein, such as patients with pelvic malignancies and pregnant patients. The asymptomatic patients show a higher incidence of isolated calf vein thrombi and of isolated femoropopliteal vein thromboses early after surgery.

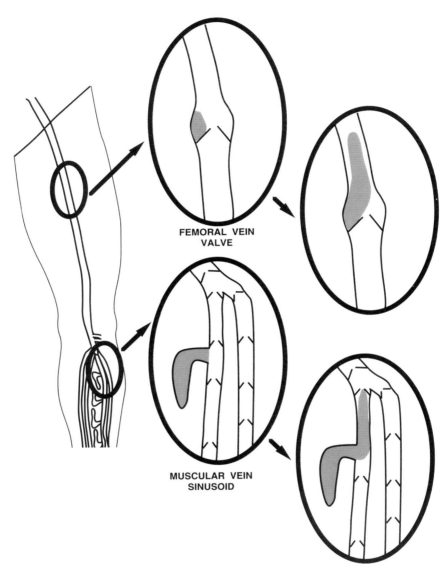

**FEMORAL VEIN
VALVE**

**MUSCULAR VEIN
SINUSOID**

Figure 2.3. Autopsy as well as postoperative studies have shown that thrombus is likely to form through one of two mechanisms. The more common pattern is early formation in the venous sinuses of the calf muscles. This is the likely site of origin of most symptomatic DVTs acquired in the outpatient population and in the majority of postoperative asymptomatic DVTs. The other location is at the venous valve of the femoral or popliteal veins. The mechanism is thought to be stagnation and aggregation of blood downstream from the valve apparatus, in the sinus of the valve. This site is often seen in bedridden patients and in patients with a hypercoagulable state or a malignancy. The latter will often have multiple discrete sites of thrombus formation.

downward to the femoral vein, affecting mostly the left side. This is due to the relative constriction of the left iliac vein caused by the crossing of the aorta or right iliac artery superior to it. In general, this slight difference in flow dynamics can account for a slightly greater incidence of left-sided thrombosis. There is also an association between prostate, bladder, and pelvic malignancies and proximal thrombosis affecting the iliac veins.

Phlegmasia cerulea dolens is a worst-case presentation and a rare complication of an episode of acute lower-extremity DVT. Venous obstruction in these cases can cause impairment of arterial supply to the leg and can lead to ischemia. If not treated by either heparinization or thrombectomy, loss of limb or even death can follow.

The incidence of upper-extremity venous thrombosis is much lower, accounting for 1% of the total episodes of DVT. Thrombosis is most often related to trauma. This includes cases referred to as "effort" thrombosis or instances of blunt or penetrating injury. Another subset includes upper-extremity thrombosis related to instrumentation and the placement of indwelling catheters. These are very commonly placed in patients with malignancies, for chemotherapy administration, or for prolonged courses of parenteral nutrition. This patient subgroup is already prone to venous thrombosis. Instances of spontaneously arising arm DVT are most often correlated with congestive heart failure, diabetes, and mediastinal obstruction by neoplasm or inflammation.

RISK FACTORS

The most common risk factor for the development of deep vein thrombosis is a previous episode of deep vein thrombosis. It has all the elements of the well-known triad attributed to Virchow: vessel wall damage, stasis of blood, and hypercoagulopathy.

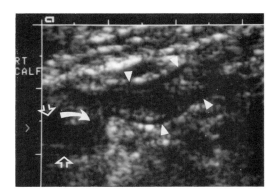

Figure 2.4. Deep venous thrombosis develops behind venous valves and within the deep muscular venous sinuses. In this oblique image, a typical muscular venous sinus containing an early thrombus (*arrowheads*) is clearly shown. It has an oblong shape reminiscent of a jalapeño pepper. The "stalk" of the sinus is not distended or deformed (*curved arrow*). This thrombus is still limited to the venous sinus and has not reached the paired posterior tibial veins (*open arrows*).

Vessel wall damage is most commonly seen following fractures. The preoperative incidence of femoral or tibial vein thrombosis in patients with fractures is attributed to this. Direct injury to the vein is also used in animal models of DVT. Disruption or modification of the endothelium is thought to be the inciting event for thrombosis.

Stasis undoubtedly contributes to the development and spread of deep venous thrombosis. The autopsy data of Sevitt and Gallagher suggest that thrombi form in the valve pockets, a zone in which slow flow predominates (Fig. 2.3). Flow within the soleal sinuses is also severely decreased during most surgical procedures, since the calf muscles are paralyzed and unable to clear the stagnant blood from the venous sinuses (Fig. 2.4).

The mechanisms responsible for hypercoagulopathy are varied. Increases in procoagulant factors that are likely to induce and help in the coagulation and thrombotic process are seen postoperatively when fibrinogen and factors II, V, VII and

XIII of the coagulation cascade increase. Deficiencies in antithrombin III, protein-C, and protein-S have also been reported to increase the risk of deep vein thrombosis. A reduction of the fibrinolytic activity of blood has also been noted in the postoperative period.

LOCATION AND PATTERN

Venous thrombi will typically form within the muscular venous plexi of the calf and spread contiguously to the tibioperoneal veins. In 20% of cases they spread to the popliteal venous segment and the superficial femoral vein, and finally involve the common femoral vein. This pattern of involvement is thought to occur in the majority of lower extremity DVT cases. On occasion, there is spread to the iliac veins and into the inferior vena cava.

Data on the distribution of deep vein thrombi have been obtained from large autopsy series. These series, performed on patients with malignancy or hospitalized for multiple trauma, show a high prevalence of thrombi within the venous plexi of the calf muscles. The number of thrombi then decrease in frequency at other sites

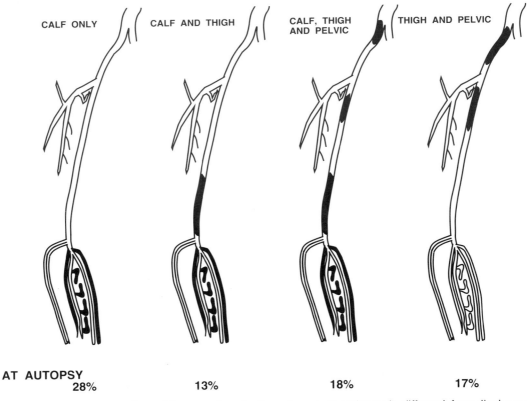

Figure 2.5. The distribution of lower-extremity thromboses at autopsy is different from that seen during venography. This reflects the fact that patients are likely to have less-extensive DVT when they are alive. Involvement of the calf veins is part of a more extensive process in eight of 10 cases. The autopsy cohort has a higher incidence of proximally located thrombi. This may reflect the patient population, which is more likely to have pelvic pathologies such as neoplastic masses or traumatic injuries. These promote stasis and are associated with local injury to the vein wall, factors known to promote thrombus growth.

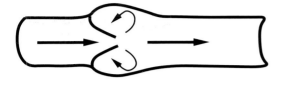

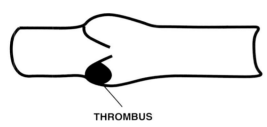

THROMBUS

Figure 2.6. A mechanism accounting for thrombus formation is summarized in this diagram. Under normal conditions, a zone of stagnation of blood flow develops at the base of the venous valve. This region is a site of early aggregation of platelets and red blood cells. The additional factors that determine why a given individual will go on to form an early thrombus are unknown.

such as the mid popliteal vein, the mid lower superficial femoral vein, the common femoral vein, and the external iliac veins (Fig. 2.5). A common denominator is that these thrombi generally arise from the sinus at the base of a venous valve. The flow dynamics due to the shape of the valve set up a zone of decreased and reversed flow at these sites (Figs. 2.6 and 2.7). This may explain why DVT is not always a unifocal disease, since thrombi can arise at multiple locations in the same patient. Patients who have had fractures of the femur with subsequent operative hip replacement or pinning are more likely to have proximal femoral vein thrombi. Similarly, patients with tibial or fibular fractures have a higher incidence of DVT. These form contiguous to the site of sur-

gery or trauma. Local injury to the wall and endothelium of the vein is thought to be the factor inciting local thrombosis.

Combined use of radioactive iodinated fibrinogen and venography has shown a prevalence of calf vein thrombi of up to 50% in the first few postoperative days. These may spread in 20% of instances into the popliteal vein and are then thought to become possible sources of pulmonary emboli. The association between pulmonary embolism and the location and type of venous thrombi has continued to generate controversy. A first approach to the problem is the belief that proximal femoral popliteal venous thrombosis alone causes pulmonary embolism. The larger caliber of these veins increases the likelihood that larger non-adherent thrombi can embolize and obstruct a large enough portion of the lungs to be symptomatic. However, it is possible for calf vein thrombi to be the source of pulmonary emboli. These are generally smaller and are less likely to be symptomatic. They are often suspected when new perfusion defects are seen on radionuclide lung scans during the postoperative period. In general, femoropopliteal vein thrombi are the more dangerous since they are more likely to embolize and to block a larger-caliber pulmonary artery. The large free-floating thrombus involving the iliac or proximal femoral vein has been considered to be at high risk for breaking off and causing pulmonary emboli. The serial use of ultrasound has shown that this is not likely the case for femoral vein thrombi, since no increased risk of embolization has been observed.

Studies looking at the location of DVT after an episode of symptomatic pulmonary embolism have shown involvement of femoral or popliteal veins in most instances. In 10 to 20% of cases, only calf vein thrombi have been observed. It has not been possible to determine whether these are the source of the emboli or what remains of a more extensive thrombosis.

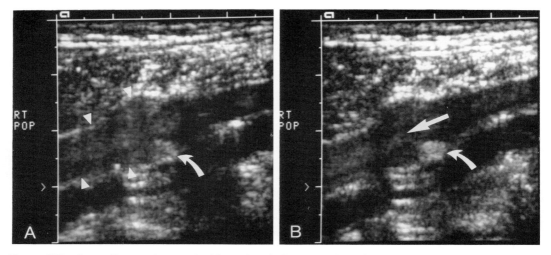

Figure 2.7. Formation and spread of thrombus is dependent on the geometry of the venous valve. A zone of stagnant blood normally forms at the base of the valve and is responsible in part for the early aggregation of red blood cells. **A,** In this first longitudinal image, the popliteal vein contains a heterogeneous conglomerate of echogenic signals (*arrowheads*). This is better seen at the base of a venous valve (*curved arrow*). **B,** This second sonogram was taken during the venous augmentation maneuver. The echogenic signals arising from the quasi-stagnant blood have almost disappeared since they are now in motion (*long arrow*). A group of red blood cells remains trapped behind the valve (*curved arrow*).

TIME COURSE

Venous thrombosis goes through different stages in its evolution. It is believed to start as an early non-obstructing thrombus forming at the base of a vein valve (Figs. 2.8 and 2.9). Poorly understood factors such as prolonged immobilization, local injury, a propensity for thrombosis, or a combination of these cause the thrombus to spread more proximally in 20% of cases. With time, involvement of the popliteal and femoral venous segments can lead to an obstructive process causing pain and lower-extremity swelling. Obstructive thrombus, by causing a relative expansion of the venous segment it involves, most likely is the source of the patient's symptoms. Non-obstructing thrombus, if it does not lyse, will often affix itself to the adjacent wall of the vein. Within 3 to 7 days, these free-floating thrombi will become adherent to the vein wall and are therefore less likely to break off and embolize.

The structure of the acutely forming thrombus is that of a loosely meshed amalgam of platelets and red cells. A matrix of cross-linked fibrin causes this structure to organize within a few hours of formation. Within a few days, local hemolysis of red cells or lysis of some of the fibrin matrix can give a heterogeneous appearance to the thrombus. Since thrombus is continuously forming, the same patient may have areas of more recent thrombosis intermixed with older-appearing thrombosis. The presence of obstructive venous thrombosis helps stimulate the development of collateral pathways for blood flow. The perforating veins that communicate between the superficial and deep veins help to shunt blood flow into the greater and lesser saphenous veins, thereby ensuring venous drainage of the lower extremity. A collateral pathway through the deep muscular branches of the thigh often forms a path between the popliteal vein and the

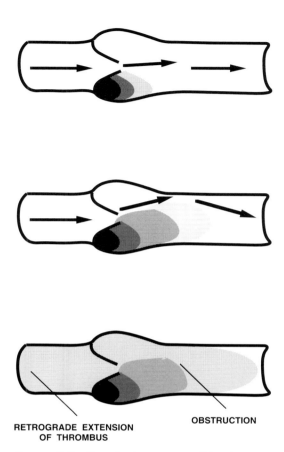

**RETROGRADE EXTENSION
OF THROMBUS**

OBSTRUCTION

Figure 2.8. The factors responsible for clot propagation are still poorly understood. However, the pattern of thrombus spread has been observed in vivo as well as at autopsy. On the top, the early thrombus continues to grow in the zone of relative stagnation at the base of the venous valve. The middle illustration shows the thrombus extending into the lumen. At this stage, it has not yet obstructed blood flow. Continued growth of the thrombus is then dependent on the interplay of many factors. Concurrent with the action of pro-coagulation factors is an opposite action of factors responsible for thrombolysis. Why one mechanism takes precedence over the other in a given individual is still unknown. The lower illustration shows one of the possible outcomes. The thrombus has continued to grow. It has also obstructed blood flow and caused thrombosis in the more distal vein.

profunda femoris vein; this pathway is potentially present in up to 50% of the population.

The venous segments that are obstructed may either slowly recanalize due to the normal fibrinolytic pathways within the body or stay permanently occluded. Partial recanalization is associated with irregularly shaped channels. The venous valves may also scar and become dysfunctional. In up to 30% of instances, the occluded segments never recanalize.

SEQUELAE

Partial recanalization of venous segments, scarring of the valve mechanism, and altered flow dynamics contribute to the development of venous insufficiency and the postphlebitic syndrome. This syndrome, in its mildest form, includes swelling and pain. The more severe forms are associated with permanent skin changes and ulceration.

Following acute DVT, 50 to 75% of patients with severe thrombosis involving the popliteal vein or above have symptoms of venous insufficiency at 5 to 6 years. Patients with thrombus limited to the calf veins have a 20% chance of developing symptoms. Control groups without documented acute DVT have up to a 14% chance of developing symptoms of vein insufficiency. This may possibly represent a bias in the selection of patients. For example, symptomatic patients suspected of having acute DVT are likely to have had symptoms due to some form of venous insufficiency that has continued to progress during the follow-up interval.

INTERVENTIONS

The current thinking on the pathophysiology of venous thrombosis favors two major strategies: prevention and treatment.

Prevention

The first interventional strategy is prevention of the development of venous

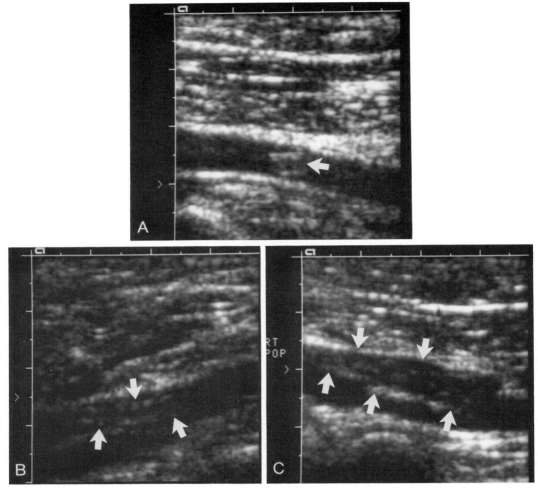

Figure 2.9. This series of images, all from the same patient, summarizes much of the evolution of an acute DVT. **A,** The first longitudinal image shows an abnormal echogenic signal at the mid popliteal venous valve (*arrow*). This finding was thought to possibly represent an early non-obstructing thrombus. **B,** A repeat sonogram was performed 2 days later. A larger echogenic collection (*arrows*) was now seen to have spread from the original thrombus. **C,** The repeat ultrasound was obtained 3 days later. On the longitudinal image, a much larger echogenic collection (*arrows*) now involves most of this popliteal segment. Progression of an early non-obstructing thrombus forming on a venous valve to a fully obstructing above-knee DVT is thought to be typical of the evolution of a DVT.

thrombosis in high-risk groups. These include postoperative patients who have undergone neurosurgical, orthopedic, or urologic procedures. Preventive measures include the use of compression stockings, intermittent pneumatic compression, or varied doses of oral and parenteral anticoagulants.

The use of these different preventive measures has been shown to significantly decrease the incidence of serious postoperative venous thrombosis. A major impact has been the decrease in the incidence of subsequent pulmonary embolization. For example, the simple use of aspirin appears to diminish the incidence of ileofemoral vein thrombosis postoperatively, although it has no effect on calf vein thrombi. The use of intermittent venous compression significantly decreases the incidence of calf vein thrombosis in controlled studies.

Treatment

The treatment of acute DVT is varied. A standard regimen is 6 months of anticoagulation with Coumadin following heparinization for 5 to 10 days.

Heparinization is well recognized as an acute intervention that decreases the likelihood of the spread of lower-extremity venous thrombosis and the likelihood of pulmonary embolization. The likelihood of pulmonary embolism is 30 to 50% in nontreated patients and decreases to 10% while under heparin treatment. This significant reduction in the number of fatal pulmonary emboli is the basic justification for the use of anticoagulants.

The subsequent use of Coumadin for a period extending from 3 to 6 months after the acute event has also been shown to reduce the incidence of recurrent venous thrombosis and pulmonary embolism. The treatment of below-the-knee (calf vein) venous thrombosis with a longer course of Coumadin administration may also decrease the recurrence rate of deep vein thrombosis.

In patients who cannot undergo long-term anticoagulation with Coumadin, the use of a percutaneously introduced inferior vena cava filter has come to replace the more aggressive and dangerous inferior vena cava interruption or plication. Percutaneous placement of these filters is needed in a minority of patients presenting with deep vein thrombosis. Follow-up examinations can be performed noninvasively to document the morbidity of the procedure. For example, a 30% prevalence of common femoral vein thrombosis has been described with placement of the larger-diameter filters. Variations on the technique of placement have been shown to decrease the incidence of these femoral vein thrombi.

More recently, a great deal of interest has been expressed in using the noninvasive sonographic examination to determine the extent of venous thrombosis during the administration of thrombolytic agents. By a judicious combination of compression ultrasound and color flow mapping, the extent of obstructive and nonobstructive venous thrombosis can be accurately mapped out. Changes subsequent to the administration of thrombolytic therapy can be followed and quantitated.

Atherosclerosis (Carotid Arteries)

INCIDENCE AND PREVALENCE

The prevalence of significant internal carotid artery stenosis is estimated partly from the incidence of stroke or transient ischemic attacks. Fifteen to 20% of patients who present with either stroke or transient ischemic attacks do not have any carotid artery pathology but are shown to have another explanation for their presenting symptoms, such as emboli arising from a cardiac source. Approximately 50% of patients have associated with their symptoms a stenotic lesion of the internal carotid artery with narrowing of the lumen diameter by more than 50%. A large proportion of patients without significant stenosis nevertheless have plaque deposition of lesser importance (Fig. 2.10). These data are somewhat skewed by the fact that symptomatic patients are being studied.

Large population surveys have become possible with the greater dissemination of high-resolution real-time sonography. For example, in subjects between 45 and 65 years of age, the prevalence of significant internal carotid artery disease with more

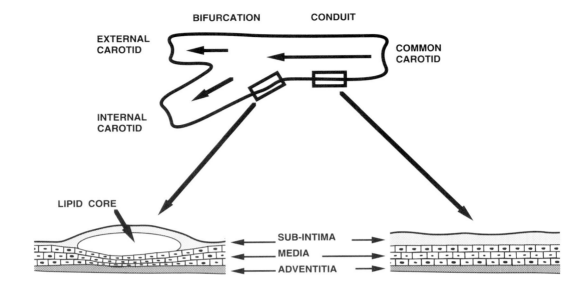

Figure 2.10. Atherosclerosis is a generalized process affecting the different arterial beds. Autopsy studies have shown that involvement of the upper abdominal aorta takes place the earliest. Carotid and coronary artery involvement occurs with a lag of 5 to 10 years. It is now believed that there may be two manifestations of atherosclerosis. The first is the traditional focal plaque that forms in the intima near arterial branch points. The second is a more subtle thickening in the wall of the arterial conduit at locations distant from any branch point or bifurcation. This thickening is superimposed on the normal age-related thickening that affects the arterial wall.

than 50% lumen diameter narrowing is approximately 5%. Lesions accounting for 25 to 50% lumen diameter narrowing are present in up to 30% of the population, and less significant, smaller focal plaques can be seen in 20 to 30% of the population.

Autopsy data have shown that atherosclerosis develops earlier in the abdominal aorta. The carotid arteries and the coronary arteries show involvement 5 to 10 years later than the aorta.

RISK FACTORS

The development of atherosclerotic plaque is related to well-studied risk factors. The commonly recognized factors include elevated cholesterol levels, cigarette smoking, diabetes, and hypertension. The LDL fraction of cholesterol is associated with plaque deposition, while HDL cholesterol seems to have a protective effect.

Constant exposure to these risk factors accelerates the development of atherosclerotic plaque and the progression to higher grade, more severe lesions that ultimately cause stenotic occlusion of the artery. These lesions may progress in the absence of any significant symptoms. Removal and control of risk factors show beneficial effects since it is now becoming recognized that plaque deposition is not necessarily irreversible. Lowering of serum cholesterol has been shown to actually halt and even reverse the development of plaque.

LOCATION AND PATTERN

The distribution of atherosclerotic changes favors the level of the carotid bifurcation in the region of the carotid bulb and extends within the first 2 cm into the origin of the internal carotid. This preferential location is thought to be secondary to the flow patterns that are established at the branching point of the internal carotid (Fig. 2.11). Although it was originally thought that zones of high shear rate could account for early plaque deposition, the current thinking is that areas of relative stagnation of blood flow are linked to the deposition of the early atherosclerotic lesions. These plaques tend to develop as small focal protuberances into the arterial lumen. They can usually be detected early by high-resolution real-time ultrasound. Attempts have been made to characterize their appearance. The more fibrous plaques tend to show echogenic signal, while the more fatty plaques and those composed mostly of smooth muscle are isoechoic. Localized areas of thrombus accumulation can also show up as isoechoic or hypoechoic. Co-existent focal stenotic lesions within the common carotid are much less common and occur in less than 5% of patients who have a high-grade stenosis in the internal carotid.

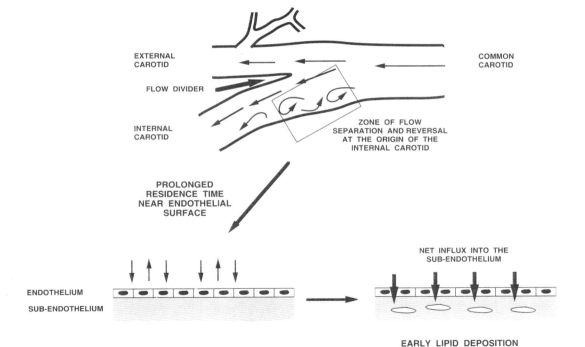

Figure 2.11. The pathophysiological mechanisms responsible for early plaque deposition have been the subject of controversy for years. It was previously thought that plaque was deposited at sites of increased shear rates. These are sites where the blood velocity changes very rapidly as a function of its distance from the artery wall; the flow divider of the common carotid artery is such a site. More recent observations suggest that early plaque forms at sites of relative stagnation or slow flow such as the far wall of the proximal internal carotid artery. A proposed mechanism for plaque deposition is summarized in this diagram. The prolonged residence time of local products generated by the endothelium might be toxic and impair lipid transport mechanisms. Another possibility is that platelet activation takes place at the site of high shear rate at the flow divider. These products then find themselves in the area of slow or reversed flow and exert a toxic effect on the endothelium.

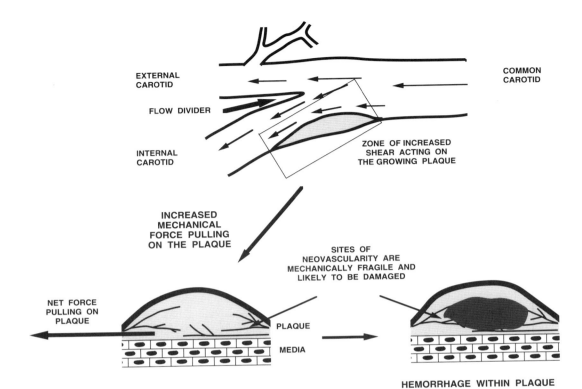

Figure 2.12. The formation of early plaques is likely promoted in zones of locally reduced blood flow. This changes once the plaque has reached a certain size. The plaque extends far enough into the lumen of flowing blood that shearing forces are exerted on it. These forces try to pull the plaque from its anchor in the artery wall. The structural strength of the plaque is decreased by the network of small vessels that develop from the vasa vasorum in the media. Local hemorrhage is likely to occur, acutely rupturing or expanding the plaque.

TIME COURSE

It is now believed that lipid deposition is not solely responsible for plaque development. The growth cycle of the atherosclerotic plaque is believed to include episodes of rupture that are followed by periods of repair. This has been seen in the carotid arteries and is believed to apply to other arterial beds as well. The early focal lesions develop at the sites of altered flow dynamics in the internal carotid. At these sites, local endothelial dysfunction occurs and somehow contributes to fat deposition, which then slowly progresses to the sub-intimal layer of the arterial wall. As the plaque takes shape it continues to grow slowly. With increasing size, new vascular channels extend from the vasa vasorum in the media of the arterial wall and develop in the base of the plaque. This neovascularity contributes to the development of an intrinsic weakness in the anchoring mechanism of the plaque. Increased shear rates are caused by blood flowing over the plaque and are accentuated by the extent to which the plaque protrudes into the lumen. These forces try to pull the plaque from the arterial wall (Fig. 2.12). The increased mechanical stress is transmitted to the base of the plaque, where damage is more likely to occur at the site of neovascularity. This local trauma can then lead to intraplaque hemorrhage. This is occasionally seen as a sonolucent area within the plaque, near the base (Figs. 2.13 and 2.14). This hemorrhage can either be self-contained or continue to actual plaque disruption (Fig. 2.15). If the plaque remains intact, it will most likely continue to grow, slowly aided by the local repair mechanism (Fig. 2.16). If there is disruption, platelets aggregate and thrombus forms at the site of exposed collagen. Persistent ulceration can then be the source of small emboli, which form at the site of the exposed plaque contents and then cause symptoms such as transient ischemic attacks (Fig. 2.17). A healing process with fibrous tissue deposition is seen in the majority of cases, however. This cycle of events may repeat many times without the patient experiencing any

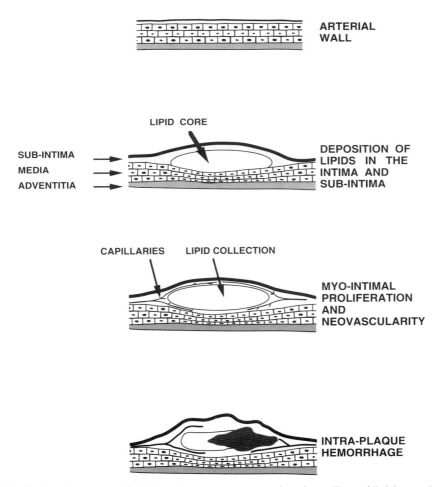

Figure 2.13. Early plaque growth takes place as a progressive deposition of lipids causing a well-circumscribed focal plaque. The development of neovascularity extending from the vasa vasorum located at the junction of the mid and outer thirds of the media helps the plaque to grow and feeds the myointimal proliferation that takes place. This slow progressive growth is almost always interrupted by an episode of intraplaque hemorrhage, so it is quite uncommon to see large, smooth-surfaced plaques. Instead, large plaques more commonly have an irregular surface and heterogeneous appearance even if they have remained asymptomatic.

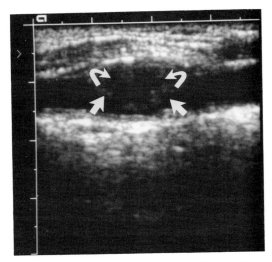

Figure 2.14. The large plaque (*arrows*) located in the carotid bulb contains a large hypoechoic region (*curved arrows*). The latter is thought to represent a large area of intraplaque hemorrhage.

symptoms (Fig. 2.18). The plaque can therefore undergo multiple similar cycles of growth, disruption, and continued growth (Fig. 2.19). Increased deposition of material causes the localized narrowing of the arterial lumen diameter to progressively increase in severity. Although symptoms can occur during any of these multiple cycles, they are more likely to occur once the plaque is larger and causes a significant narrowing of the internal carotid lumen (Fig. 2.20). If disruption occurs at these later stages when the plaque already obstructs a significant portion of the arterial lumen, thrombus formation appears to be more likely and more extensive. This increases the likelihood of embolization or occlusion.

SEQUELAE

The two major clinical outcomes of internal carotid stenosis are transient ische-

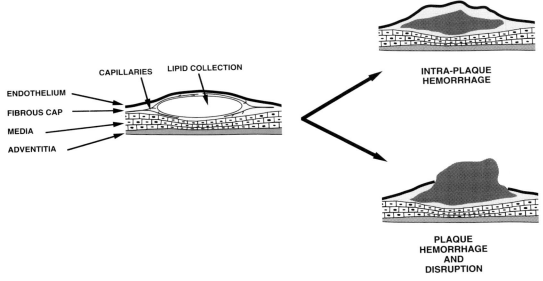

Figure 2.15. The early plaque is found in the intima and consists of a lipid core. It is surrounded by small capillaries, which grow from the outer portion of the media (vasa vasorum). These fragile vessels are prone to rupture and hemorrhage. The two most common outcomes are contained hemorrhage and plaque rupture. The first is likely to remain asymptomatic. Symptomatic individuals are likely to have had a complete plaque disruption. The presence of a disrupted plaque need not imply the presence of symptoms. It is likely that the acute hemorrhage will remain asymptomatic and unnoticed by the patient.

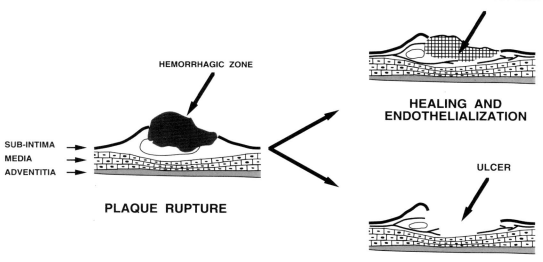

FIBROUS ZONE

HEMORRHAGIC ZONE

HEALING AND
ENDOTHELIALIZATION

SUB-INTIMA

MEDIA

ADVENTITIA

ULCER

PLAQUE RUPTURE

PERSISTENT
ULCERATION

Figure 2.16. The sequelae of an acutely ruptured plaque have yet to be studied in any systematic way. It appears that, of the two possible outcomes—healing or persistent ulceration—healing is by far the most likely. The surface of the plaque occupied by the hemorrhage will slowly heal by forming a fibrous zone equivalent to a small scar. Persistent ulceration is much less common. If it is present, then symptoms of transient ischemic attack or amaurosis fugax are quite likely.

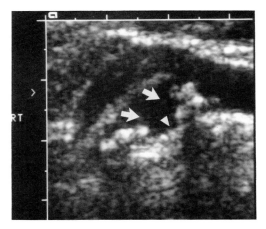

Figure 2.17. The sonographic diagnosis of plaque ulceration is difficult and often unreliable. These ulcers are more likely to be present in the more complex and extensive plaques. Calcification is often present, making it more difficult to image the plaque. It is uncommon to be able to clearly delineate a discrete ulcer as shown here (*arrows*). A common difficulty is in differentiating an ulcer from a normal portion of the artery wall lying between two discrete plaques. An ulcer is more likely if the floor of the segment in question extends down into the media of the artery wall (*arrowhead*).

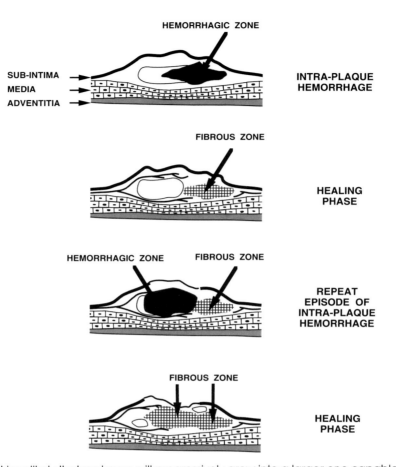

Figure 2.18. It is unlikely that a plaque will progressively grow into a larger one capable of causing a hemodynamically significant stenosis. Evidence gathered from studies of the coronary arteries suggests that plaques may undergo a series of growth cycles interrupted by episodes of hemorrhage and repair. This hypothesis is summarized in this diagram. It is still unclear how many of these cycles take place before the lesion either becomes the source of symptoms or progresses to cause a hemodynamically significant stenosis. With each of these cycles, the surface of the plaque is more and more likely to show an irregular contour. Similarly, plaques that have undergone multiple cycles of growth and repair are likely to appear heterogeneous on the ultrasound images.

mic attacks (TIAs) and stroke. Progression of internal carotid plaque and stenosis is currently believed to culminate in either or both of these clinical symptoms. The rate of stroke or TIA in patients without active intervention is a function of the severity of the stenosis. Patients without significant stenoses have a low likelihood of developing a stroke or TIA over a 1-year period. Patients with documented narrowing of the internal carotid are much more

likely to develop either of these. Finally, the TIA is often viewed as a herald of impending stroke. This is most often the case in patients with a documented high-grade stenosis of the carotid.

INTERVENTIONS

Surgical intervention with endarterectomy remains the principal means of treating symptomatic high-grade stenosis of

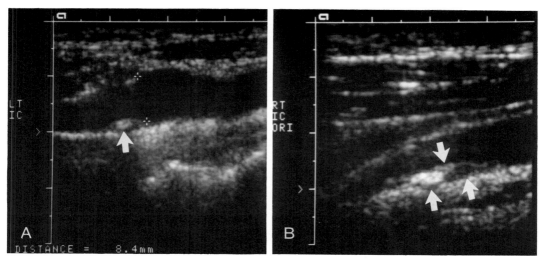

Figure 2.19. **A,** Development of an early heterogeneous plaque is most likely secondary to fibrosis at the site of intraplaque hemorrhage. This plaque at the origin of the internal carotid artery has a central area of increased echogenicity likely to have evolved from such an event (*arrow*). **B,** This moderately large plaque (*arrows*) at the origin of the internal carotid artery is characteristic of a heterogeneous composition and mild surface irregularity. According to the current concepts of plaque evolution, it is likely that this plaque has undergone at least one previous episode of intraplaque hemorrhage.

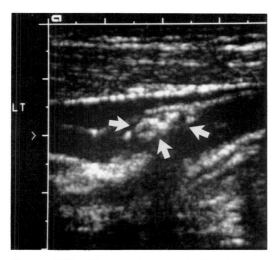

Figure 2.20. Plaque characterization is done by comparing the sonographic texture of the plaque with respect to the surrounding soft tissues. In this case, a plaque (*arrows*) located in the carotid bulb has a heterogeneous appearance. Areas of increased echogenicity are intermixed with isoechoic areas.

the extracranial carotid branches. Complication rates remain low and overall morbidity is lower than when treatment is withheld in *symptomatic* patients with high-grade stenosis. Recurrence of stenosis can occur at a rate of 5 to 10% in the first year following the procedure. This is due to fibrointimal hyperplasia rather than recurrence or progression of atherosclerosis.

According to preliminary findings from the North American Symptomatic Carotid Endarterectomy trial (NASCET), surgical intervention is currently indicated for symptomatic high-grade stenosis above 70% lumen diameter narrowing. When a high-grade stenosis is detected in an asymptomatic patient, the current belief is that surgical intervention should be withheld until symptoms develop. The morbidity associated with the operative intervention (endarterectomy) is slightly greater than that of simple observation if the lesion remains asymptomatic. Progression in the severity of these high-grade stenoses or a high diastolic velocity detected by Doppler while the patient remains asymptomatic may ultimately be used to identify patients at more immediate risk of developing TIA or stroke. Finally, if symptoms of transient ischemia develop in a patient with a high-grade stenosis, there is a high likelihood of a stroke occurring during the ensuing months.

The coexistence of coronary and carotid artery disease makes it likely that patients undergoing cardiothoracic surgery will have a significant stenosis of the internal carotid. Prophylactic endarterectomy, if it is performed, is reserved for higher-grade stenoses above 75%.

More recently, the use of balloon angioplasty has been proposed as a means of alleviating high-grade stenosis of the internal carotid. Reported technical success rates are high. The issue currently being addressed is whether the acute risk of embolization to the vessels during angioplasty is worse than the morbidity related to operative interventions.

Atherosclerosis (Lower Extremity)

INCIDENCE AND PREVALENCE

The incidence and prevalence of lower-extremity atherosclerosis is even harder to determine than for the carotid artery. This is in part due to the abundant collateral arterial network that can develop concomitant with the progression of significant arterial stenosis or occlusions of the lower-extremity arteries. Arteriographic studies performed on patients with significant coronary artery disease or significant carotid artery disease show a high prevalence of significant peripheral arterial narrowings and claudication.

No structured noninvasive surveys using ultrasound have yet been performed to evaluate the distribution of disease in the general population. Self-administered questionnaires such as the Rose questionnaire have suggested that the prevalence of claudication in all individuals is close to 2%. Based on measurements of the ankle-brachial ratio—a value less than 0.8 serving as a diagnostic threshold—the prevalence of disease is approximately 5% in patients between 55 and 75 years of age. It is believed that one-third to one-half of patients with abnormal hemodynamics consistent with peripheral arterial stenoses do not have symptoms of claudication.

LOCATION AND PATTERN

Atherosclerotic plaque within the peripheral arteries of the leg preferentially affects the branch points along the length of the popliteal and femoral arteries. Significant narrowings are most likely to occur at the junction of the distal superficial femoral artery and the popliteal artery. This preferential distribution of significant high-grade stenosis in the region of the adductor canal has been verified by both angiographic and autopsy series. Additional involvement of one of the distal calf arteries (either anterior tibial, posterior tibial, or peroneal arteries) is also common (Fig. 2.21). More peripheral involvement of the calf arteries is normally seen in patients with diabetes mellitus and less often in non-diabetics. Preferential involvement of the aorta and iliac arteries is more common in younger (45- to 55-year-old) women. The likelihood of obstructive lesions is increased by a smoking history.

Buerger's disease, although commonly associated with atherosclerosis, is a diffuse inflammatory response that affects the arterial wall. It preferentially affects males over females (10:1) and is directly linked to cigarette smoking. It affects the small vessels of the calf first and then spreads more proximally to the popliteal and femoral ar-

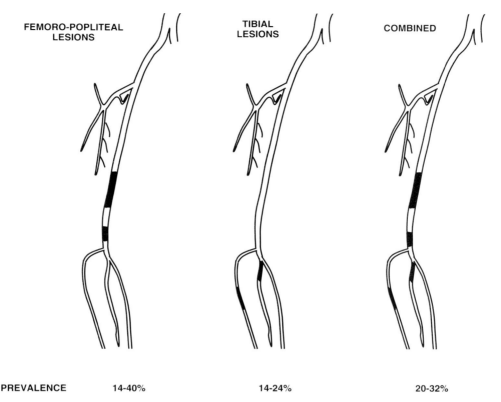

FEMORO-POPLITEAL LESIONS	TIBIAL LESIONS	COMBINED

| PREVALENCE | 14-40% | 14-24% | 20-32% |

Figure 2.21.   The distribution of significant lower-extremity arterial lesions (defined as more than 50% lumen narrowing or total occlusion) has been mostly determined from arteriographic studies of preoperative patients. As shown in this diagram, most of the lesions are located in the femoral and popliteal arteries. Isolated tibial artery lesions are more commonly seen in diabetics and, on occasion, in patients with Buerger's disease. Although not indicated here, coexistent aortoiliac lesions can be seen in 10 to 20% of these extremities. They can also be an isolated finding, more commonly appreciated in middle-aged women.

teries. It is also referred to as thromboangiitis obliterans and affects the upper as well as the lower extremity.

Aneurysmal disease or arteriomegaly is often associated with atherosclerosis. Recent studies suggest that, in up to 40% of patients, atherosclerosis is only an associated process. The underlying causative mechanism is an inherent genetic weakness in the arterial wall. The presence of aneurysms tends to be multifocal in the same patient. For example, a popliteal aneurysm can be associated with a contralateral aneurysm in up to 50% of cases. Co-existent aortic aneurysms are seen in 30% of instances. The progressive ballooning out of the arterial wall perturbs flow dynamics and is conducive to the deposition of thrombus. Progression of thrombus is likely to cause either distal embolization or total occlusion. The likelihood is then very high that amputation will be needed.

TIME COURSE

Claudication does not necessarily appear when significant arterial lesions or occlusions are present in an extremity. This is in part due to the development of extensive collateral arteries that supply the more distal arteries, either via collaterals established through the profunda femoral branch or from higher collaterals arising from the superficial femoral artery and communicating either directly to the popliteal arterial segment or to the infrapopliteal tibial branches.

Progression of symptoms is observed in approximately 60% of patients who are observed without intervention. Up to 30% of patients will remain asymptomatic over a 3- to 5-year period if no surgery is performed. Actual regression of symptoms can occur in up to 10% of patients. This may be due to adaptive changes due to collateral development and partly to decreases in levels of activity. Actual exercise programs have recently been shown to decrease the extent of symptomatic claudication. The promotion of newer and larger collateral channels is thought to explain the improvement of these patients.

SEQUELAE

Ultimately, the progression of arterial stenosis leads to total occlusion and associated thrombosis of arterial segments that are not necessarily involved by hemodynamically significant stenosis. The zone or extent of thrombosis is partly defined by the extent of collateral vascularization. The thrombosis tends to extend proximally to the next major collateral or deep feeding branch. The development of additional lesions and the progressive narrowing of the arterial tree at multiple sites ultimately leads to rest ischemia and to gangrene, since the collaterals are also affected by the disease process. Amputation then becomes the ultimate endpoint. This pattern has been markedly influenced by the development of newer surgical procedures. Once surgery is performed and the dysfunctional diseased segments have been bypassed, symptomatic relief is often achieved for the patient's lifetime. The presence of concomitant significant atherosclerotic lesions in the coronary and carotid arteries are more likely to cause patient mortality. This often occurs before disease of the lower extremity can again progress enough to cause irreversible tissue injury to the limb.

INTERVENTIONS

Multiple strategies have been developed to bypass the occluded arterial segments and to perfuse the distal portions of the extremity. This not only prevents resting ischemic pain but also interrupts the normal progression towards ischemia, gangrene, and ultimately amputation. These include a variety of surgical alternatives and newer percutaneous interventions.

Synthetic grafts made of Dacron are commonly used in the pelvis for aortoiliac or aortofemoral bypass. Dacron or polytetrafluoroethylene (PTFE) are likely to be used in the axillofemoral or femoro-femoral bypass procedures. PTFE is the material still commonly used for the above-the-knee bypass procedures. The development of newer bypass techniques now permits revascularization down to the tibial and peroneal arteries. Bypass to these below-the-knee arteries is achieved using reversed vein segments or, more recently, the in situ approach. Patency rates of these bypass grafts are now greater than 80% at 5 years. Unfortunately, the patients who undergo peripheral arterial revascularization have a high long-term morbidity. This high rate is due to associated coronary or cerebral vascular events. It is now common to see patients die of stroke or myocardial infarction with patent and functional bypass grafts.

Grafts that are likely to fail between the second month and second year following surgery are most likely affected by fibrointimal hyperplasia. This pathophysiologic process represents a proliferation of the smooth muscle cells, which causes progressive narrowing of the lumen of the vein graft. These lesions are most likely to occur at the site of anastomosis, including the 2 cm proximal and distal to the actual surgical anastomosis. If they are detected and corrected before graft thrombosis occurs, the patency rate of the graft returns to normal, i.e., up to 80% at 3 to 5 years.

The use of non-surgical interventions has increased over the last 20 years. Newer approaches such as angioplasty, atherectomy, and laser angioplasty are becoming more important. Percutaneous angioplasty has become an accepted alternative to bypass surgery whenever short segmental stenoses are identified. A balloon catheter is inserted percutaneously and is inflated across the site of narrowing. This locally disrupts the plaque and part of the underlying artery wall. This remodeled arterial lumen is then considered repaired. The long-term success rates are then greater than 70%. The technique does not perform as well for segmental occlusions of greater than 4 cm, with patency rates of 40 to 60% currently being reported. Percutaneous atherectomy physically removes portions of atherosclerotic plaque. Lesions are first crossed, a small centering balloon is then inflated at a fraction of the pressure used for angioplasty, and the plaque is slowly trimmed away by back and forward motion of a rotating blade. The success rate appears to be the same as for angioplasty.

Laser angioplasty is performed by delivering a large amount of energy to an arterial lesion via a high-intensity beam of laser photons. There are two implementations of this type of intervention. The first uses the laser energy to heat a metal tip, which "cooks" the obstruction. The utility of this approach is marginal. It does not seem to perform better than more traditional angioplasty. The second application more recently introduced, is the use of selected laser frequencies to vaporize constitutive elements of the atherosclerotic plaques.

All of these percutaneous interventions have a high re-stenosis rate (30% at 1 year) caused by the same pathophysiologic mechanism that affects bypass vein grafts—fibrointimal hyperplasia. This remains the major limitation to the use of these techniques.

SUGGESTED READINGS

Browse N. Diagnosis of deep-vein thrombosis. Br Med Bull 1978;34:163–167.

Browse NL, Thomas M. Source of non-lethal pulmonary emboli. Lancet 1974;1:258–259.

Cronenwett JL, Warner KG, Zelenock GB, et al. Intermittent claudication. Current results of nonoperative management. Arch Surg 1984;119:430–436.

Haimovici H. Patterns of arteriosclerotic lesions of the lower extremity. Arch Surg 1967;95:918–933.

Hertzer NR, Beven EG, Young JR, et al. Coronary disease in peripheral vascular patients. A classification of 1000 coronary angiograms and results of surgical management. Ann Surg 1984;199:223–233.

Imparato AM, Kim GE, Davidson T, Crowley JG. Intermittent claudication: its natural course. Surgery 1975;78:795–799.

Imparato AM, Riles TS, Mintzer R, Baumann FG. The importance of hemorrhage in the relationship between gross morphologic characteristics and cerebral symptoms in 376 carotid artery plaques. Ann Surg 1983;197:195–203.

Kalebo P, Anthmyr BA, Eriksson BI, Zachrisson BE. Phlebographic findings in venous thrombosis following total hip replacement. Acta Radiol 1990;31:259–263.

Kannel WB, Shurtleff D. The natural history of arteriosclerosis obliterans. Cardiovasc Clin 1971;3:37–52.

Karino T, Motomiya M. Flow through a venous valve and its implication for thrombus formation. Thromb Res 1984;36:245–257.

Kistner RL, Ball JJ, Nordyke RA, Freeman GC. Incidence of pulmonary embolism in the course of thrombophlebitis of the lower extremities. Am J Surg 1972;124:169–176.

Leahy AL, McCollum PT, Feeley TM, et al. Duplex ultrasonography and selection of patients for carotid endarterectomy: plaque morphology or luminal narrowing? J Vasc Surg 1988;8:558–562.

Liu GC, Ferris EJ, Reifsteck JR, Baker ME. Effect of anatomic variations on deep venous thrombosis of the lower extremity. AJR 1986;146:845–848.

Lusby RJ, Ferrell LD, Ehrenfeld WK, Stoney RJ, Wylie EJ. Carotid plaque hemorrhage. Its role in production of cerebral ischemia. Arch Surg 1982;117:1479–1488.

Morris GK, Mitchell JR. Evaluation of ^{125}I fibrinogen test for venous thrombosis in patients with hip fractures: a comparison between isotope scanning and necropsy findings. Br Med J 1977;1:264–266.

Nylander G, Olivecrona H. The phlebographic pattern of acute leg thrombosis within a defined urban population. Acta Chir Scand 1976;142:505–511.

Sevitt S, Gallagher N. Venous thrombosis and pulmonary embolism: A clinico-pathological study in injured and burned patients. Br J Surg 1961;48:475–489.

Solberg LA, Eggen DA. Localization and sequence of development of atherosclerotic lesions in the carotid and vertebral arteries. Circulation 1971; 43:711–724.

Soskolne CL, Wong AW, Lilienfeld DE. Trends in pulmonary embolism death rates for Canada and the United States, 1962–87. Can Med Assoc J 1990;142:321–324.

Watt JK. Arterial occlusion in the lower leg. Br Med J 1966;547:18–20.

CHAPTER THREE

Efficacy of Vascular Diagnostic Tests

Introduction

The diagnostic accuracy of vascular sonography has mostly been established by comparative studies against gold standard examinations. The two traditional methods of vascular diagnosis are performed by injecting iodinated contrast material into the vessel to opacify the contents of the lumen of either the artery (arteriography) or the vein (phlebography or venography). Radiographs are taken while the contrast material is being injected. These two methods have, by default, become the gold standard examinations against which the noninvasive vascular tests need to be validated.

VENOGRAPHY

Venography (phlebography) is well recognized as the gold standard examination for making the diagnosis of acute deep vein thrombosis. Its status as a gold standard examination may, under certain circumstances, be questioned. For example, the two most reliable diagnostic criteria used to classify an examination as positive for the presence of deep vein thrombosis are the abrupt termination of the column of contrast within the lumen of the vein

(cut-off sign) and the presence of a distinct filling defect. A good proportion of examinations (10%) will have long portions of the venous channels that are difficult to fill with contrast. Successful opacification of these segments, which may or may not contain thrombosis, is dependent on the persistence of the operator and the use of special approaches such as placing tourniquets over the calf and thighs, repositioning the patient, and massaging the calves. In certain cases, full opacification of all venous segments is not possible. Approximately 5% of venograms are considered to be technically unsuccessful. Therefore, when comparing the results of a noninvasive test against this gold standard, account should be taken of the number of successful examinations and of the diagnostic criteria used. This may not be as critical for assessing the diagnostic accuracy of the test, i.e., answering the question is clot present or absent? These technically limited examinations cannot be used when evaluating for the presence of calf vein thrombosis or when determining the extent of the thrombosed venous segments. Nonopacified segments may still be free of thrombus yet fail to opacify.

The ultimate gold standard against which examinations are compared is the autopsy. Correlations between venography and autopsy have been unreliable and difficult to perform due to the dynamic nature of deep vein thrombosis. Venous channels patent 1 or 2 days before the autopsy may yet become occluded in the interval of time to death. Venograms performed on a cadaver may show opacified segments that would not be seen if the patient were alive.

ARTERIOGRAPHY

The situation in peripheral arterial disease is somewhat more complicated. Arteriography is a definite gold standard for making the diagnosis of occlusive arterial disease. However, it is recognized that real-time sonography is better suited to diagnose the presence of popliteal aneurysms and to evaluate their extent. This high accuracy has been correlated against operative findings and surgical pathology specimens. There are many instances when the popliteal arterial segments opacify normally during arteriography despite the presence of an aneurysm. This is due to the presence of laminated thrombus lining the aneurysm wall. Although arteriography is recognized as a gold-standard in peripheral arterial disease, it is also limited by the fact that it cannot be used to evaluate the perivascular spaces for the presence of masses. Even when evaluating arterial segments, poor radiographic technique can hide possible lesions due to poor timing between contrast injection into the artery and subsequent radiographic filming. This has been the source of significant overestimation of the extent of occluded arterial segments during peripheral arteriography.

The issue of selecting the proper gold standard examination is made more difficult by the presence of newer imaging techniques such as intravenous digital subtraction angiography and intraarterial digital subtraction angiography. Although the digital subtraction techniques are by

themselves of diagnostic quality, their accuracy is not as great as that of a standard cut film arteriogram. For example, the intravenous digital subtraction angiograms used to opacify the vessels of the neck and to diagnose the presence of carotid or vertebral artery disease has a 15% rate of uninterpretable studies due to motion artifact or vessel overlap. Validating Doppler or color Doppler sonographic examinations for the detection of significant carotid disease against this gold standard would not be desirable.

Intraarterial digital subtraction techniques involve placing a catheter at the origin of the artery of interest. Lower concentrations of contrast material are needed and the examination length is dramatically shortened. There is, however, a loss in resolution. Most of the current validation studies for Doppler sonography of the carotid arteries are performed against this gold standard. The more traditional contrast arteriogram is more likely to be used in the peripheral arteries.

DEFINITION OF TERMS

Given the availability of a gold standard examination, the efficacy of a noninvasive vascular examination is normally evaluated by determining parameters such as sensitivity, specificity, positive predictive value, negative predictive value, true positive, true negative, false negative, true negative rates, and likelihood ratio. These have been traditionally used for this purpose and should be available for all tests. They give an overall appreciation of how well a noninvasive test performs its diagnostic task.

The sensitivity of a diagnostic test is its ability to detect the presence of a disease process. Truth, or the presence of the disease process, is normally defined by means of a positive gold standard examination. An example is the use of carotid sonography to make the diagnosis of significant narrowing of the internal carotid artery. The sensitivity (or true positive rate) is defined as the number of times this test is positive divided by the total number of subjects evaluated who are known to have the disease process by angiography. In this case, disease is defined as a 50% or greater narrowing of the lumen diameter of the carotid artery. Angiography is considered the gold standard examination.

The specificity is defined as the number of times the test is negative or gives a negative result (true negative) divided by the number of patients who are free of disease. For example, the specificity of duplex sonography for the detection of internal carotid artery disease is defined as the number of patients who, by sonography, have a peak systolic velocity of *less than 1.25 m/sec.* The number of these patients divided by the total number of patients without a significant stenosis (<50% lumen diameter narrowing) defines the specificity of this test.

Continuing with our example on the evaluation of duplex sonography, the accuracy of the examination is calculated by adding the true positive and true negative examinations and dividing this total by the total number of patients who have had both angiography and duplex sonography. This calculated accuracy is dependent on the number of patients with the disease process (disease prevalence) in the cohort being studied. For example, in 100 patients, if the disease prevalence is low (i.e., 10%), a sensitivity of 90% and specificity of 80% will give an overall accuracy of 81%. If disease prevalence is 60%, then a sensitivity of 90% and specificity of 80% will give a higher accuracy for the test (i.e., 54 + 32 or 86%). This effect is summarized in Tables 3.1 to 3.3.

Data from comparative validation studies can also be used to determine the ability of the examination to diagnose or exclude disease. These parameters are the positive and negative predictive values of the examination respectively. These relationships, when applied to a well-defined

Table 3.1.
Parameters Used for Determining Diagnostic Accuracy: Disease Prevalence of 10%

Sensitivity	:	9/10	:	90%
Specificity	:	72/90	:	80%
Accuracy	:	81/100	:	81%
Positive predictive value	:	9/27	:	33%
Negative predictive value	:	72/73	:	99%
Likelihood ratio	:	9/10 × 90/18	=	4.5

	GOLD STANDARD		
	Positive	Negative	TOTAL
SONOGRAPHY			
Positive	9	18	27
Negative	1	72	73
TOTAL	10	90	100

Table 3.2.
Parameters Used for Determining Diagnostic Accuracy: Disease Prevalence of 30%

Sensitivity	:	27/30	:	90%
Specificity	:	56/70	:	80%
Accuracy	:	83/100	:	83%
Positive predictive value	:	27/41	:	66%
Negative predictive value	:	56/59	:	95%
Likelihood ratio	:	27/30 × 70/14	=	4.5

	GOLD STANDARD		
	Positive	Negative	TOTAL
SONOGRAPHY			
Positive	27	14	41
Negative	3	56	59
TOTAL	30	70	100

Table 3.3.
Parameters Used for Determining Diagnostic Accuracy: Disease Prevalence of 60%

Sensitivity	:	54/60	:	90%
Specificity	:	32/40	:	80%
Accuracy	:	86/100	:	86%
Positive predictive value	:	54/62	:	87%
Negative predictive value	:	32/38	:	84%
Likelihood ratio	:	54/60 × 40/8	=	4.5

	GOLD STANDARD		
	Positive	Negative	TOTAL
SONOGRAPHY			
Positive	54	8	62
Negative	6	32	38
TOTAL	60	40	100

patient population, can predict how well the test performs in triaging patients with disease from those without. The positive predictive value of a test is defined as the true positive number divided by the total number of positive and negative sonographic examinations. The negative predictive value is defined as the true negative number divided by the total number of positive and negative sonographic examinations.

All of these parameters are dependent on disease prevalence or the makeup of the population studied in the laboratory. A tertiary referral laboratory is more likely to see a high prevalence of disease, whereas a community-based clinic is likely to see a low disease prevalence. These parameters summarize how well a laboratory functions but do not give any insight as to how likely a patient with an elevated value on Doppler sonography is of having a significant stenosis.

Sample calculations with the example given above show that the positive and negative predictive values are 33% and 99% respectively when disease prevalence is 10%. These change to 87% and 89% respectively when disease prevalence is 60%. In both cases, the sensitivity and specificity are the same. A useful parameter for determining how good a test result is at predicting that a given patient has a disease process is the likelihood ratio. It is defined as the true positive ratio divided by the false positive ratio. It is not dependent on disease prevalence. In summary, a patient with a positive Doppler examination is 4.5 times more likely to have the suspected disease process (i.e., significant internal carotid artery stenosis).

Venous Thrombosis

VENOGRAPHY

The gold standard examination for excluding or confirming the presence of deep vein thrombosis (DVT) is phlebography. Phlebography consists of the injection of contrast material within the veins of the upper or lower extremities and subsequent x-ray filming over these anatomic regions. The opacified lumen of the draining veins is recorded on the radiograph. Failure to opacify a given venous segment can be due to the presence of deep vein thrombosis or to technical factors causing suboptimal distribution of the contrast material. This is often due to the presence of collateral venous channels or to communication with the superficial draining veins. Acute thrombosis is diagnosed whenever the abrupt termination of the contrast column by an intraluminal mass or the presence of a distinct filling defect within the lumen of the vein is seen.

There are many variations on the technique used to opacify the veins. Some require tourniquets located at the calf and thighs. Placing the patient supine may help opacify the deep veins of the calf. In the early 1970s a practical approach to performing phlebography using a tilt table was described. In the mid-1980s, the agent used was changed from the more standard contrast material to either noniodinated or dilute contrast material to diminish the associated risk of postprocedure phlebitis, which occurred in approximately 1 in 30 patients.

The test does carry with it potential complications. These are due either to local irritation such as cellulitis, chemical phlebitis, or rarely, skin necrosis. The incidence of mild allergic reactions, including urticaria, varies from 3 to 10%. More severe reactions, although rare, can occur in 1 in 200 to 1 in 1,000 cases. Anaphylaxis and death are rarely reported, occurring in less than 1 in 10,000 cases.

Care must be taken to properly opacify the deep veins of the calf. Normally, the needle used to inject the contrast material is placed within a superficial pedal vein. The normal plantar arch has a communicating vessel that fills the deeper portion of the posterior tibial and dorsal veins. The use of tourniquets is encouraged either to limit the flow of contrast material through the superficial system or to help the opacification of partly obstructed segments within the deep calf veins.

Phlebography has, by default, become the gold standard examination against which the accuracy of all noninvasive tests is determined. It does, however, have an observer variability of 10%. Although postmortem phlebograms could be correlated against direct pathological examination of the veins, this has limited value since most of the venographic technique is altered in vivo by the dynamic changes that continuously occur in the flow patterns within the venous system. These are caused by preferential flow through collateral branches that developed following previous episodes of deep vein thrombosis and by pressure changes in the calf during muscle contraction.

PLETHYSMOGRAPHY

Plethysmography, in its varied forms, has been the cornerstone of the noninvasive techniques used to diagnose acute deep vein thrombosis. There are two broad categories of plethysmography: measurement of *volume outflow* dynamics and determination of altered *blood flow patterns*.

Impedance or pulse-volume plethysmography basically relies on measuring the effects of venous outflow obstruction (Fig. 3.1). A cuff is inflated for a predetermined amount of time. The rate of filling within the deep veins of the thigh and calf are measured using either a partly inflated blood pressure cuff (pulse volume), a strain gauge, or impedance measurements (impedance plethysmography). Impedance plethysmography has been extensively used for making the diagnosis of deep vein thrombosis. Poor filling of the deep veins is normally ascribed either to a chronic venous thrombosis or to failure of the patient to relax his or her calf muscles (Fig. 3.2). Following deflation of the cuff, blood flow and venous return increase as the blood trapped in the leg or arm now empties. Loss of normal outflow is normally ascribed to an obstructive process such as an acute deep venous thrombus (Fig. 3.3). Extrinsic obstruction of venous outflow due to a mass, pregnancy, or right-sided heart failure can perturb the normal venous emptying dynamics and possibly be misdiagnosed as a venous thrombosis.

Phleborheography is a technique that relies on detecting normal alterations in venous blood flow in response to either respiration or maneuvers that accentuate emptying of the calf veins (Fig. 3.4). A series of partly inflated cuffs are placed over the foot, calf, thigh, and abdomen. Alterations in normal flow suggest the presence of obstruction to the veins. The limitations of the technique are similar to those of plethysmography. Performing the examination is more labor intensive since many more cuffs need to be placed and adjusted by the technologist.

The sensitivity, specificity, and overall accuracy of these techniques have been estimated to be above 90%, although those of phleborheography may be lower. However, biases have been introduced in the evaluation of the accuracy of these techniques since the populations studied have predominantly suffered from obstructive (symptomatic) deep vein thrombosis.

Outpatients and hospitalized patients who manifest symptomatic deep vein thrombosis have a high likelihood of having occlusive thrombus. Under these circumstances, the techniques perform with a sensitivity above 90% for the presence of femoral or popliteal vein thrombosis. The sensitivity is slightly less for strain gauge plethysmography than for impedance plethysmography. In asymptomatic post-

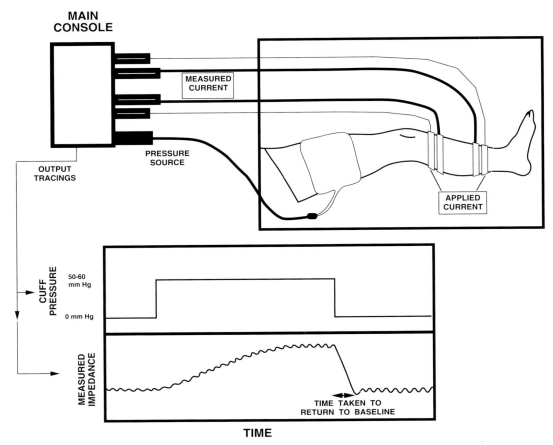

MAIN CONSOLE

MEASURED CURRENT

PRESSURE SOURCE

OUTPUT TRACINGS

APPLIED CURRENT

CUFF PRESSURE

50-60 mm Hg

0 mm Hg

MEASURED IMPEDANCE

TIME TAKEN TO RETURN TO BASELINE

TIME

Figure 3.1. The impedance plethysmogram (IPG) has been the standard noninvasive examination for detecting the presence of acute deep vein thrombosis for many years. Changes in calf volume are measured during the inflation and deflation of a pressure cuff placed over the proximal thigh. The normal response is an increase in volume to a steady value over a 1- to 3-minute interval. Following cuff deflation, the trapped blood rapidly empties through the patent venous channels.

operative patients with above-knee thrombosis, the sensitivity of the technique drops precipitously to below 70%. This is a reflection of the large proportion of patients who have nonobstructive thrombus.

Calf vein thrombosis is difficult to detect with all of the plethysmography techniques. Obstructive thrombosis, if it involves more than two of the paired venous systems, can impair blood flow sufficiently to be detected. Overall, in symptomatic patients with obstructive calf vein thrombosis the sensitivity may approach 40 to 50%. In the early postoperative population, in whom nonobstructive thrombosis predominates, the sensitivity for detecting calf vein thrombosis is 20% or less.

TIME COURSE

The natural history of deep vein thrombosis is such that collateral venous channels develop rapidly. Within a few weeks, 20% of impedance plethysmograms performed have returned to normal. By 2 months, 60% of the examinations have returned to normal. A patient who has had an episode of deep vein thrombosis and who is suspected of having a second episode of acute DVT can have the diagnosis made by impedance plethysmography with a sensitivity of 70 to 80%.

DOPPLER (CW)

Doppler sonography has been used for evaluating of the presence of deep vein thrombosis using mostly nonimaging CW pencil probes operating at a frequency of 10 MHz. The probe is positioned over the common femoral, proximal superficial femoral, popliteal, and posterior tibial veins. Standard maneuvers are performed

to establish patency at these venous segments. Respiratory variation normally causes a cyclical variation in blood flow velocity. Squeezing the lower calf causes emptying of some of the blood pooled in the veins. The acceleration of blood flow is then detected as a "swishing" sound on the audio channel of these probes. Loss of these responses is considered a positive examination. The technique requires considerable operator experience and can be quite accurate. It performs best in symptomatic patients with obstructive deep vein thrombosis. On occasion, a negative test is obtained when a superficial or deep collateral vein is sampled instead of the deep vein. Nonobstructive deep vein thrombo-

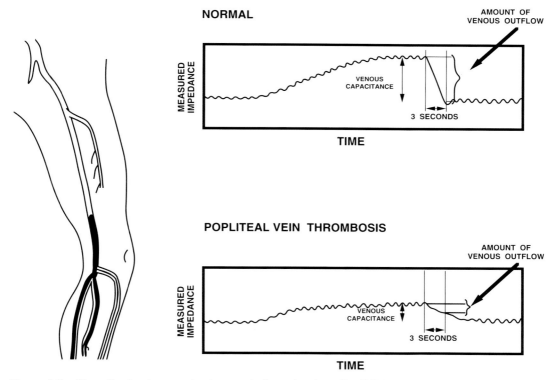

Figure 3.2. The effects of an acute deep vein thrombosis on the IPG tracing are twofold. The acute thrombus fills in and replaces the volume normally occupied by blood. The venous capacitance, or the amount by which the calf veins fill while the cuff is inflated, is therefore decreased. The thrombus itself also acts as an obstruction to the egress of blood. This decreases the amount of blood that leaves the calf once the pressure cuff is deflated.

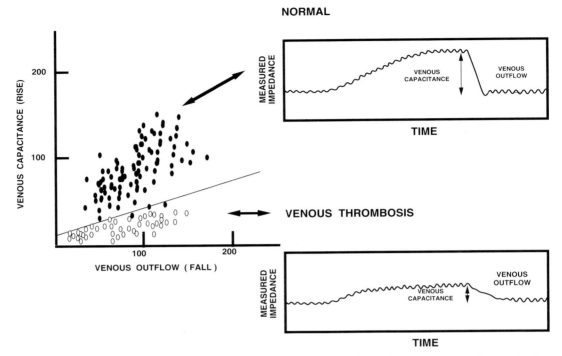

Figure 3.3. The test is normally performed with the patient being asked to relax the leg while the leg is slightly elevated. Voluntary contraction of the muscles can cause false positive results. Up to three attempts are made to obtain a normal result. If one normal result is obtained it is always kept. The definition of normal and abnormal have been established from a curve of the response (filling and emptying) of lower extremities with and without DVT. Points falling below the line on the graph are considered to be indicative of acute DVT.

sis is likely to be missed. Similarly, the test has poor specificity and many false positives can be caused by an extrinsic obstructive process within either the thigh, the pelvis, or the abdomen. Elevated right-sided heart pressures will also blunt the normal flow responses.

I-125 FIBRINOGEN SCANNING

Fibrinogen binds to actively forming thrombus. Iodinated fibrinogen scanning is quite reliable for detecting calf vein thrombi that form postoperatively (Fig. 3.5). It does, however, suffer from many

limitations. It is unreliable in the thigh. It is also likely to give false positive results over areas of inflammation. The technique is currently investigational in the United States, since costs linked to the use of blood products forced commercial distribution to cease in early 1990.

Sensitivity for forming calf thrombi has been reported to be between 70 and 100%. It is much lower and, in fact, is considered to be unreliable in the thigh. A major limitation of the technique is the need to perform serial daily measurements, since abnormal uptake is defined as a greater than 20% elevation in count rate that persists for more than 2 days.

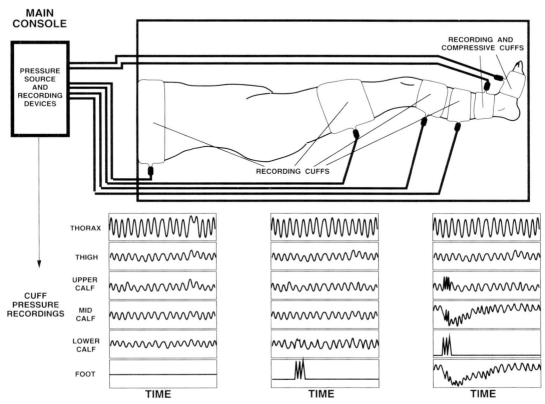

Figure 3.4. The phleborheogram is normally performed with a series of six cuffs. The one in the thorax is used to monitor respirations. The ones on the thigh and the proximal and mid calf are also recording cuffs. The lower calf cuff and the foot cuff are also used to cause increased blood flow when inflated rapidly. The normal baseline recording (*left*) shows respiratory waves transmitted all the way into the lower calf. A recording is also made when the foot cuff is rapidly filled (*center*). This increases venous return and should not have any effect on the more proximal tracings. In case of an obstruction secondary to DVT, the tracings from the more proximal cuffs would show an elevation in signal. This would be seen to the cuff contiguous with the proximal extent of the thrombus. A third recording is also made with the lower calf cuff being rapidly inflated (*right*). This causes a decrease in foot volume and affects the proximal and mid calf cuffs. Again, the extremity involved with DVT would show an elevation in the tracing to the level of the obstructing thrombus. The definition of a normal PRG includes a normal baseline and the presence of respiratory waves. Their absence is the main criterion for making the diagnosis of acute DVT.

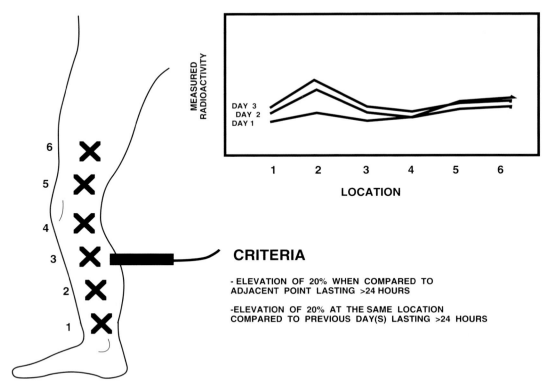

Figure 3.5. The iodinated fibrinogen (I-125 fibrinogen) test is performed following the intravenous injection of approximately 100 microcuries of the radioactive compound. The amount of radioactivity accumulating in the legs is then measured over consecutive days. This test assumes that the compound has been injected as a blood clot is forming. It is therefore best suited for the postoperative detection and monitoring of calf vein DVT. It does not perform well for monitoring the thigh since the veins are too deeply located. The commercial distribution of this compound has recently ceased in the United States.

Carotid Stenosis

ARTERIOGRAPHY

Direct injection of contrast material into the carotid artery was performed as a standard diagnostic test during the 1950s and 1960s. Opacification of the major branches of the carotids was achieved and used to diagnose the presence of significant stenosis. The technique's contribution evolved into a diagnostic test as well as a road map to help plan the operative approach whenever carotid endarterectomy was contemplated. First introduced in 1954, carotid endarterectomy was a driving force for the dissemination and technical improvements in arteriography. The ability to map out the extent and severity of carotid stenosis was essential before any operative repair was attempted.

The diagnostic uses of carotid angiography were not limited to carotid atherosclerotic disease. Cerebral angiography had other applications such as mapping the location of intracerebral aneurysms, determining the presence of arterial malformations, and aiding in the diagnostic workup of stroke.

Validation of the arteriographic technique was performed with the aid of surgical pathology samples obtained during carotid endarterectomy.

The direct puncture into the carotid artery carries a 5% risk of either local intimal injuries, embolization, or hematoma. Stroke or cerebral vascular accidents (CVAs) were noted in a surprisingly small population of patients (i.e., 1 to 2%).

In an effort to reduce the local complication rate, a less direct method of performing the arteriogram came into favor. The standard approach is now made from the femoral artery using long polyethylene catheters with predetermined shapes. These catheters are advanced into either the proximal aortic arch or at the origin of the carotid. The technique relies on the use of rapid film changers and small focal point biplane arteriographic tables to obtain high-resolution images of the carotid bifurcations. Local complication rates at the groin entry sites are in the 1 to 2% range, and the risk of stroke is diminished to less than 0.5%.

Less invasive approaches were proposed and implemented in the mid-1970s. Computer-assisted methods were used to sequentially acquire a series of images following a large injection of contrast material into either a central vein or the right atrium. These images were then processed and subtracted from a background image with no contrast in the artery, and the subtracted image then showed the opacified artery. These intravenous digital subtraction angiograms are performed by rapidly injecting contrast medium (30 to 50 cc) into the inferior vena cava (IVC), superior vena cava (SVC), or right atrium. Comparative sensitivity and specificity for the detection of significant narrrowings at the internal carotid are approximately 90% when compared to standard high-quality angiograms. Poor patient cooperation or other technical factors give a 10 to 15% rate of unreliable and indeterminate studies. Two views are required to diagnose a significant carotid lesion. A large amount of contrast material is often necessary to obtain these and to overcome overlapping vessels from the right and left sides of the neck.

The newer approach to this technique is the digital acquisition of images following intra-arterial contrast medium injection. The advantage is a decreased catheter residence time in the proximal common carotid. This decreases the likelihood of embolic phenomena and associated stroke or transient ischemic attack (TIA). Although currently the diagnostic gold standard, the digital technique has a resolution that is slightly less than that of standard carotid angiography. Although this does not adversely affect the overall diagnostic accuracy, the loss in resolution makes the examination slightly less reliable for the detection of ulceration and smaller irregularities in the wall of the arteries. Grading of very high-grade stenosis is also slightly less reliable. Determination of the presence of the subtotal occlusions (pseudoocclusion or 99% stenosis) of the internal carotid artery requires the use of prolonged contrast agent injection and delayed films using standard cut-film angiography.

OCULOPLETHYSMOGRAPHY

The need to screen patients noninvasively and atraumatically for the presence of hemodynamically significant stenosis was partly driven by the availability of a "cure" for the symptomatic high-grade stenosis. Carotid arteriography, which carries with it a small yet non-negligible morbidity, can then follow only if there is a high likelihood of finding a lesion amenable to endarterectomy.

The basic physiologic principle on which this screening test is based is the detection of a significant pressure drop in the cerebral circulation.

Oculoplethysmography (OPG) detects the hemodynamic effects of a significant carotid artery stenosis as a decrease in the pulse pressure wave that reaches the ocular globe. In one form (OPG-Zira), a small suction clip is positioned on the cornea and the arrival time of the pulse pressure wave is measured at both ocular globes and compared to an external reference point such as the ear lobe (Fig. 3.6). A significant delay of greater than 5 msec in the arrival time of the pulse pressure wave suggests the presence of a significant obstructive lesion within the carotid artery on that side. The technique is quite accurate for the detection of significant lumen diameter narrowing of the internal carotid artery of greater than 75%. Potential problems arise when significant bilateral internal carotid artery stenoses are present. The

technique cannot differentiate between significant obstructive lesions within the internal carotid artery territory, the ophthalmic branches, the common carotid, or even the right innominate artery.

Another implementation of this principle is the ocular plethysmogram (OPG-Gee) (Fig. 3.7). Here, negative pressure is applied to both ocular globes by suction cups placed on the corneas. Increasing the negative pressure leads to a loss in the pulse transmitted to the ocular globe. Slow release of the negative pressure results in the return of the pulse pressure wave. A difference in the return of the pressure wave between both globes suggests the presence of a significant stenosis. Symmetric disease can often be underestimated. Similarly, the level of obstruction cannot be determined with any anatomic accu-

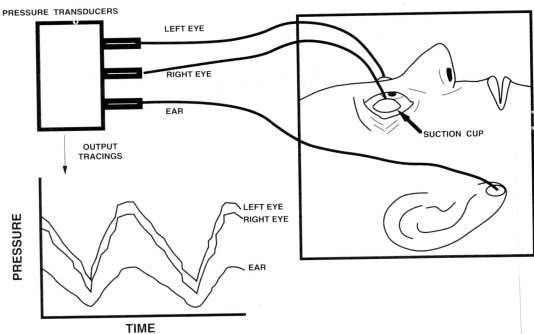

Figure 3.6. The oculoplethysmograph also comes as another slightly different variant: the Zira method. The pressure cups placed on the eyes have only a small amount of negative pressure applied to them (40 to 60 mm Hg). Tracings are made of the arterial waveform at both ocular globes and with an ear lobe as a reference point. A delay in the waveform of 5 msec is considered to be indicative of the presence of a significant carotid lesion.

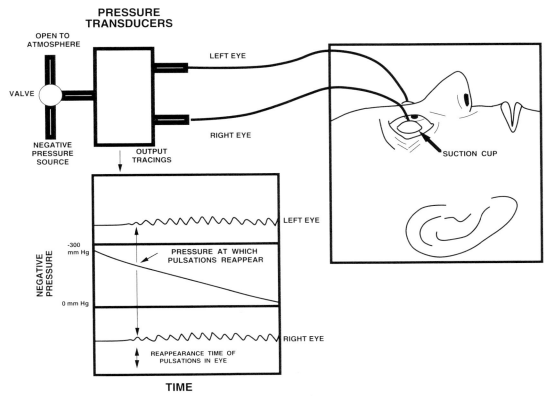

Figure 3.7. The oculoplethysmograph is used to measure pressure differences caused by proximal arterial lesions. These develop when a stenosis reaches a 75% or greater lumen diameter narrowing in one of the two carotid arteries. In the Gee method, a negative pressure of 300 mm Hg is applied to small suction cups placed on the outer aspect of the eye. This negative pressure occludes blood flow through the retina from the ophthalmic artery. The pressure is then slowly released and the time at which arterial pulsations reappear in the eye is measured. A significant lesion of the common, internal, or ophthalmic artery will cause a pressure difference in the reappearance of these pulsations.

racy. The accuracy of the technique is similar to oculoplethysmography using OPG-Zira.

A variant of this plethysmographic approach is to directly measure the pulse arrival time in the arteries surrounding the ocular globe. Although slightly safer, since the anaesthetized cornea need not be put in contact with a foreign body, it is less reliable since the arterial branches around the ocular globe are quite tortuous and the cross-collaterals can be quite numerous.

PERIORBITAL DIRECTIONAL DOPPLER

There are multiple anastomotic pathways between the internal carotid circulation and the external carotid circulation around both ocular globes. These potential collateral pathways are such that the preferential pattern of blood flow is from the internal circulation outward into the external carotid branches. A Doppler pencil probe placed on either the supraorbital or the frontal branches will normally show this outward direction of blood flow (Fig. 3.8). Compression at selected points on

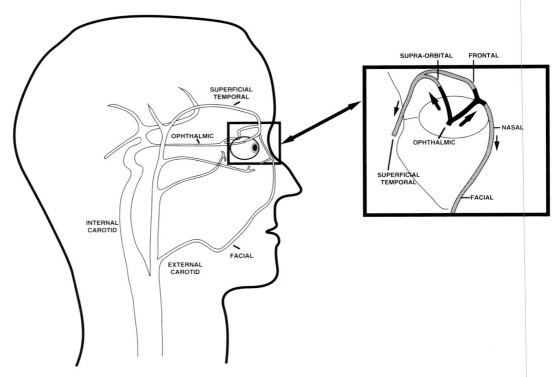

Figure 3.8. The use of periorbital Doppler signals to detect significant carotid stenoses is best suited to very high-grade stenoses of 90% lumen diameter narrowing or greater. The periorbital vessels act as a watershed area with competitive flow being directed outward from the ophthalmic artery and inward from the facial and superficial temporal arteries. The prevalent direction of blood flow is outward. This is normally measured using a 10- to 20-MHz directional Doppler pencil probe at the supraorbital and frontal branches.

the temporal branch of the external carotid, the facial artery, or the mandibular branches should normally cause either an increase in the outward flow of blood or no significant change.

The presence of a significant carotid artery stenosis causes the flow pattern within these periocular branches to change. The direction of flow is now directed inward toward the ocular globe (Fig. 3.9). Application of external pressure on the temporal, facial, or mandibular branches normally abolishes the flow signal (Fig. 3.10). These changes are normally present in higher-grade stenosis and more commonly with greater than 90% lumen diameter narrowing. The specificity of the test is quite high (90%) while the sen-

sitivity improves as the severity of the stenosis progresses above 90% lumen narrowing.

OCULAR DOPPLER

Direct measurement of the direction of flow within the ophthalmic branch can be done by placing an ultrasonographic transducer over the globe. The direction of blood flow through this vessel is then measured. The maneuvers described above can also be applied. This approach may have potential biological effects due to energy deposition in the retina by the ultrasonographic beam. Performing this test requires a large amount of patient cooperation.

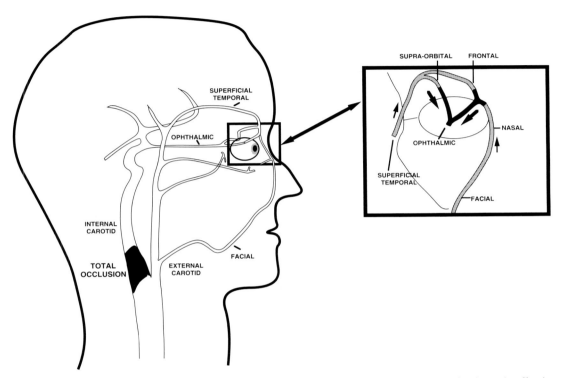

Figure 3.9. The normal outward direction of blood flow reverses when a high-grade stenosis affects the internal carotid. Flow is then directed inward through the facial and superficial temporal arteries into the supraorbital, frontal, and nasal branches to finally reach the ophthalmic artery. The ophthalmic artery will then often feed the intracranial branches through the upper portion of the internal carotid.

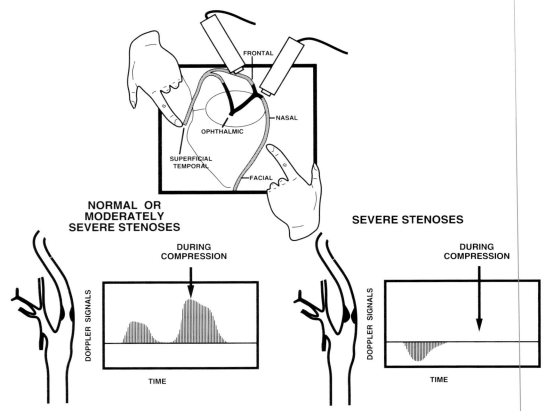

Figure 3.10. In addition to noting the direction of blood flow, the periorbital Doppler examination is performed with the aid of two additional maneuvers. The preauricular branch of the superficial temporal artery and the facial artery are compressed while the Doppler signals are listened to. The normal response is either no change in the Doppler signals or an increase in their intensity. The abnormal response is a loss of the Doppler signal.

Peripheral Arterial Stenosis

ARTERIOGRAPHY

Contrast injection into the peripheral arteries and subsequent x-ray filming was first performed in the 1940s. Clinical peripheral arteriography was first performed, and is still performed in a few institutions, following the translumbar placement of a needle through the soft tissues of the back. The catheter directly enters the abdominal aorta. Contrast material is subsequently injected. A single long focal film of the leg or a series of films taken at multiple stations along the length of the

leg are then taken to fully visualize the peripheral arterial tree. Validation of this arteriographic technique has been performed on cadavers and by correlating arteriographic findings against those obtained from surgical specimens. The latter has been limited, since it is hard to justify the need for full surgical exposure and arteriotomy over long portions of the arteries. Selective cannulation of the femoral artery using a beveled needle (i.e., the Seldinger approach) further simplified peripheral arteriography. Improvements in filming technique such as rapid film changers and the dissemination of mechanized tables (step tables) permit filming to be efficiently performed at different levels of the leg during the same injection of contrast material.

Intravenous digital angiography is less commonly used. As with the carotids, large amounts of contrast are often necessary to image even small segments of the limb arteries. Digital subtraction angiography is more often used in conjunction with an intraarterial catheter. This permits the rapid filming and review of regions of concern. It is more useful as a method of assessing progress during percutaneous interventions.

The arteriogram is still viewed as the gold standard examination and as the only suitable road map for possible surgical correction. These procedures include endarterectomy and vascular bypass with either synthetic material or autologous vein. The increasing use of peripheral balloon angioplasty, atherectomy, laser angioplasty, and thrombolysis will most likely lead to a more cost-effective approach to patient management. Triaging patients to either treatment approach will require accurate mapping of the severity and length of lesions within the peripheral arterial tree. For example, stenotic lesions of less than 4 cm in length within the superficial femoral artery are amenable to angioplasty and show high patency rates (80% at 5 years), while lesions longer than 4 cm do worse (40 to 60% patency at 5 years). Although this has been the realm of angiography, Doppler sonography now promises to make a significant contribution to the diagnostic workup.

PLETHYSMOGRAPHY

Pulse volume recording is a basic technique used for the detection of significant peripheral arterial disease (Fig. 3.11). A partly inflated blood pressure cuff is used to detect volume changes caused by the arterial pulsations at the different levels of the lower or upper extremity. Tracings of these volume changes can then be used to detect the presence of significant arterial stenosis or occlusions (Fig. 3.12). The loss of the normal pulse wave contour suggests early disease. Progressive smoothing of the pulse contour tracing with a loss of the amplitude of the waveform parallels worsening arterial disease. The severity and extent of these lesions cannot, however, be accurately mapped out anatomically (Fig. 3.13). Pulse volume recordings are normally performed by placing blood pressure cuffs at at least 3 to 4 levels in the lower extremities and 2 to 3 in the upper extremities.

Sensitivity of the technique by itself is 80% for peripheral arterial disease. It is most often used as an adjunct to segmental pressure measurements and is especially useful in patients in whom noncompliant and stiff arteries make pressure measurements unreliable (i.e., diabetes).

SEGMENTAL PRESSURES

In the early 1970s, the need to noninvasively screen patients prior to arteriography led to the creation of the noninvasive laboratory. The simplest noninvasive technique used to detect evidence of peripheral arterial disease is the ankle-brachial ratio (Fig. 3.14). The systolic pressure in an arm is compared to the systolic pressure measurements made with a blood pressure cuff placed around the calf. The systolic blood pressure in the arm is used as the denominator. The blood pressure in the calf vessels is measured with a Doppler probe to detect flow signals within the dorsalis pedis or posterior tibial artery. This systolic pressure is used as the numerator. A normal result is a ratio above 0.9. Between 0.8 and 0.9 lies an indeterminate zone where the presence of peripheral arterial disease is quite likely. Between 0.6 and 0.8, claudication is likely and arteriography will show moderately severe pe-

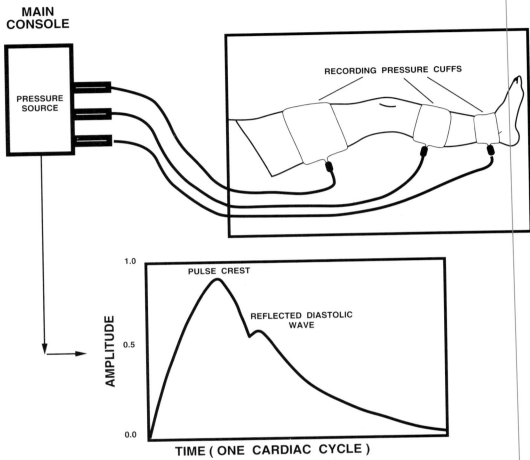

Figure 3.11. The pressure-volume recorder (PVR) consists of a series of partly inflated cuffs positioned over the calf and thigh. The amount of pressure is kept at a standard value between 50 and 70 mm Hg. The arterial tracings recorded from these cuffs have a typical appearance with a period of rapid rise, a peak, a diastolic wave, and a slow decline. Since the system is partly calibrated, changes in the amplitude of the curve can be used to diagnose the presence of significant arterial lesions. The loss in tracing amplitude occurs distal to the obstructed arterial segment. Most of the diagnostic uses of these recordings rely on a change in the shape of the PVR tracing, with loss of the diastolic wave being the best indicator.

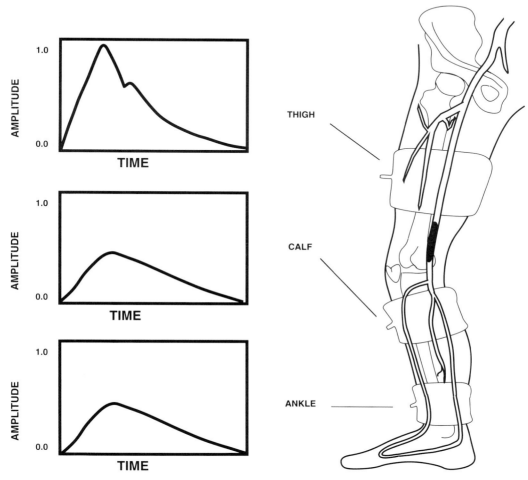

Figure 3.12. The presence of a significant arterial lesion will cause the PVR tracing to become more symmetrical. Loss of the diastolic wave is one of the earliest changes to occur. At the next level of severity, the peak amplitude decreases mildly and there is a significant decrease in the slope of the signal rise. Finally, the amplitude of the signal decreases progressively as the extent of peripheral disease worsens. Although the level of the obstructive arterial process can normally be identified, its length or severity cannot be accurately predicted.

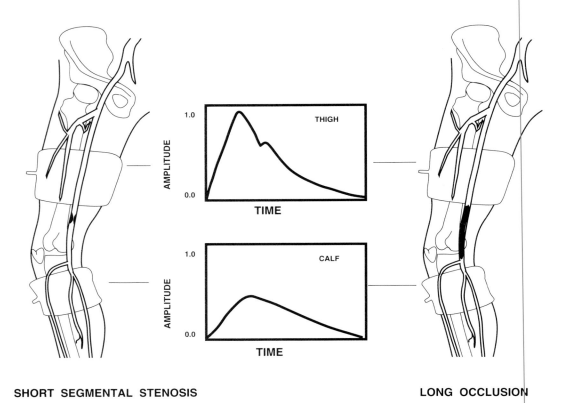

SHORT SEGMENTAL STENOSIS

LONG OCCLUSION

Figure 3.13. Although the PVR tracings are very similar, the two lesions shown are very different. The one on the left is a high-grade stenosis amenable to angioplasty. The lesion on the right is a long occlusion, which may be treated with a more aggressive percutaneous intervention but is more likely to undergo bypass surgery.

ripheral arterial disease. More severe segmental disease normally corresponds to a ratio between 0.4 and 0.6. Rest ischemia and severe symptoms are normally seen when the ankle-brachial index is below 0.4.

The ankle-brachial index offers a rough screen for the presence of significant stenotic lesions anywhere in the arterial circuit feeding the extremity being examined (Fig. 3.15). Multiple blood pressure cuffs can also be positioned along the extremity to determine at what level the actual pressure drop occurs (Fig. 3.16). For example, a pressure drop above 20 mm Hg in the thigh suggests aortic or iliac arterial occlusions. A drop at the thigh corresponds to femoral or popliteal artery dis-

ease. The thigh cuffs must be of sufficient diameter to properly occlude the arteries when they are inflated. A significant pressure drop of greater than 20 mm Hg or a loss of 0.2 unit in the ankle-brachial ratio between two different levels normally signifies significant segmental disease (Fig. 3.17).

The sensitivity and specificity of the test have recently come into question. Overall accuracies of approximately 80% have been reported. However, the test performs quite poorly when concomitant femoropopliteal and aortoiliac artery disease are present. The specificity drops abruptly to less than 50% when both processes are present. Again, the extent and severity of the lesions cannot be measured. Severe se-

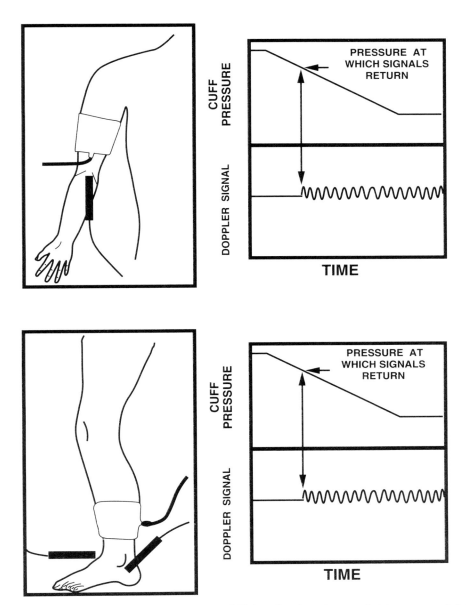

Figure 3.14. The ankle-brachial pressure index (ABI) is a simple yet very reliable means of detecting the presence of significant peripheral arterial lesions. A Doppler probe is used to detect the reappearance time of blood flow. This corresponds to the systolic pressure in the artery studied. The determination is performed in both arms at the level of the brachial artery. A significant difference between both arms is indicative of an upper-extremity arterial lesion. The dorsalis pedis and the posterior tibial arteries are then both sampled. An absent dorsalis pedis pulse can be seen in 8% of normals. The ABI is calculated by dividing the systolic pressure determined in the dorsalis pedis or posterior tibial by that measured in one arm. The expected value is normally 1.1. Values below 0.9 are indicative of lower-extremity arterial disease.

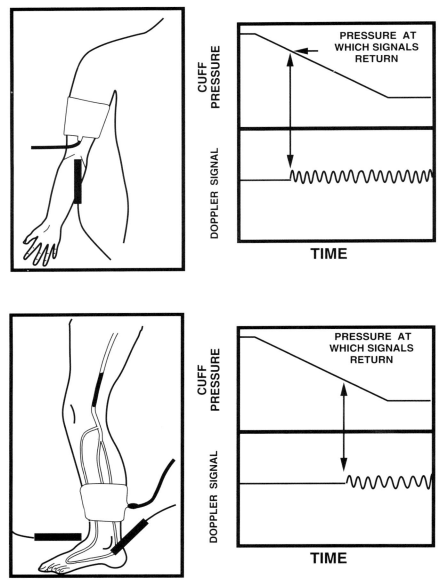

Figure 3.15. The ABI is decreased whenever a significant narrowing or occlusion is present in the arteries connecting the heart to the ankle. It is not possible to determine the length, location, or severity of the obstructive lesions. In general, however, the more depressed the ABI, the more severe the extent of peripheral arterial lesions. The ABI may not be depressed in individuals with poorly compliant vessels despite the presence of significant lesions. This is more likely in diabetics, who commonly have calcified arteries.

MAIN CONSOLE

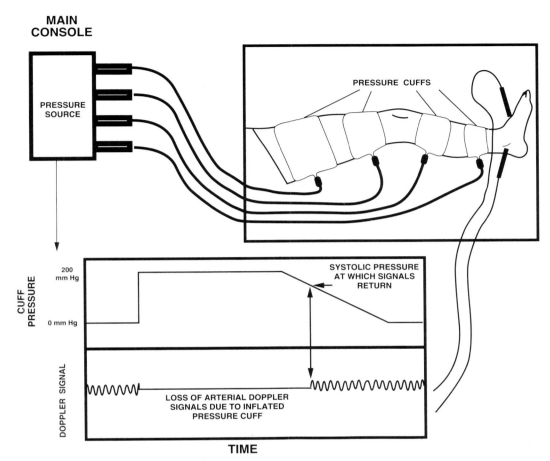

Figure 3.16. The use of segmental pressures is a refinement in the ABI measurement discussed above. Multiple pressure cuffs are sequentially inflated and the systolic pressure is measured by the reappearance time of the Doppler waveform in the dorsalis pedis or posterior tibial artery. A decrement in pressure of 20 mm Hg between two levels is considered to be evidence of a significant arterial lesion (stenosis or occlusion) in the lower segment. The results of the segmental pressure measurements can also be expressed as a ratio with the brachial artery pressure. A decrement of 0.15 in this modified ABI is then considered to be evidence of a significant lesion.

rial focal lesions amenable to angioplasty or long segment occlusions amenable to bypass surgery can give similar segmental blood pressure measurements. These cannot be differentiated on the basis of this noninvasive test alone.

The ankle-brachial ratio is often used for serial monitoring of peripheral arterial disease. The reproducibility of the technique is such that a drop of 0.15 mm Hg is considered to be significant.

DOPPLER (CW)

The continuous-wave Doppler probe is mostly used to interrogate the distal pulses. It is used in association with the blood pressure cuff to detect the reappearance of the pulse pressure wave. Rough

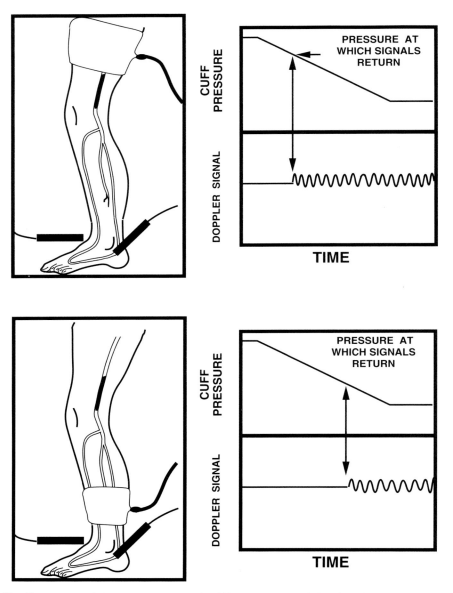

Figure 3.17. The segmental pressures can detect the presence of significant segmental disease by showing a pressure drop of at least 20 mm Hg between two pressure cuffs. This diagram shows how a low femoral lesion would be detected using the segmental pressure measurement. The decrement in pressure takes place between the thigh and the upper calf pressure cuffs. This same pressure decrement is maintained between the thigh and the lower calf cuffs, since there are no intervening arterial lesions in the tibioperoneal arteries.

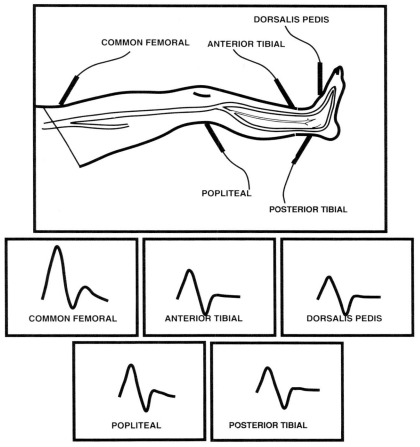

Figure 3.18. Small hand-held Doppler probes can be used to record arterial waveforms at the different levels of the extremity. The output of these probes is a "mean" velocity and not a spectral display. This "mean" waveform is recorded from different levels in the leg and displayed on a paper chart recorder. They are not accurately calibrated, so only a subjective evaluation is performed of the appearance of the arterial waveform.

characterization of the audio signal can be used to determine the severity of the stenosis.

WAVEFORM ANALYSIS

Actual measurement of the waveform of the Doppler probe can be used, as is the case with the pulse volume recording, to detect evidence of peripheral arterial disease. The normal Doppler waveform has a triphasic pattern in the peripheral arteries of the arm and leg (Fig. 3.18). With severe occlusion or ischemia, the early diastolic reversal of flow is lost and a more monophasic pattern of blood flow emerges (Fig. 3.19). This pattern is quite similar to what is seen following exercise or following the administration of a vasodilator. It is due to the marked peripheral vasodilation caused by poor inflow of oxygenated blood. In response to proximal obstruction, the peripheral arterial and capillary beds dilate and create a low-resistance system. The level at which the waveform loses its normal biphasic or triphasic pattern normally

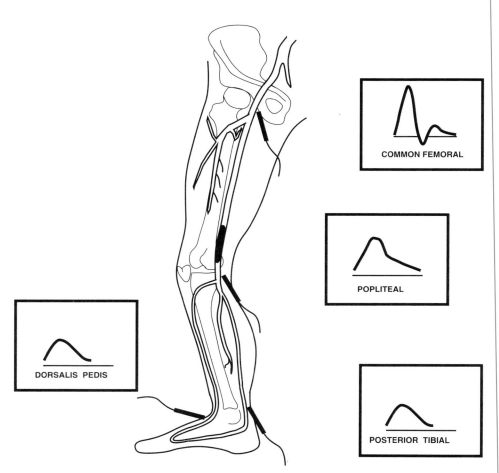

Figure 3.19. The presence of an arterial lesion (stenosis or occlusion) is normally inferred when the Doppler tracing shows one of the following changes: a loss of the normal triphasic waveform, the presence of a monophasic waveform, and a loss in the amplitude of the signal. These changes reflect the homeostatic readjustment taking place to compensate for the decreased delivery of oxygenated blood to the peripheral limb. When the transducer is inadvertently placed over a lesion, the velocity tracing will be elevated if it is a stenosis and absent if it is an occlusion. This technique is of special utility in patients whose calcified vessels preclude the use of segmental pressure measurements.

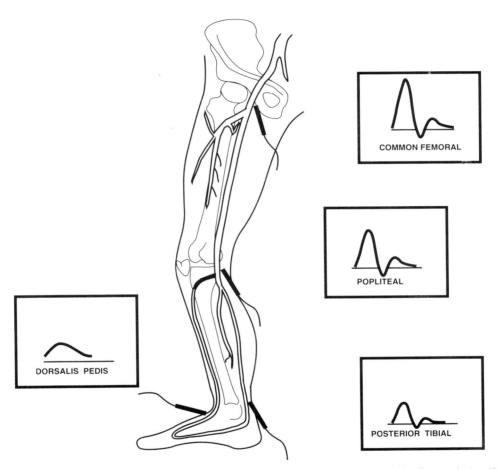

Figure 3.20. The peripheral Doppler tracings can be selectively applied to the anterior tibial/dorsalis pedis and the posterior tibial arteries. They can therefore also detect the presence of significant disease in either of these arteries.

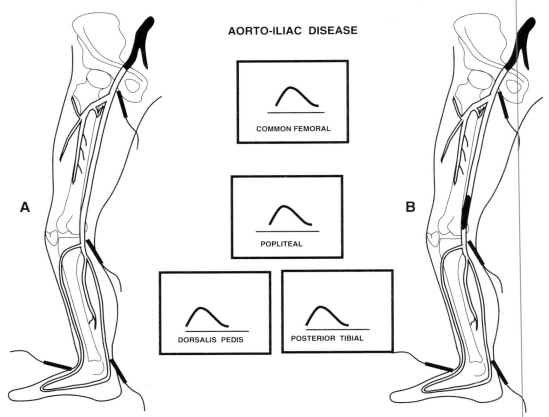

AORTO-ILIAC DISEASE

COMMON FEMORAL

POPLITEAL

DORSALIS PEDIS

POSTERIOR TIBIAL

A

B

Figure 3.21. Peripheral Doppler tracings, PVR tracings, and segmental pressure measurements share a common limitation. The concomitant presence of severe aortoiliac disease interferes with the accuracy of the tracings made farther down in the limb. In the case of the peripheral Doppler tracings, a marked loss in signal amplitude and a persistent monophasic waveform are seen in the arteries distal to an aortoiliac occlusion (**A**). The additional presence of a popliteal occlusion (**B**) does not cause any additional changes in the already markedly abnormal tracings. This tandem lesion would therefore have been missed.

reflects the site of obstruction (stenosis or occlusion) (Fig. 3.20). Absence of flow signals at a given location can normally be ascribed to a total occlusion. Difficulties can arise, however, in differentiating between smaller peripheral collateral arteries and a diseased larger arterial branch. This is most likely to occur at the level of the popliteal fossa. The sensitivity and specificity of these tests are reported to be about 70 to 80%. Actual localization of the lesion is unreliable. All of these limitations are accentuated in the presence of concomi-

tant aorto-iliac occlusions (Fig. 3.21). The technique is very operator dependent.

There is an important difference between the waveform generated by the hand-held pencil probes and the spectral waveform analysis possible during duplex sonography. The older generation devices generate a waveform that is roughly proportional to the mean velocity of blood. The spectral waveform seen with Doppler imaging shows the full distribution of the motions being detected. For this reason published values of velocity are often discordant, with the older-generation devices reporting lower velocity values (see Fig. 1.31).

Summary

Before the introduction of vascular sonography, it was not possible to gain an exact anatomic localization of the extent and character of thrombosis in acute DVT or to determine the length and severity of obstructive arterial lesions in the peripheral arteries.

The noninvasive techniques mentioned in this chapter have slowly decreased in importance. Sonography has completely replaced all other noninvasive tests. For the presence of acute deep vein thrombosis, Doppler sonography is now the examination of choice for detecting internal carotid stenosis. Sonographic imaging has also gained importance for monitoring the

results of surgical or interventional revascularization procedures.

SUGGESTED READINGS

Baker JD, Dix DE. Variability of Doppler ankle pressures with arterial occlusive disease: an evaluation of ankle index and brachial-ankle pressure gradient. Surgery 1981;89:134–137.

Bernstein EF. Noninvasive diagnostic techniques in vascular disease. 2nd ed. St. Louis: CV Mosby, 1982.

Campbell WB, Cole SEA, Skidmore R, Baird RN. The clinician and the vascular laboratory in the diagnosis of aortoiliac stenosis. Br J Surg 1984;71:302–306.

Chikos PM, Fisher LD, Hirsch JH, Harley JD, Thiele BL, Strandness DE Jr. Observer variability in evaluating extracranial carotid artery stenosis. Stroke 1983;14:885–892.

Martin KD, Patterson RB, Fowl RJ, Kempczinski RF. Is the continued use of ocular pneumoplethysmography necessary for the diagnosis of cerebrovascular disease? J Vasc Surg 1990;11:235–243.

Slot HB, Strijbosch L, Greep JM. Interobserver variability in single-plane aortography. Surgery 1981;90:497–503.

Yao ST. Haemodynamic studies in peripheral arterial disease. Br J Surg 1970;57:761–766.

CHAPTER FOUR

Neck Arteries

Incidence and Clinical Importance

The prevalence of significant internal artery stenosis is related to patient age, sex, and risk factors such as smoking and hypercholesterolemia. Screening using ultrasound puts the prevalence of greater than 50% narrowing of the carotid at approximately 3 to 7%. The lower number applies to the younger subset, whereas in the older population it can reach up to 7%.

The presence of significant carotid artery stenosis has been causally related to the subsequent development of stroke and cerebrovascular events. Recent data from the North American Symptomatic Carotid Endarterectomy Trial (NASCET) have supported the belief that the presence of symptoms in a patient with a significant carotid stenosis ($\geq$70% lumen diameter narrowing) normally warrants surgical correction by endarterectomy. The presence of asymptomatic significant carotid artery stenosis remains a controversial management problem. It is recognized that once symptoms develop in a patient with a significant stenosis, there is a high incidence of stroke, estimated at a 4 to 6% annual rate. The relative risks of surgical

endarterectomy are then less than the risk of conservative medical management. There is also an increasing belief that patients with high-grade stenosis (>75% lumen diameter narrowing) undergoing a prolonged surgical procedure such as coronary artery bypass surgery should have a prophylactic endarterectomy in an effort to prevent the high likelihood of perioperative stroke.

Carotid Artery

NORMAL ANATOMY AND TECHNIQUE

Two-dimensional gray-scale imaging is used to identify the location and course of the carotid branches. Distinguishing between the internal and external carotid branches is normally accomplished with the aid of duplex sonography or color Doppler flow imaging.

The left common carotid artery normally arises directly from the aortic arch (Fig. 4.1). The origin is only occasionally visualized by sonography. On occasion, the left common carotid shares a common trunk with the subclavian, but the general rule is for the subclavian and common carotid to have separate origins. On the right side, the subclavian and common carotid

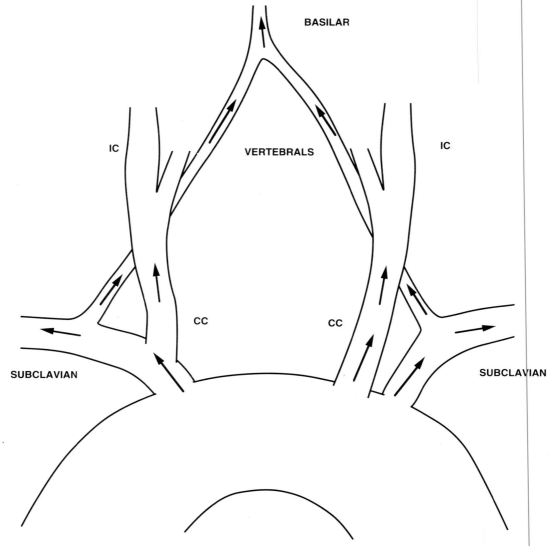

Figure 4.1. The internal carotid and the vertebral arteries are the major vessels supplying the brain. Flow in both systems has a low-resistance waveform with persistent flow throughout diastole. The vertebrals originate from the subclavian arteries and join together to form the basilar artery. The basilar artery and the internal carotid arteries communicate with each other at the base of the brain in the circle of Willis.

both originate from a common innominate or brachiocephalic artery. They then branch. The innominate artery is normally visualized by sonography.

The common carotid artery courses in the soft tissues of the neck, deep to the platysma and the sternocleidomastoid muscles. The vessel is in close proximity to the jugular vein, which lies superficial to it. The common carotid is a tubular structure that measures between 6 and 8 mm in diameter. Near the junction of the middle and distal third of the neck, the vessel dilates into the common carotid bulb. From this arise two major branches, the internal and external carotids. The internal carotid normally lies posterior and somewhat lateral, whereas the external carotid artery is more medial and anterior. In a small percentage of persons, this normal relationship is reversed with the internal carotid being seen more medially. Under such circumstances, the internal carotid will ultimately return to a more lateral location before entering the internal carotid artery canal at the base of the skull. The internal carotid does not have any branches in the neck. Near the common carotid bulb a superior thyroidal branch can occasionally be seen near the junction of the common and external carotids. The external carotid artery has multiple branches, which can be seen on careful examination of the artery. This is facilitated by color Doppler imaging. These side branches may be more difficult to perceive when significant carotid artery atherosclerotic disease and increased vessel tortuosity are present. The flow divider is defined as the portion of the arterial wall lying between the external and internal carotids at their origin.

Our standard imaging protocol for examining the carotid artery system is as follows (Fig. 4.2): a slow transverse scan is performed from the lowest portion of the neck, just superior to the clavicle, to a point 4 to 6 cm above the bifurcation, near the angle of the jaw. This scan helps to perceive any changes in the course of the carotid and to determine the extent and location of plaque deposition within the common and internal carotid branches. Atherosclerotic change is more likely to occur near the origin of the internal carotid or within the carotid bulb. Subjective quantitation *of stenosis less than 50%* is facilitated by this transverse view. This is partly due to the fact that plaque is often eccentric and favors the lateral and posterior walls of the carotid. Focal stenoses at the origin or in the middle of the common

carotid are much less common than internal carotid plaque, occurring in less than 2% of patients with significant stenoses of the carotid arteries. The wall of the common carotid is often diffusely thickened in patients with severe plaque deposition or stenosis of the internal carotid. This diffuse thickening is increasingly believed to be a marker for the atherosclerotic process.

The transducer is then rotated longitudinally for measurements of the Doppler spectral waveform. Imaging is normally performed with the head rotated medially away from the side being imaged by approximately 45°. The transducer is placed either anterior near the junction of the perceived sternocleidomastoid muscle or in a more lateral and posterior location using the jugular vein as an acoustic window for better appreciation of the carotid walls. These longitudinal images are taken at the level of the carotid bulb and the internal carotid to better characterize any plaque previously seen during the transverse scan. The transducer and vessel walls are kept as parallel to each other as possible. This helps to delineate the layers of the arterial wall and to visualize any plaque deposits (Fig. 4.3). These same longitudinal projections are also the most useful when performing either duplex sonography or color Doppler mapping. Although it is possible to obtain flow information with the transducer transverse to the artery, the transducer must be slightly angled with respect to the vertical to emphasize the signals arising from moving blood. This is used in combination with duplex sonography to sample the Doppler waveform and to distinguish the internal from the external carotid in cases of ambiguous anatomy. This imaging approach often helps to identify sites of high-grade stenosis of either the internal or external carotid in the patient with extensive calcified plaque. Transverse color flow mapping is useful in following tortuous arteries as they meander in the neck and

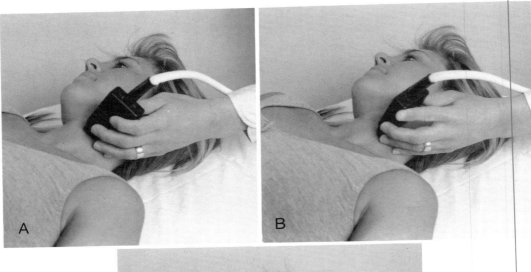

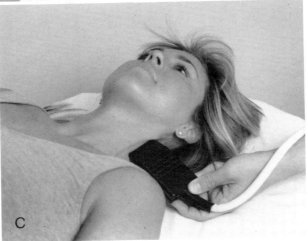

Figure 4.2. The evaluation of the carotid artery system is normally performed in three steps. **A,** A transverse scan is performed from the level of the clavicle, moving upward to the level of the angle of the jaw. This gives a rapid appraisal of the course of the common carotid and its major branches. It is also useful in assessing the distribution of asymmetric plaque. **B,** The standard position of a transducer is from an anteromedial approach. The head is rotated slightly away from the transducer. **C,** On occasion, it may be difficult to visualize the carotid artery. This is especially true in patients with shorter necks. A slight variation in imaging position with the transducer situated more posteriorly and laterally with the head rotated either in a neutral position or slightly toward the transducer is sometimes useful.

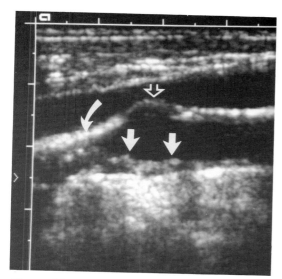

Figure 4.3. The early plaque (*arrows*) tends to have a smooth surface and a mildly hyperechoic texture. It is homogeneous and often located in the carotid bulb (*open arrow*) just proximal to the origin of the internal carotid artery (*curved arrow*). It can become quite large before reaching hemodynamic significance, since the region of the carotid bulb has the largest diameter of any of the carotid artery segments.

appear to intersect the internal jugular vein and its branches.

Transverse images are normally displayed according to the standard sonography convention, that is, with the image on the screen oriented as if the observer were looking up at the patient from their feet. Longitudinal images are displayed with the more distal (toward the head) segment of the carotid at the left of the screen as if the observer were looking at the patient from the right side.

On occasion, it may be difficult to visualize portions of the internal and external carotid and to follow them as continuous structures. The image gap which is created can easily hide the presence of high-grade stenosis. These gaps more often occur when there is calcified plaque or when the bifurcation lies deep in the soft tissues of the neck. Placing the transducer in a

posterolateral position on the neck and then asking the patient to turn his or her head toward the side being imaged will often open a new acoustic window (see Fig. 4.2C). The success of such a maneuver is explained by the fact that it gives a new imaging window to the artery than what can be achieved from the anterior approach. This helps circumvent the loss of image detail caused by the thickest component of an eccentric, calcified plaque.

DIAGNOSTIC CRITERIA (DOPPLER)

The normal flow patterns within the common, internal, and external carotid branches give a typical appearance on the Doppler spectral waveform (Fig. 4.4). In distinction to flow in the peripheral arteries, the carotid branches have forward flow during the duration of the cardiac cycle (Fig. 4.5). Flow reversal (flow away from the head) is uncommon and more likely to occur in patients with regurgitation of the aortic valve (Fig. 4.6).

In the internal carotid, the low vascular resistance of the intracerebral branches leads to a mostly monophasic flow pattern with strong systolic and diastolic flow throughout the cardiac cycle. The contour of the waveform tends to be smooth. Peak systolic velocities are normally 0.6 to 1.0 m/sec. In younger patients the spectrum may show a "bouncy" appearance, with multiple small reflections seen in systole and early diastole.

The external carotid artery has a more pulsatile pattern of blood flow. This is a reflection of the increased resistance of the multiple smaller branches supplying both the neck and the face. Flow is mostly antegrade, with a smaller diastolic component being appreciated. The increased pulsatility is caused by reflection of the pressure waveform against the multiple branches that arise from the external carotid. The peak systolic velocity will often show a spike that can easily be accentuated when

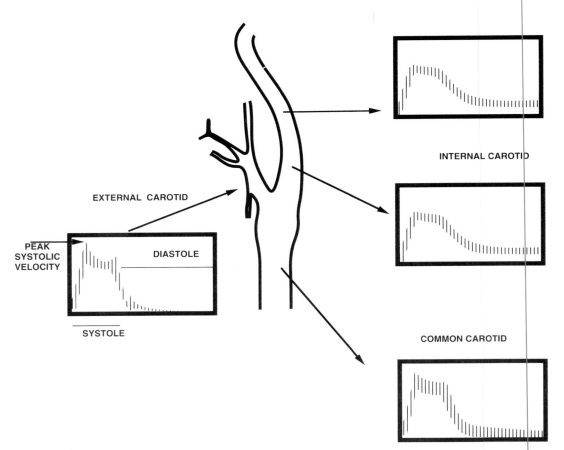

Figure 4.4. The Doppler velocity waveforms obtained in the various branches of the carotid artery are slightly different. In general, they all have forward flow throughout the cardiac cycle, with the external carotid more likely to have low velocities near the end of diastole. The waveform in the external carotid is also more "bouncy," with a sharp peak in systole. The internal carotid has a smoother-appearing Doppler waveform. Flow persists throughout diastole. The common carotid shares the appearance of both its branches by having the "bouncy" systolic appearance of the external carotid and the persistent diastolic flow of the internal carotid.

the sensitivity (gain) of the Doppler signal is set too high.

The flow pattern within the common carotid combines the characteristics of both the internal and external circulations. The flow pattern within this branch shows a mixture of the pulsatility of the external carotid with the stronger diastolic flow seen within the internal carotid.

The internal carotid waveform can show a pattern closer to that of the external carotid following carotid endarterectomy. The cause of this "externalization" of the waveform is poorly understood. In the younger patient population, it is quite common to have increased pulsatility within the internal carotid artery. The appearance can be quite similar to that seen in the external carotid of an older patient. However, imaging of the external and common carotids shows them to share this more pulsatile appearance as well.

A zone of flow separation typically occurs at the origin of the normal internal carotid (Fig. 4.5**D**). This is caused by the loss of normal structured laminar flow or parallel flow present in a straight conduit such as the common carotid. The geometric branching of the common carotid into external and internal branches is the source of this flow pattern. It is not due to compliance of the vessel or the pulsatile nature of blood flow. The zone of flow reversal is located in the internal carotid artery opposite the flow divider and can be seen with either duplex sonography or color Doppler imaging of normal subjects and of flow phantoms emulating the carotid branches. The size of this zone varies as a function of the relative amount of blood flowing through the internal and external carotid branches. Vessel compliance

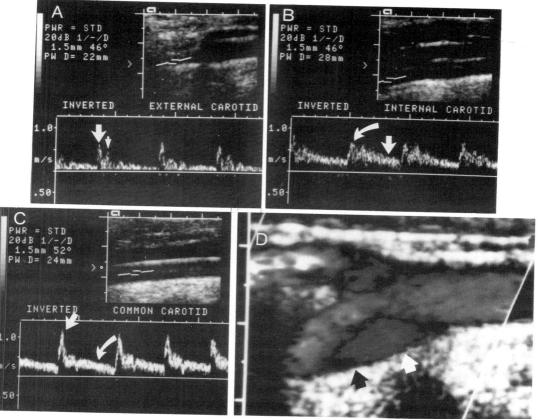

Figure 4.5. **A,** The normal-velocity waveform within the external carotid artery has a strong early systolic pulsatile waveform (*arrows*) with a variable amount of diastolic flow. **B,** The internal carotid artery waveform has a low resistance pattern with higher-velocity diastolic flow (*arrow*). It also has a smoother appearance and a less pulsatile shape to the early systolic portion. **C,** The Doppler velocity waveforms within the common carotid show a mixture of the patterns within the external and internal carotid arteries. The pulsatile appearance of the external carotid (*arrow*) is shared with the lower-resistance pattern of the internal carotid (*curved arrow*). **D** (see color plate II), This color image of the normal carotid bifurcation shows the normal phenomenon of flow reversal encoded as blue signals in the proximal internal carotid artery (*arrows*). The blue at the origin of the external carotid artery corresponds to the combined effect of a change in direction of the vessel with respect to the color Doppler window as well as the presence of a small area of flow reversal. Helical flow is not directly visualized on this color Doppler image, which displays the magnitude of the mean velocity parallel to the color Doppler window.

and the pulsatile nature of blood flow are secondary factors that may affect the size of this zone. Loss of this zone of flow reversal has been proposed as a sign of early atherosclerotic change. It is unclear whether this finding might be of diagnostic value. The site of early deposition of carotid atherosclerotic plaque does correspond to this zone of flow reversal (see Fig. 2.11). This observation has lent strong support to the hypothesis that stagnation of metabolic products and their interaction with the endothelium of the carotid wall are important for the future development of early atherosclerotic lesions.

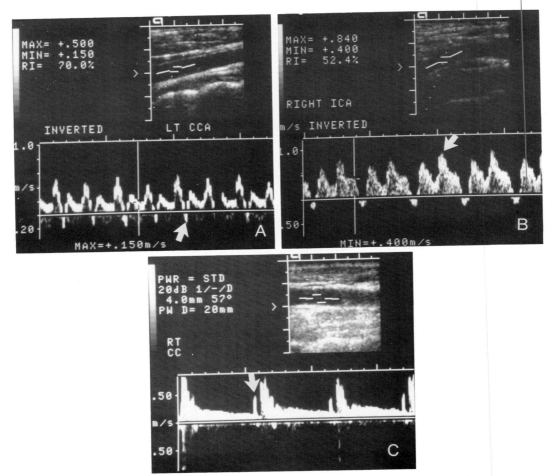

Figure 4.6. The normal Doppler waveform can be affected by a variety of pathological processes not related to the carotid arteries. **A,** This patient has a cardiomyopathy associated with aortic insufficiency. This has significantly perturbed the normal waveform. The peak systolic velocity is depressed (0.5 m/sec) due to the decreased cardiac output. Early diastolic flow reversal is taking place (*arrow*) due to aortic valve insufficiency. **B,** Bigeminy, or the presence of alternating normal and ectopic beats, has created this waveform. The normal beat (*arrow*) has a higher peak systolic velocity due to a more effective contraction of the left ventricle of the heart. **C,** The early systolic portion of this waveform is altered by the presence of an aortic dissection. Early systolic flow is being compromised (*arrow*) by the distending false lumen of the dissection.

FLOW PATTERNS AT STENOSIS

Significant obstructive lesions of the carotid arterial system tend to develop at the origin of the internal carotid artery. Although plaque deposits form within the common carotid bulb, the larger diameter of this portion of the common carotid makes it less likely that the plaque will grow rapidly enough to cause a hemodynamically significant stenosis to develop at this site. Given similar growth rates, progressive deposition of atherosclerotic plaque in the proximal internal carotid wall leads to earlier disturbances in flow. These can be seen as a typical progression by Doppler sonography. As the stenosis evolves to occupy approximately 20 to 30% of the lumen diameter, the measured velocity spectrum shows a wider or broader distribution in the velocity of blood cells. This corresponds to a loss in the laminar pattern of blood flow. It is measured on the Doppler waveform as spectral broadening. Although present even at lower grades of lumen diameter narrowing, this finding is poorly reproducible. It depends on the size of the Doppler sample gate and on whether sampling is performed at or slightly beyond the zone of narrowing. It is therefore an unreliable means of quantitating the severity of the developing stenosis.

As the stenosis reaches hemodynamic significance (50% lumen diameter narrowing), a more consistent elevation in the velocity of red cells across the stenosis is normally detected (Fig. 4.7). This is measurable as an 80% increase in the *peak systolic velocity* of the internal carotid artery compared to the ipsilateral common carotid. This corresponds to an increase in the mean velocity of approximately 40%. A peak systolic velocity above 1.25 m/sec is recognized as a good indicator of significant narrowing of the internal carotid. On CW Doppler, this translates to a frequency shift of 4000 Hz when a carrier frequency of 4 MHz is used. Red cells tend to move at the same velocity at the site of maximal narrowing or the throat of the stenosis. The laminar pattern of blood flow is lost. Beyond the throat of the stenosis, this fast motion of the red cells can remain coherent and starts to appear as a jet (see Fig. 1.43). The sampled spectral window of this jet is very sharp, with most of the cells moving at the same velocity. A zone of turbulence or broadening of motion of the red cells is normally seen at the edges and just beyond this jet as the rapidly moving blood cells dissipate their energy (Fig. 4.8). This broadening effect on the Doppler spectrum is partly a reflection of the location and size of the Doppler gate used to sample the moving blood and of the severity of the stenosis. A wider sampling gate accentuates the relative amount of spectral broadening. With progressively severe stenosis, the actual jet of blood carries the red blood cells, which are now moving at higher velocities, farther beyond the actual point of maximal stenotic narrowing (Fig. 4.9). This jet can extend over distances up to 1 cm if the lesion is symmetric or 0.5 to 1 cm if the lesion is asymmetric. The velocity of blood within this jet can be measured and used to estimate what the peak systolic velocity would be at the stenosis proper. This strategy is often used when calcified plaque surrounds the point of maximal stenosis (Fig. 4.10). The jet tends to direct itself preferentially in one direction and to hit the wall of the carotid in the same spot. A zone of flow reversal normally starts to form just beyond the stenosis once the amount of lumen diameter narrowing reaches 50% (Fig. 4.11). This is accentuated for stenoses above 75% and is seen mostly during systole. The zone of flow reversal occupies the remaining volume of the artery not occupied by the "jet" proper, and turbulence forms distal to the zone over which the velocity jet is dissipating its energy. This occurs 1 to 2 cm from the stenosis proper.

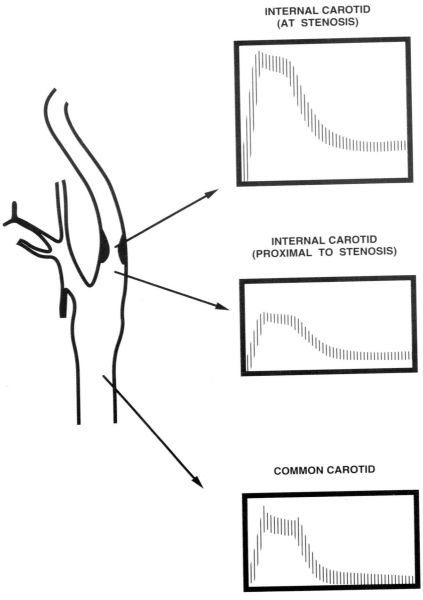

**INTERNAL CAROTID
(AT STENOSIS)**

**INTERNAL CAROTID
(PROXIMAL TO STENOSIS)**

COMMON CAROTID

Figure 4.7. The Doppler waveform at the site of a significant stenosis of the internal carotid artery will normally show an increase in the peak systolic velocity as well as the peak end-diastolic velocity. For most moderate to severe stenoses (50 to 75% lumen diameter narrowing), the effects of the stenosis on the proximal internal carotid and the common carotid are minimal.

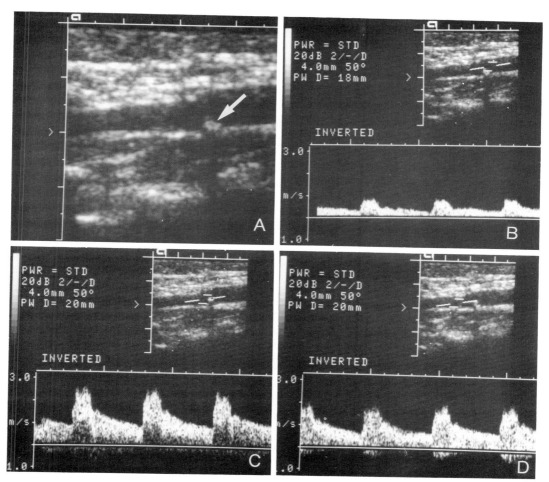

Figure 4.8. **A,** The presence of significant stenosis of the internal carotid artery is often missed on real-time two-dimensional sonography. The internal carotid artery distal to a small focal plaque at its origin (*arrow*) appears free of any obstructive lesion. **B,** Sampling of the Doppler velocities proximal to the focal plaque reveals a normal peak systolic velocity of less than 1.0 m/sec. **C,** Insonation slightly beyond the focal plaque reveals a marked increase in peak systolic velocities to 2.7 m/sec. This increase is at a site that appeared normal on the two-dimensional gray-scale image. **D,** Insonation slightly downstream from this point shows persistent elevation of the peak systolic velocity to 2.0 m/sec. The waveform at this level suggests turbulence.

The measured peak velocity has shown a close correlation with the severity of lumen diameter narrowing once a stenosis is greater than 50%. This does not correspond to an actual measurement of *volume* flow, but only to the *velocity* of moving blood. The velocity at a stenosis is proportional to the degree of lumen diameter narrowing until a degree of stenosis of 90% is reached. The relationship between Doppler frequency shift and stenosis severity holds best for lesions between 50 and 90% lumen diameter narrowing. An additional index of high-grade stenosis of the internal carotid is the elevation in the peak end-diastolic velocity at the stenosis. We have found that a peak end-diastolic velocity above 0.8 m/sec is an excellent indicator of

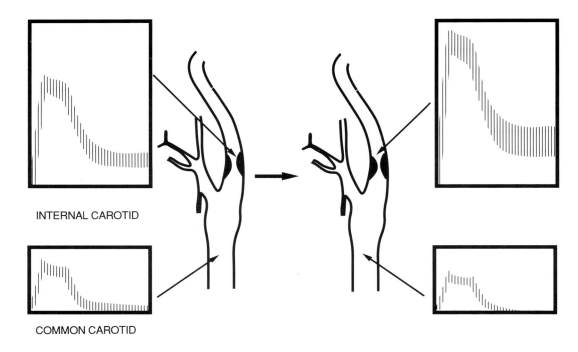

INTERNAL CAROTID

COMMON CAROTID

INCREASED SEVERITY OF INTERNAL CAROTID STENOSIS

Figure 4.9. The peak systolic velocity measured at an internal carotid artery stenosis increases as the severity of the stenosis increases. This is the basis for the use of Doppler waveform analysis for the detection and grading of carotid stenoses. Blood flow velocity in the ipsilateral common carotid artery is also affected. Both the peak systolic velocity and the diastolic flow will also decrease. This effect is more obvious for the more severe internal carotid stenosis. This finding, when present, is strong evidence for the presence of a high-grade internal carotid stenosis.

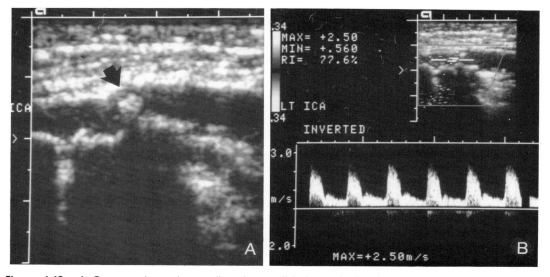

Figure 4.10. A, On occasion, a large, discrete carotid plaque is clearly seen on gray-scale imaging and appears to occlude the lumen of the internal carotid artery almost completely (*arrow*). **B,** The corresponding Doppler waveform sampled at the site of narrowing suggests that a high-grade stenosis is in fact present but that the artery is far from being subtotally obstructed. Based on the peak systolic velocity, a 75% stenosis is in fact suspected.

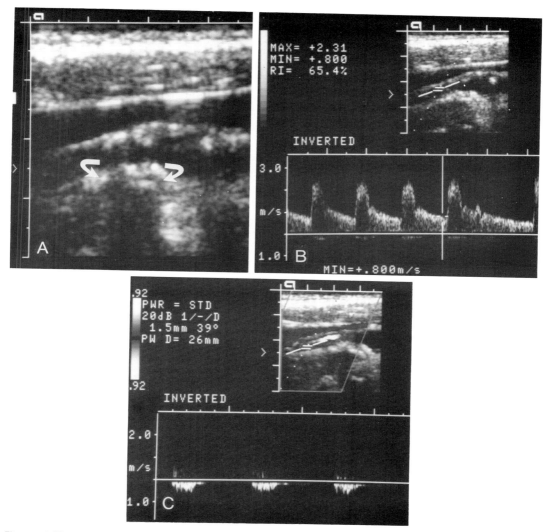

Figure 4.11. A, The two-dimensional image at the origin of the internal carotid artery shows a zone of signal loss due to the presence of a calcified plaque (*curved arrows*). **B,** The Doppler spectral waveform obtained within the velocity jet shows a peak systolic velocity of 2.3 m/sec, suggestive of a stenosis of 75% lumen diameter narrowing. **C,** Sampling of the signals within the lumen of the artery along the far wall of the internal carotid shows a corresponding zone of signal reversal distal to the stenosis and outside the flow jet caused by the focal stenosis.

a stenosis of greater than 75% lumen diameter narrowing. A peak end-diastolic frequency shift of 6.5 KHz (which corresponds to 1.4 m/sec assuming 60° insonation and a 5-MHz carrier frequency shift) has helped to identify a subgroup of patients with narrowing of the lumen diameter by 75% who are also at high risk for subsequent stroke. This observation suggests that the internal carotid peak end-diastolic flow velocities may hold more prognostic information than the measured peak systolic velocities.

Stenosis of greater than 95% narrowing of the lumen diameter can cause the actual volume flow of blood to decrease to the extent that the peak systolic velocities drop. Measurement of the peak velocity may therefore miss significant lesions since it may falsely be lower than expected. A simple way around this problem is to look at the size of the color flow lumen. A small-diameter, poorly visualized lumen suggests this possibility. Another way to overcome the problem is to use an adjunctive test such as periorbital directional Doppler signals (PDDS). These will likely be abnormal at such a high grade of stenosis.

The beginning sonographer may have great difficulty distinguishing an artery that is without significant stenosis from one that is subtotally occluded. Both may show depressed velocities. The first step to help differentiate between these two pos-

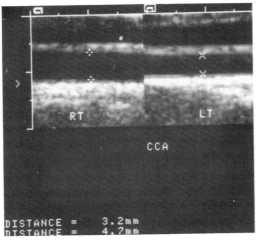

Figure 4.12. The normal diameter of the carotid arteries tends to be between 5 and 6 mm. In smaller females, the carotids often have a smaller diameter, as shown on the left of this figure where the diameter is measured at 4.7 mm. Measurements of the contralateral left common carotid artery show it to have an even smaller diameter (3.2 mm) because of a traumatic occlusion of the ipsilateral internal carotid artery many years before. The discordance in diameters is adaptive in that the intracerebral arterial branches are mostly fed by the right carotid system through the circle of Willis.

sibilities is to evaluate the opposite carotid artery to judge whether the flow patterns are similar, possibly due to a low cardiac output secondary to congestive heart failure or aortic stenosis. The second step is to evaluate the diameter of the artery comparing it to the opposite side and to the expected value of 6 mm (Fig. 4.12). Color Doppler can be used to fully visualize the extent of flow in the artery lumen by decreasing the velocity range of the color window. The arterial lumen will then be filled with color signals and be quite reassuring. Using duplex sonography, the gate must be moved slowly along the length of the artery. The greater the diameter of the artery, the lower the velocity of the signals detected. This simple rule explains why low flow signals are sometimes seen in the carotid branches. This applies to almost all patients when sampling Doppler signals from within the carotid bulb. Since the common carotid dilates at the bulb, velocity readings obtained here are often lower than anywhere else in the carotid system. This is often observed despite the presence of what may appear to be a significant buildup of atherosclerotic plaque.

Depressed velocities in the internal carotid should suggest the possibility of a high-grade obstruction in the intracranial portion of the internal carotid (Fig. 4.13). In the younger patient, the possibility of a spontaneous or traumatic dissection should be considered (Fig. 4.14). In the older patient, a stenotic lesion of the carotid near the siphon is a rare but likely explanation. The diastolic component of the internal carotid waveform is so depressed that it may in fact disappear. The presence of a high-grade stenosis of the internal carotid also has an effect on the blood flow of the ipsilateral common carotid artery. With stenosis of sufficient severity, mostly above 75%, the velocity in the common carotid will perceptibly decrease (Fig. 4.15). With these high-grade stenoses, the diastolic velocity of blood

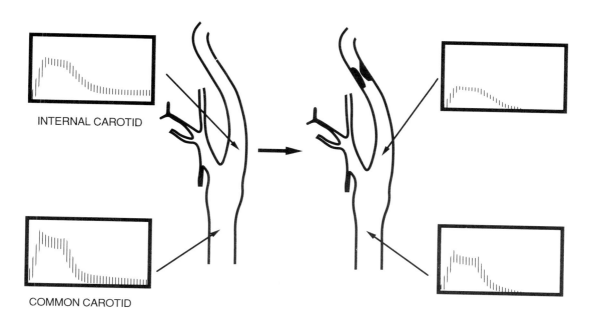

INTERNAL CAROTID

COMMON CAROTID

HIGH-GRADE STENOSIS OF INTRACRANIAL INTERNAL CAROTID

Figure 4.13. The internal carotid artery has no other branches before the level of the ophthalmic artery. It behaves as a conduit vessel. The presence of a high-grade stenosis in the intracranial portion of the internal carotid will therefore affect the blood flow velocity measured proximally. This is seen as a reduction in the peak systolic velocity and a loss of the diastolic component of blood flow.

flow may actually be so severely reduced that it falls below the sensitivity of the spectrum analyzer. This is more likely to be detected when comparing with the contralateral common carotid artery. A compensatory increase in velocity is in fact occasionally seen in the common carotid opposite the side with an internal carotid stenosis.

Common carotid stenoses are uncommon in the segment extending from 2 cm distal to the origin of the common carotid from the aorta to 2 cm proximal to the carotid bulb (Fig. 4.16). Grading of the severity of a stenosis is normally accomplished by using a ratio of the peak systolic velocity at the lesion to that at a point where there is normal blood flow (Fig. 4.17). Doubling of this ratio suggests a greater than 50% stenosis, while tripling suggests a greater than 75% stenosis. Even less

common are lesions affecting the origin of the common carotid artery. When severe enough, these cause a decrease in the velocity of the common carotid and the external and internal branches (Fig. 4.18). The diastolic velocity increases out of proportion, so the calculated resistive index measured in all carotid branches is decreased.

Ipsilateral high-grade lesions of the external carotid artery can affect the velocity of blood in the internal carotid. The velocity of blood is artificially increased in the internal carotid since most of the blood flow is going into the internal carotid. This becomes noticeable only if the external carotid has high-grade (75%) stenosis.

Contralateral high-grade lesions of the common or internal carotid cause an increase in blood flow through the opposite carotid system (Fig. 4.19). This is an attempt to compensate for the decreased in-

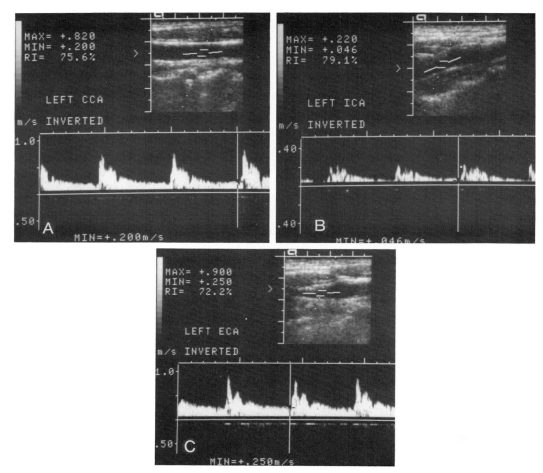

Figure 4.14. Depressed velocity signals in the internal carotid artery can be secondary to a high-grade stenosis located in the intracranial portion of this artery or to poor inflow. The latter can be caused by a stenosis at the origin of the common carotid or innominate artery or secondary to a depressed cardiac output. **A,** In this case, common carotid velocity profiles are slightly decreased and the artery has a relatively normal diameter. **B,** The internal carotid artery has a depressed Doppler velocity signal with a peak systolic velocity of 0.22 m/sec. This finding is compatible with a subtotal occlusion above the region accessible by Doppler velocity sampling. This patient had a dissection of the internal carotid artery. The artery was still maintaining very slow antegrade flow. **C,** Despite the relative occlusion of the internal carotid artery by the dissection, the external carotid artery has a normal peak systolic velocity. The diastolic component of the waveform does show some characteristics of the internal carotid artery with evidence of increased diastolic flow.

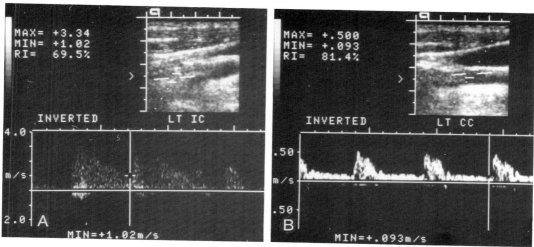

Figure 4.15. It is often quite difficult to clearly delineate the locations of the internal and external carotid branches on two-dimensional imaging. **A,** This image was obtained with the aid of color Doppler mapping to position the Doppler gate and to angle correct parallel to the color flow lumen. The Doppler waveform at this level shows a peak systolic velocity of 3.3 m/sec, corresponding to a stenosis greater than 75%. On the gray-scale image, the actual lesion or the lumen of the internal carotid is not clearly visualized. **B,** Sampling of the common carotid proximal to the bifurcation reveals a peak systolic velocity of 0.5 m/sec compared to a peak systolic velocity of 0.8 m/sec on the opposite side. This finding is also suggestive of the presence of a high-grade stenosis in the internal carotid.

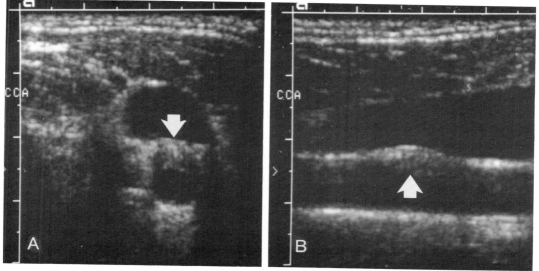

Figure 4.16. Isolated plaques involving the common carotid are somewhat rare. More often, they are seen in association with hemodynamically significant stenoses of the internal carotid artery. **A,** This transverse image of the common carotid reveals a solitary plaque (*arrow*). **B,** The accompanying longitudinal image shows the eccentric plaque (*arrow*), which appears to protrude into the wall of the common carotid.

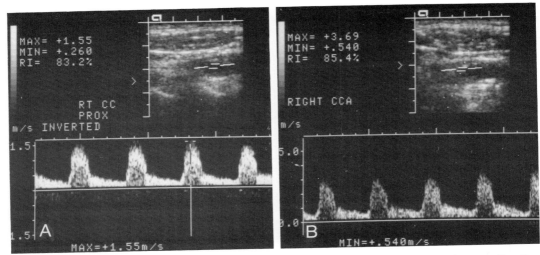

Figure 4.17. Focal high-grade lesions involving the common carotid artery are rarely seen. Grading of the stenosis is normally accomplished with the aid of the peak systolic velocity ratio. **A,** The peak systolic velocity of the common carotid artery proximal to the site of maximal abnormality is shown in this first image. The peak systolic velocity is 1.55 m/sec. This elevation in the peak systolic velocity is due to diffuse thickening and narrowing of the common carotid artery wall. **B,** Sampling of the peak systolic velocity in closer proximity to the common carotid bifurcation shows a value of 3.69 m/sec. This finding suggests a significant (greater than 50%) stenosis of the common carotid artery.

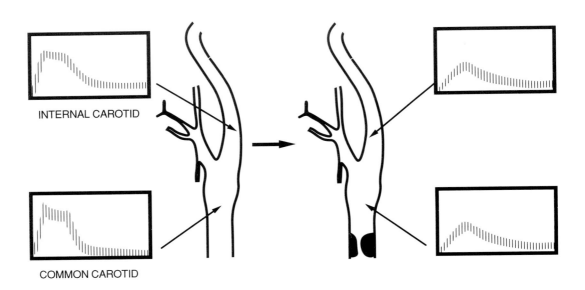

INTERNAL CAROTID

COMMON CAROTID

EFFECT OF CAROTID INFLOW RESTRICTION

Figure 4.18. This diagram summarizes the effects of an inflow restriction in the carotid artery system. Because of the poor inflow, there is a reactive vasodilation of the distal branches of the internal carotid and of the external carotid. This causes a reduction in the velocities on the side of the obstruction and a relative increase in the amount of blood flow during diastole.

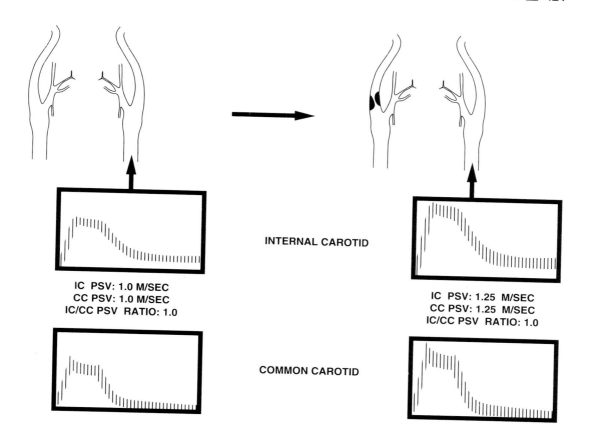

IC PSV: 1.0 M/SEC
CC PSV: 1.0 M/SEC
IC/CC PSV RATIO: 1.0

INTERNAL CAROTID

IC PSV: 1.25 M/SEC
CC PSV: 1.25 M/SEC
IC/CC PSV RATIO: 1.0

COMMON CAROTID

CONTRALATERAL HIGH-GRADE INTERNAL CAROTID STENOSIS

Figure 4.19. The effect of a contralateral high-grade stenosis on the opposite carotid is an increase in blood flow and therefore the velocity of flowing blood. This effect tends to be minor in most instances. Use of the peak systolic velocity ratio compensates for this situation.

flow on the diseased side. The velocity ratio of the internal carotid to the common carotid is normally not affected and is used to grade stenosis severity. The opposite occurs on the side of the high-grade lesion (Fig. 4.20). Since the inflow is decreased, the expected absolute increase in velocities is blunted. This problem can also be dealt with by the use of the peak systolic velocity ratio. The peak systolic velocity ratio is calculated in the following way. The point of maximal velocity increase in the internal carotid is measured from the Doppler

spectrum. A measurement is also taken in the common carotid 2 to 4 cm proximal to the carotid bulb. If there is a coexistent common carotid focal stenosis, a nonstenotic segment with normal flow is used as the site for sampling the common carotid Doppler waveform. The ratio of the peak systolic velocity of the internal carotid to that of the common carotid should be less than 1.8. Values above this are consistent with significant (>50% diameter) narrowing of the internal carotid artery. The peak systolic velocity ratio is useful

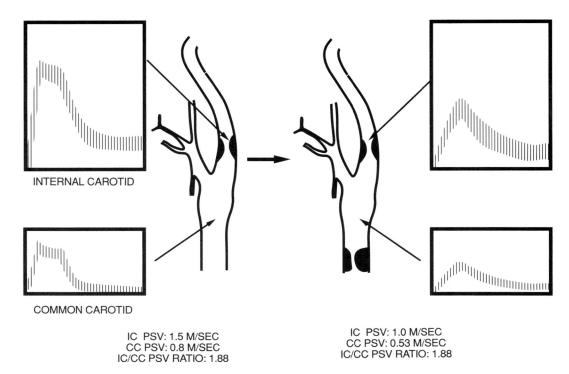

INTERNAL CAROTID

COMMON CAROTID

IC PSV: 1.5 M/SEC
CC PSV: 0.8 M/SEC
IC/CC PSV RATIO: 1.88

IC PSV: 1.0 M/SEC
CC PSV: 0.53 M/SEC
IC/CC PSV RATIO: 1.88

Figure 4.20. A high-grade stenosis may easily be masked by the depressed velocities caused by a proximal common carotid stenosis. In this case, the expected peak systolic velocity corresponding to a 50 to 60% stenosis is 1.5 m/sec. A peak systolic velocity of only 1.0 m/sec is obtained when the effects of a proximal common carotid stenosis come into play. A means of compensating for this problem is to rely on the peak systolic velocity ratio. As shown here, it compensates for the effects of the inflow problem. It is also a useful way of correcting for patients with low cardiac output due to aortic valve stenosis or heart failure.

whenever flow delivery to the common carotid artery is decreased (Fig. 4.21). This is likely to occur due to systemic depression of the cardiac output due either to heart failure or to restrictive lesions of the aortic valve. A high-grade stenosis of the origin of the common carotid or an outflow obstruction caused by a stenosis of the internal carotid above the normal imaging range—in the cranium—can also depress blood flow in the carotid system. The velocity ratio is useful in most of these instances. However, it is unreliable for grading the severity of internal carotid artery stenosis when an intracranial lesion coexists.

Increased carotid artery blood flow velocities are normally seen in children and adolescents. Systemic states such as hyperthyroidism or exercise also artificially increase carotid blood flow velocities. Finally, the carotid contralateral to an obstructive lesion will normally show increased blood flow. This is likely due to the increase in blood delivery needed to supply intracranial as well as extracranial collateral branches that form to compensate for the effects of the stenosed opposite artery. Other pathophysiologic states may affect the flow profile in the internal carotid. The most common is the presence of an arrhythmia. The ectopic beat is likely to

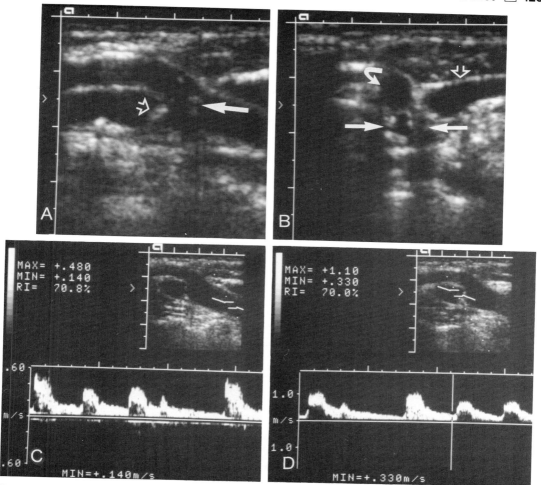

Figure 4.21. **A,** This two-dimensional real-time image shows irregular plaque in the common carotid bulb (*arrow*) as well as at the origin of the internal carotid artery (*open arrow*). The normal relationship of the carotid arteries is reversed when imaging from this lateral position with the external carotid artery lying superiorly closer to the transducer. The plaque within the common carotid has the appearance of nonanchored or floating plaque. **B,** Transverse imaging shows that the apparent occlusion at the origin of the internal carotid artery corresponds in fact to a stenosis of approximately 50% (*arrows*). The jugular vein is shown to the right of the image (*open arrow*), while the external carotid (*curved arrow*) lies superior to the internal carotid. **C,** Doppler spectral analysis in the common carotid artery shows evidence of an arrhythmia with alternating cycles of peak systolic velocity of 0.48 m/sec and 0.35 m/sec. **D,** Imaging at the site of maximal narrowing in the internal carotid artery shows a peak systolic velocity of 1.1 m/sec alternating with peak systolic velocities of 0.8 m/sec. This example again summarizes the technical difficulties in relying on only longitudinal imaging to assess carotid artery stenosis near or above 50% lumen diameter narrowing. The use of the peak systolic velocity ratio is recommended specifically in patients who have a significant arrhythmia. In this case, a peak systolic ratio of 2.2 is consistent with a 60% narrowing of the internal carotid artery. An estimate of a peak systolic velocity ratio of close to 3 would have been obtained if the improper cardiac cycle had been analyzed. Conversely, a peak systolic velocity of 1.1 m/sec is not suggestive of a significant narrowing of the internal carotid artery. Without the velocity ratio, the lesion would have been missed in this patient with a low cardiac output due to a cardiomyopathy.

show decreased velocity due to the transient decrease in cardiac output. Working out the presence of stenosis in any of the above always requires an overall appreciation of what carotid flow looks like on both sides. The size of the common carotid must be factored in.

Although peak systolic velocity has long been used to detect and grade carotid artery stenosis, other derived parameters are quite useful. As mentioned above, the peak diastolic velocity is a useful marker of more severe stenoses (Fig. 4.22). The peak

systolic and peak diastolic velocity ratios perform somewhat similarly (Fig. 4.23). A recently proposed ratio of the peak systolic internal carotid artery velocity divided by the common carotid peak end-diastolic velocity (Fig. 4.22) relies on the fact that not only does the peak systolic velocity increase at the internal carotid stenosis, but the decreased blood flow in the ipsilateral common carotid causes a decrease in the diastolic velocity (Fig. 4.24). Although all these parameters can be useful, we have tended to use the peak systolic velocity

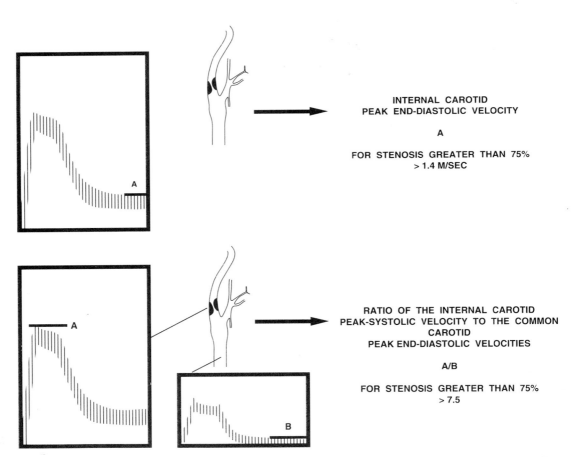

Figure 4.22. The peak end-diastolic velocity measured at the point of a suspected internal carotid artery stenosis is a parameter that is gaining in popularity. It appears to give more consistent results for stenoses above 75% lumen diameter narrowing. An uncommonly used ratio is the peak systolic velocity of the internal carotid artery divided by the common carotid end-diastolic velocity. This ratio also works best for stenoses above 75%. It will give inconsistent results due to the fact that the end-diastolic velocity of the common carotid often may not be accurately measured.

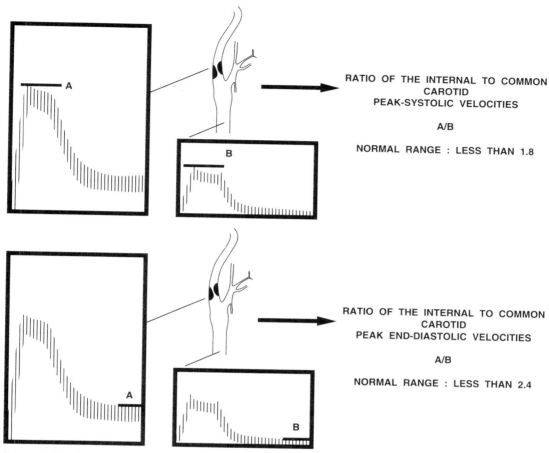

RATIO OF THE INTERNAL TO COMMON
CAROTID
PEAK-SYSTOLIC VELOCITIES

A/B

NORMAL RANGE : LESS THAN 1.8

RATIO OF THE INTERNAL TO COMMON
CAROTID
PEAK END-DIASTOLIC VELOCITIES

A/B

NORMAL RANGE : LESS THAN 2.4

Figure 4.23. Two parameters derived from the Doppler velocity waveforms have shown themselves to be quite useful. The first and more useful is the peak systolic velocity ratio. The highest peak systolic velocity in the internal carotid is used as the numerator. The peak systolic velocity of the common carotid measured 2 to 4 cm from the carotid bulb is the denominator. The common carotid peak systolic velocity is measured proximal to any stenosis in the mid or distal common carotid. The second parameter is the ratio of the diastolic velocities of the internal to common carotid arteries. This ratio is less reliable, since the end-diastolic velocity of the common carotid may sometimes be so depressed as to be not measurable.

supplemented by the peak systolic velocity ratio when needed. An added advantage of the peak systolic velocity is its greater reproducibility. This makes it an ideal choice for following patients at risk of showing progressive narrowing of their carotids, for example following endarterectomy (Fig. 4.25).

FLOW PATTERNS AT STENOSES OR BENDS

Turbulence is commonly seen in the internal carotid and common carotid. Following endarterectomy, the loss of the normal endothelial lining leads to a disruption of the normal laminar contour of

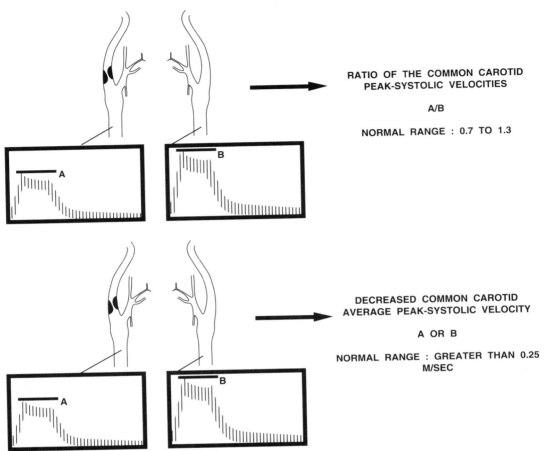

Figure 4.24. The effects of a high-grade internal carotid artery stenosis are felt at the level of the common carotid. The peak systolic velocity decreases, reflecting an overall decrease in blood flow on the affected side. Two methods are used to quantitate this effect. The first is the ratio of the peak systolic velocities between the right and left sides. This should normally be between 0.7 and 1.3. Detection of stenoses above 50% lumen diameter narrowing is possible but with a sensitivity between 30 and 40%. The peak systolic velocity may also be decreased below 0.25 m/sec. This criterion has a poor sensitivity of between 20 to 30%.

blood flow and to randomization of the motion of blood flow near the arterial wall. This can cause an artificial elevation in the velocity of blood. This loss of the normal laminar blood flow pattern can also be seen beyond a sharp bend in the artery. Relatively increased velocity is seen along the outside of the curve, while slower velocities are seen along the inner aspect of the curve. On average, the velocity across the cross section of the vessel in the curve

is similar to that within a straight segment either proximal or distal to it. Angle correction for determining the velocity of blood flow should be made with the assumption that blood flow at least midway into the arterial curve is parallel to the wall. We normally put the Doppler gate angle correction parallel to the inner wall of the vessel. This rule is broken if there is a stenosis just proximal to the bend. The angle correction should be made by aligning the cursor parallel to the jet of blood exiting the stenosis. All of these corrections are facilitated by the use of color Doppler flow mapping. Without it, the sonographer must somehow visualize the flow jet in his or her mind based on the knowledge of these hemodynamic patterns.

Diagnostic Accuracy

The diagnostic accuracy of Doppler sonography for detecting significant inter-

nal carotid artery stenosis is greater than 90%. These estimates apply to CW Doppler measurements performed with a non-imaging pencil probe, to duplex sonography, and to color Doppler sonography. A greater diagnostic accuracy is hard to reach since there are uncertainties in the "gold standard" carotid arteriograms against which Doppler sonography is validated. Inherent limitations in the reproducibility of Doppler sonography, linked to angle correction and uncertainties when large calcified plaques are present, also

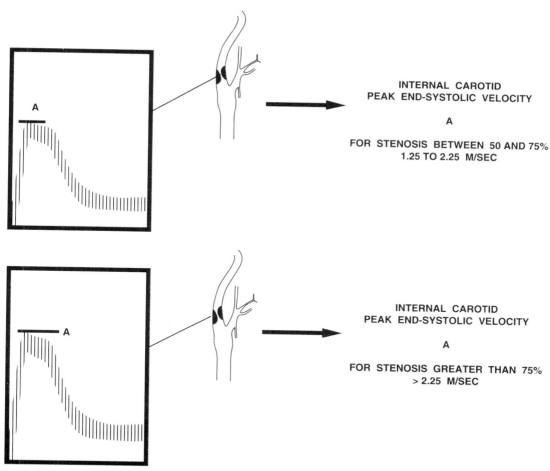

Figure 4.25. Internal carotid stenosis can be graded in categories of severity using the peak systolic velocity. A velocity between 1.25 and 2.25 m/sec corresponds to a 50 to 75% lumen diameter narrowing. A value above 2.25 m/sec is indicative of a stenosis greater than 75%.

contribute to decrease the diagnostic accuracy of the test.

A common error during the Doppler sonographic examination is confusion of the external and internal carotid branches. Simple percussion of the temporal artery preauricular branch will cause oscillations in the external carotid flow profile (Fig. 4.26). This is more easily perceived when there is a severe lesion within the external or internal carotid branch. If the lumina of the external and internal carotids are widely patent, these oscillations are likely to be transmitted into the internal carotid through the open common carotid (Fig. 4.27). With significant stenosis involving the origin of the external carotid, this maneuver causes very prominent amplitude oscillations on the Doppler spectrum since they are less likely to be transmitted backward into the common and internal carotids (Fig. 4.28). In fact, this maneuver performs best when it is most needed, i.e., in cases with a high-grade stenosis of the external carotid mimicking an internal carotid lesion (Fig. 4.29).

Duplex sonography performs poorly for detecting the presence of two types of lesions. The first is an ulcerated plaque and the second, high-grade or subtotal occlusions of the internal carotid. The presence of ulcerated plaques within the internal carotid were originally thought to be detectable with sensitivities above 80%. In our experience, carotid sonography probably detects plaque ulceration with a sensitivity of approximately 40%. However, the sensitivity for detection with carotid angiography is not much better and is estimated to be between 60 and 70%. The ultimate gold standard examination is pathologic examination of the specimen. Difficulties in obtaining these and in properly preparing carotid arteries following surgical removal limit the number of studies that have evaluated the accuracy of sonography and angiography for detecting this type of lesion.

Extremely high-grade stenotic lesions of the internal carotid, the so-called pseudoocclusions, are difficult to detect. These lesions cause such a reduction in blood flow velocity that the Doppler gate may inadvertently miss the zone of the slow flow in a small residual lumen. The ability to detect this type of lesion has improved somewhat with color Doppler flow mapping (Fig. 4.30). No large series are currently available that have studied the accuracy of color Doppler mapping for clarifying this diagnosis. It should, however, be remembered that this type of lesion is also very difficult to unmask by arteriography. It requires prolonged injection of contrast in the artery and prolonged filming. This should be done using the more traditional contrast angiogram and not digital subtraction angiography. The distinction between internal carotid occlusion (Fig. 4.30) and pseudoocclusion is important, since surgical repair of the former tends to fail while the latter is quite successful.

Complete occlusions of the common carotid are rare but offer a difficult imaging challenge (Fig. 4.31). If the internal carotid is shown to be open, the likelihood of surgical repair is high (Fig. 4.32). Patency at the level of the carotid bulb is normally ensured, since blood flow is directed through from collaterals joining the external carotid. These include the superior thyroidal branch, which communicates to the common and external carotid junction as well as the facial and temporal branches.

Measuring the color flow lumen can also be used to grade stenosis severity (Fig. 4.33). This approach is very dependent on the color Doppler encoding algorithm and can give quite different results, which vary between imaging devices. This application remains a possible future contribution of improved color Doppler imaging devices and will likely perform best for

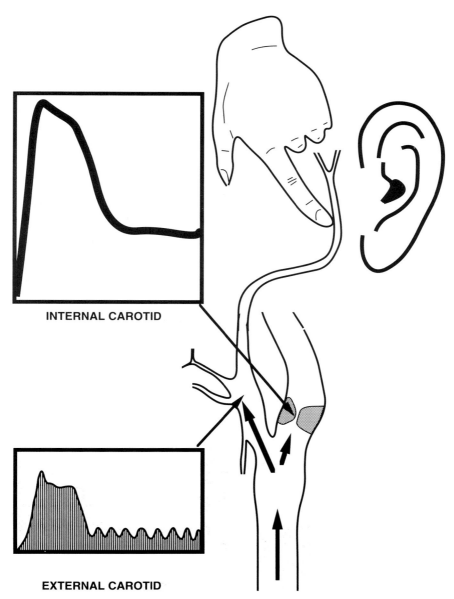

INTERNAL CAROTID

EXTERNAL CAROTID

Figure 4.26. The temporal tap maneuver is performed by having the sonographer press up and down on the preauricular branch of the temporal artery. This is easily identified by feeling for a pulse just in front of the ear canal. These oscillations are transmitted to the more proximal external carotid and not to the stenotic internal carotid. These oscillations in the spectrum may be transmitted backwards into the common and internal carotid arteries of normal bifurcations.

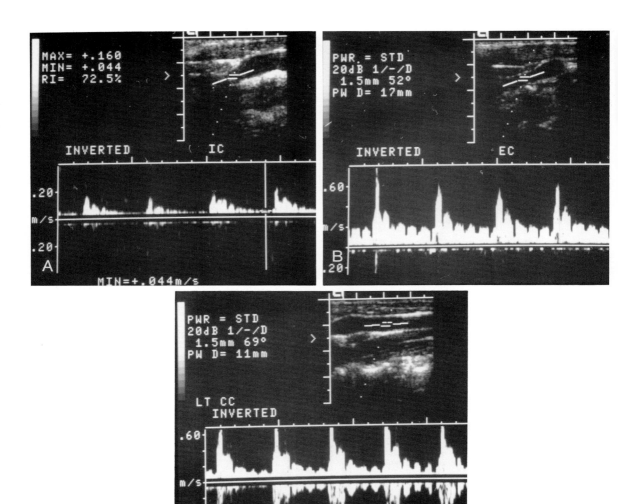

Figure 4.27. Percussion of the temporal artery normally causes oscillations in the Doppler waveform of the external carotid artery. This maneuver works best when there is a significant stenosis at the origin of the external carotid artery. These oscillations can, however, be transmitted into the common and internal carotid arteries whenever the bifurcation is relatively free of disease. **A,** In this example, a subtotal occlusion of the internal carotid artery has caused a significant drop in velocities at the origin of the internal carotid. **B,** The percussion maneuver has been applied to the preauricular branch of the temporal branch, and oscillations have been transmitted to the external carotid. **C,** These oscillations have also been transmitted to the common carotid. A similar effect can be observed in a totally normal carotid bifurcation. The maneuver is most effective at identifying *the external carotid,* since the oscillations will always be more pronounced when it is stenosed.

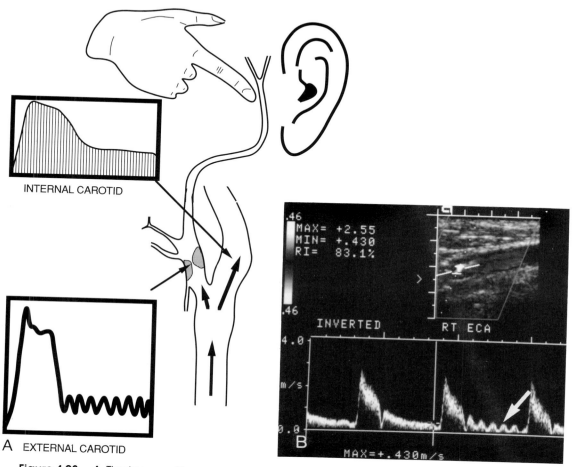

INTERNAL CAROTID

A EXTERNAL CAROTID

Figure 4.28.   A, The temporal tap maneuver works best in the one instance where it is most needed: confirming that the site of a stenosis is in the external and not the internal carotid artery. High-grade external carotid artery stenoses are often detected in patients who present with the physical finding of a bruit. The waveform is often indistinguishable from that of a stenosed internal carotid. Application of the temporal tap maneuver confirms the location of the stenosis. The oscillations are almost never transmitted proximal to the stenosis. **B,** The effectiveness of the temporal tap maneuver is maximal when the external carotid artery has a stenosis. As seen here (*arrow*), the oscillations in the Doppler waveform obtained at the origin of the external carotid artery are very prominent. The presence of an external carotid stenosis in the absence of an internal carotid lesion is considered a benign finding.

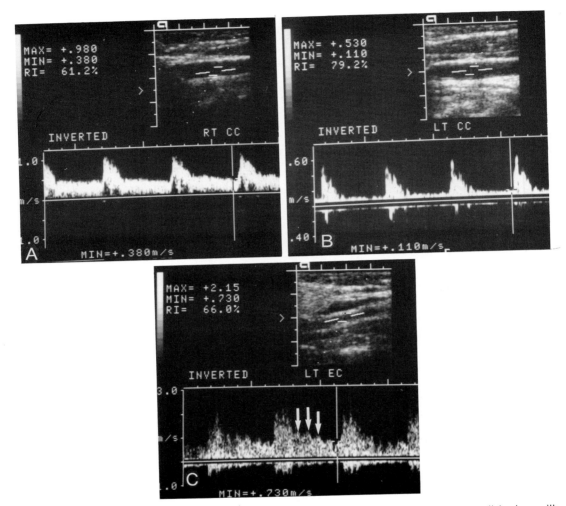

Figure 4.29. **A,** This first figure shows normal flow velocity within the right common carotid artery with a peak systolic velocity of 0.98 m/sec. **B,** The opposite carotid shows a depressed peak systolic velocity of 0.53 m/sec. This carotid also has a relatively depressed component of diastolic flow, reflecting mostly the pattern expected from an external carotid artery. This waveform is in fact due to the combination of obstruction of the internal carotid artery and moderately severe stenosis of the external carotid artery. **C,** The Doppler waveform of the external carotid artery confirms a mild to moderate stenosis of the external carotid artery with a peak systolic velocity of 2.15 m/sec. The appearance of the waveform emulates that of the internal carotid artery with a strong diastolic component. The nature of the vessel, however, is confirmed by the transmission of oscillations during the temporal tap maneuver (*arrows*). The internal carotid artery was totally occluded, thereby explaining the depressed common carotid artery velocities shown in **A.**

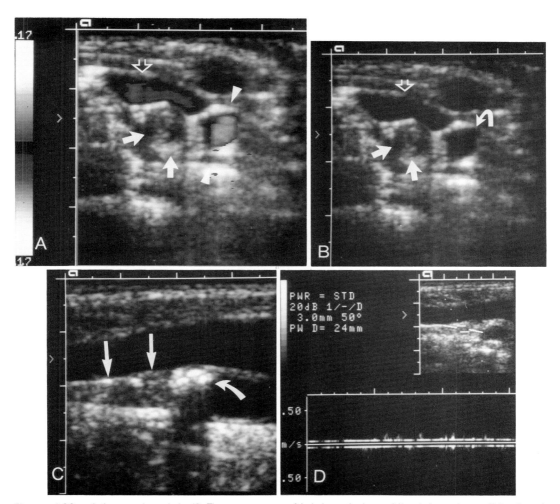

Figure 4.30. **A** (see color plate II), The presence of total occlusion of the internal carotid artery is normally suspected when extensive echogenic material is present within the lumen of the artery. There are no color signals in the occluded internal carotid (*arrows*). The external carotid is located medially (*arrowheads*). The velocity scale and sensitivity of the color Doppler map are set such that flow signals are seen in the jugular vein (*open arrow*). **B,** The thrombus is also shown on transverse gray-scale imaging of the internal carotid artery (*arrows*). The internal jugular vein lies superiorly (*open arrow*) and the external carotid artery lies to the side (*curved arrow*). **C,** On longitudinal imaging the extensive deposition of echogenic material within the internal carotid (*arrows*) is appreciated. A plaque (*curved arrow*) lies at the origin of the internal carotid artery. The internal jugular vein lies superiorly. **D,** Confirmation of the total occlusion is made by positioning the Doppler gate over the site of suspected occlusion. The sensitivity of the Doppler sampling has been set high enough so that the baseline signals due to the noise generated by the Doppler analyzer are seen at the bottom of the Doppler tracing. **E** (see color plate II), Subtotal occlusion or pseudoocclusion of the internal carotid artery has traditionally been a difficult diagnosis to make by noninvasive techniques. Color Doppler imaging has improved the ability to distinguish between total occlusion and subtotal occlusion. The proximal internal carotid artery is shown lying underneath the internal jugular vein (*IJV*). A faint color lumen connects the proximal internal carotid (*arrowheads*) to the more distal internal carotid (*open arrow*).

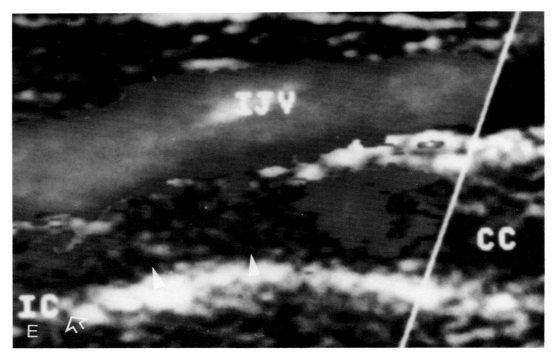

Figure 4.30. E.

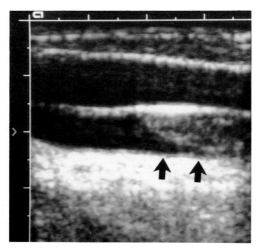

Figure 4.31. Acute thrombosis within the common carotid artery is an uncommon event. In this example, the leading edge of a dissection arising from the root of the aorta has extended into the innominate artery reaching the right common carotid. The edge of the dissection contains thrombus (*arrows*) and is partly obstructive of the common carotid lumen.

stenoses of less than 50% diameter narrowing.

For many years our laboratory has relied on CW Doppler measurements (at 4 MHz) to grade the severity of internal carotid artery stenosis. The measurements that follow are the CW frequency shift, the estimated percent diameter stenosis, and the corresponding pulsed Doppler velocity.

CW Doppler	% Stenosis	Pulsed Doppler m/sec
5,000	50	1.3
6,000	55	1.6
7,000	60	1.9
8,000	65	2.2
9,000	70	2.5
10,000	80	2.8
12,000	85	3.4
14,000+	90+	4.0

We have recently come to favor categorizing disease severity according to the peak systolic velocity as follows: less than 50%

stenosis for a peak systolic velocity less than 1.25 m/sec, 50 to 75% stenosis for velocity between 1.25 and 2.25 m/sec, 75 to 90% stenosis for a velocity between 2.25 and 3.25 m/sec, and more than 90% stenosis for a velocity of 3.5 m/sec or higher.

DIAGNOSTIC CRITERIA (PLAQUE)

The real-time component of the duplex sonogram is used to diagnose carotid plaque when there is less than 50% lumen diameter narrowing. In essence, whenever the Doppler spectrum does not show a >50% stenosis, the percentage of lumen diameter narrowing is subjectively estimated by combining the information on cross-sectional and longitudinal images taken from that portion of the artery (Fig. 4.34). Although cross-sectional imaging in the transverse plane may offer better delineation of asymmetric and eccentric

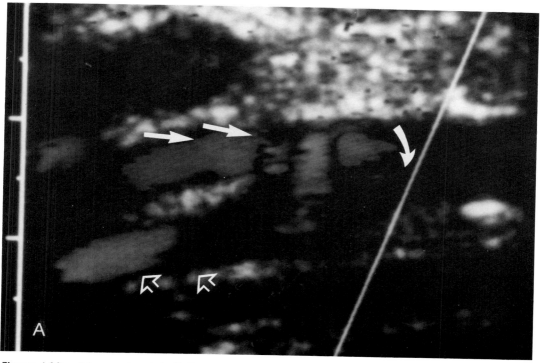

Figure 4.32. **A** (see color plate II), This totally occluded common carotid artery is devoid of any flow signals. The external carotid artery has reconstitution of flow through cross-communicating collaterals from the superior thyroidal plexus. This is encoded as reversed (blue signal) flow (*arrows*). Flow then reaches the common carotid artery bulb (*curved arrow*). It has a normal direction in the internal carotid artery (*open arrows*). **B,** Complete thrombosis of the common carotid artery is occasionally seen. This pathologic entity is normally confirmed by the presence of echogenic material within the common carotid. **C,** Confirmation of the occlusion must be obtained by a combination of color Doppler imaging as well as direct insonation using the Doppler gate. The gain settings must be set sufficiently high so that signals due to the electronic noise show up above the baseline of the waveform (*arrow*). **D,** The internal carotid has depressed antegrade flow. This is due to the retrograde flow down the external carotid artery into the region of the common carotid bulb, which reestablishes antegrade flow in the internal carotid. Under these circumstances Doppler signals are often of low amplitude and difficult to detect. Additional care is required for confirming this diagnosis.

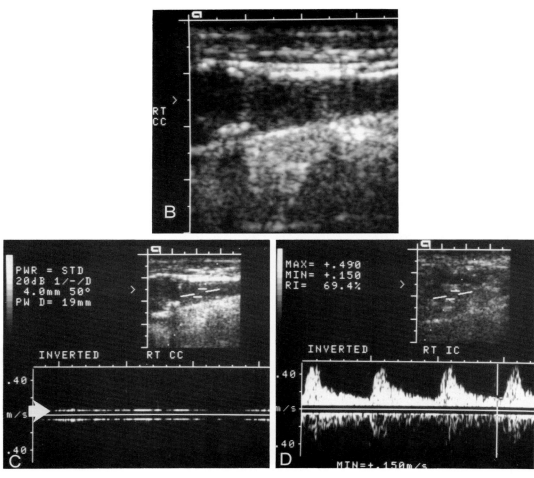

Figure 4.32.   B to D.

plaques, the physics of ultrasound make it difficult to resolve the edges of the more lateral aspects of the artery. For better resolution, a linear array transducer is used to image parallel to the axis of the vessel. Although this may systematically overestimate the severity of the lesion, it offers the best delineation of plaque length and thickness.

Sizing of carotid plaque can be performed either by considering the protuberance or amount of thickening of the wall or by determining the residual lumen of the vessel. The length of the lesion is roughly

quantitated. We have come to favor measurement of plaque thickness taken from images acquired with the transducer in the standard orientation (Fig. 4.35). Residual lumen diameter measurements show more variability (Fig. 4.36). This type of study is gaining importance for evaluating the growth or regression of atherosclerotic plaque.

SURFACE CHARACTERISTICS

The characterization of plaque surface is gaining in clinical importance. Early ca-

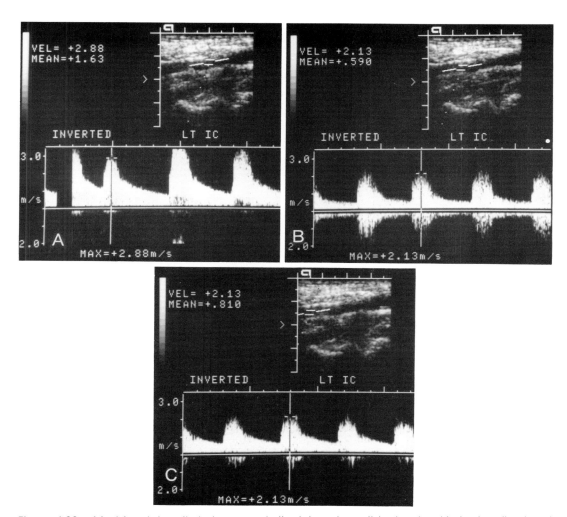

Figure 4.33. Most focal stenotic lesions seen in the internal carotid artery tend to be localized and less than 0.5 cm in length. Long, diffuse narrowing of the internal carotid artery is normally seen following endarterectomy. **A,** In this first image, the proximal portion of the internal carotid artery has a peak systolic velocity of 2.8 m/sec, suggesting a stenosis greater than 75%. **B,** Sampling of the peak systolic velocity 1 cm distal to this point shows evidence of turbulence and a peak systolic velocity of 2.13 m/sec. **C,** Sampling 1 cm farther downstream or 2 cm away from the original site of flow abnormality again shows persistent elevation of the peak systolic velocity and the presence of turbulence. **D** (see color plate II), The presence of a long, diffuse stenosis of the internal carotid artery secondary to fibrointimal hyperplasia is easily identified by color Doppler imaging. The stenotic lesion narrowing is easily recognized on the color Doppler image (*arrows*). The echogenic material corresponds to fibrointimal hyperplasia.

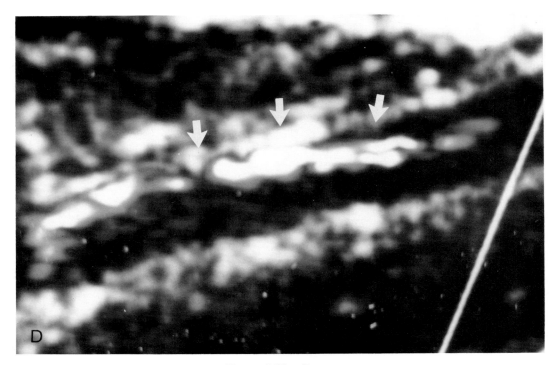

Figure 4.33.   D.

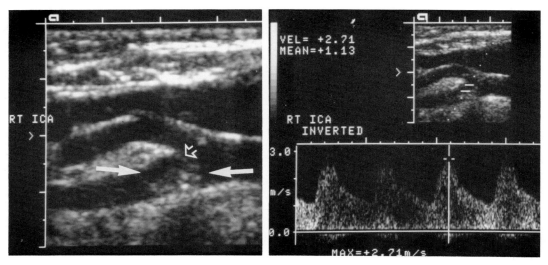

Figure 4.34.   A, A high-resolution sonogram of the carotid bifurcation shows an isoechoic plaque (*arrows*), which does not appear to seriously compromise the lumen of the internal carotid artery (*open arrow*). The hypoechoic component of the plaque is unfortunately not shown on the gray-scale image. **B,** The corresponding Doppler sonogram shows a high-grade flow abnormality with a peak systolic velocity of 2.7 m/sec—roughly equivalent to an 80% diameter stenosis.

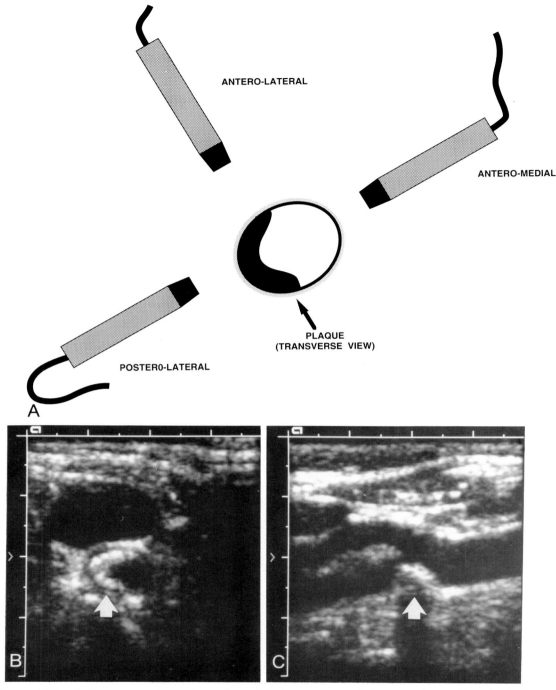

Figure 4.35. A, The asymmetric nature of carotid plaque accounts for many inconsistencies in its appearance in longitudinal images of the same patient. This diagram shows the location of the transducer used to image the plaque shown in the following images. **B,** The deposition of atherosclerotic plaque tends to occur in an asymmetrical fashion. This first transverse view of the origin of the internal carotid shows a well-circumscribed plaque located more laterally (*arrow*). **C,** An anteromedial location of the transducer gives the appearance that the plaque is preferentially located on the far wall (*arrow*). **D,** A more anterior location of the transducer shows both the near-wall and far-wall elements of the plaque (*arrows*). **E,** A more lateral location of the transducer has the effect of giving the appearance of a plaque that is mostly located on the near wall (*arrow*). **F,** The important finding for this patient is the normal Doppler velocity waveform, which excludes the presence of any significant stenosis secondary to the presence of this plaque.

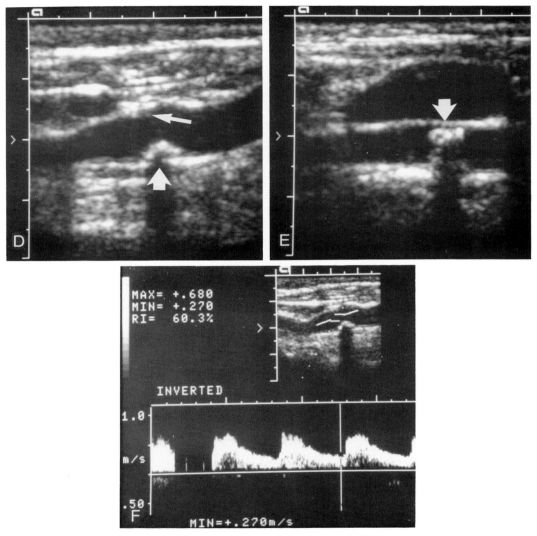

Figure 4.35.   D to F.

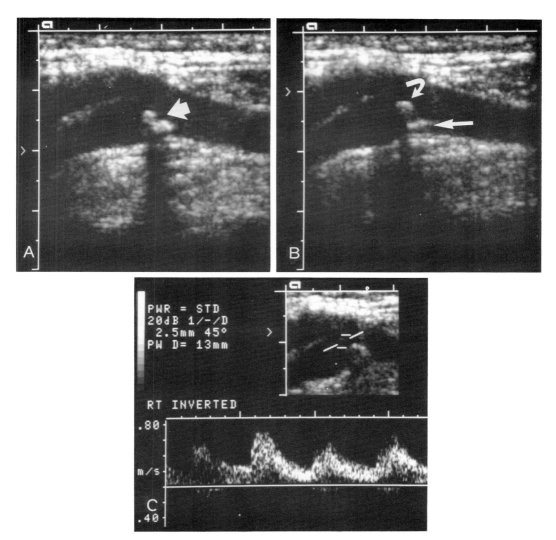

Figure 4.36. High-resolution imaging has significant limitations for gauging the severity of carotid plaque deposition. Significant errors are made in estimating the percentage of narrowing caused by a partly calcified carotid plaque. **A,** This first longitudinal image shows an irregular plaque located on the far wall and protruding into the lumen of the internal carotid (*arrow*). **B,** A slightly different projection of the same artery shows the plaque to have an element (*curved arrow*) disconnected from an apparent anchoring point (*arrow*). This type of plaque is often called a "floater." **C,** Both of these images suggest that the plaque is severe enough to have caused at least a 50% narrowing of the internal carotid. The corresponding Doppler waveform does not confirm this impression, however. **D,** The findings seen in both images are explained by the relative placement of the transducer with respect to the plaque. The first estimate of carotid stenosis severity should be made with the Doppler velocity waveform. If the peak systolic velocities are below 1.25 m/sec, then the visualized plaque is not severe enough to have caused a hemodynamically significant stenosis. It can then be graded visually as less than 50%. If velocities are greater than 1.25 m/sec, then the peak velocity is used to grade stenosis severity.

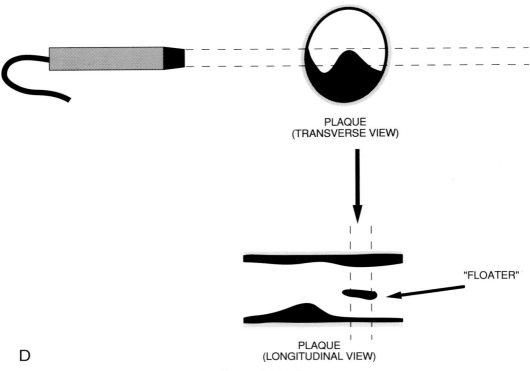

D

Figure 4.36. D.

rotid lesions tend to show a smooth surface due to the proliferation of smooth muscle cells that come from the media into the intima and the deposition of fat in the intima. These lesions, as they expand, are more susceptible to developing internal zones of hemorrhage (Fig. 4.37). At worst, the plaque may fracture and break open. In cases where the hemorrhage is contained, it is likely that the healing process with fibrosis and calcification will form a focal dense lesion in the plaque. The fibrotic healing process can then cause an irregular surface to form if the plaque has ruptured (Fig. 4.38). Calcification may develop along the luminal edge of the plaque. In time, it is believed that this leads to the development of more dense and irregular appearing surfaces. The significance of these more irregular surfaces is unclear. Differentiation between a healed plaque with an irregular surface and a plaque that has recently ruptured and is actively aggregating platelets at the exposed collagen surfaces is almost impossible by sonography. Ulceration, a marked gap within the plaque extending into the exposed collagen of the artery wall, is known to cause platelet aggregates, which can subsequently embolize. Although larger ulcerations of plaques can be readily identified, the smaller ulcers are almost impossible to reliably detect and quantify by sonography.

MORPHOLOGY

Plaque is normally characterized by its sonographic appearance. In density, plaque can be hypoechoic, isoechoic, or hyperechoic compared to the surrounding soft tissues. The hyperechoic plaque is

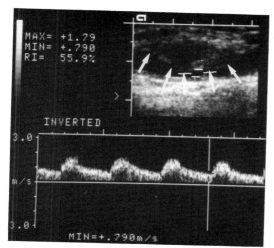

Figure 4.37. This large sonolucent plaque (*arrows*) appears to subtotally obstruct the lumen of the proximal internal carotid artery. The peak systolic velocities of 1.79 m/sec suggest that the imaging plane used overestimates the size of the asymmetric plaque and the relative stenosis.

commonly associated with a large amount of fibrous material. Mixtures of smooth muscle cell and cholesterol are thought to cause a hypoechoic or isoechoic appearance. This appearance is also similar to that of thrombus or fibrointimal hyperplasia, a reactive response of the artery wall seen following endarterectomy.

Plaque with relatively homogeneous texture and without elements of different echogenicity are normally referred to as homogeneous. When elements that are either hyperechoic or hypoechoic share the volume of the plaque, it is characterized as heterogeneous. A plaque that has a sonolucent zone near its base is thought to contain a small hemorrhage. A focal hyperechoic zone in the midst of the plaque likely represents healing or a fibrotic reaction at the site of a previous hemorrhage.

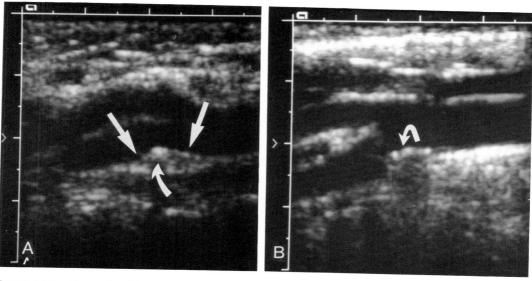

Figure 4.38. The natural history of carotid plaques is believed to include a stage when areas of hemorrhage are thought to heal by fibrosis. **A,** A small focal zone of increased echogenicity (*curved arrow*) is located at the top of a broader carotid plaque (*arrows*). Although partly conjectural, this zone of fibrosis may represent the site of a previous intraplaque hemorrhage. **B,** According to the same theory of plaque evolution, larger areas of the plaque surface may undergo this same process. This plaque shows a more extensive change along its outer surface (*curved arrow*). The surface is more irregular, as if there had been more extensive damage to the plaque. This may have occurred either as one episode or as many smaller events. In both cases, the underlying plaque appears isoechoic.

CALCIUM

Calcium deposition is detected as an area of acoustic shadowing. It is a category of plaque characterization separate from the others. Calcium can obscure visualization of the artery lumen and limit the evaluation of stenosis severity in up to 10% of bifurcations. This is more likely if the shadowing is greater than 1 cm in length. Strategies to surmount the calcified plaque are based on the knowledge that high-grade stenoses normally perturb blood flow patterns for 1 to 2 cm downstream from the lesion. By judiciously angling the color Doppler window, it is possible to peek underneath the calcium deposits to verify the existence of high-grade stenosis. However, it may not be possible to accurately grade the severity of the stenosis but rather to make a statement suggesting its presence or absence.

DIAGNOSTIC ACCURACY (PLAQUE)

Monitoring of early atherosclerosis and quantitating the extent of the disease process before a lesion becomes hemodynamically significant is now being done by sonography. The pathophysiologic mechanism responsible for CVA or stroke is thought to be related to the carotid circulation in up to 80% of occasions. In 15 to 20% of instances, other sources such as emboli from the heart are thought to be responsible. However, recent studies have shown that in up to 50% of cases of stroke and transient ischemic attack, the lesion present in the internal carotid artery has less than a 50% lumen diameter narrowing.

The possibility that active plaques that are not yet hemodynamically significant can cause strokes has lead to increased interest in characterizing plaques by their morphology and surface appearance. The early plaque that is about to hemorrhage is now thought to be a homogeneous or slightly heterogeneous plaque that is iso-echoic except for a small hypoechoic zone near its base. This hypoechoic region is thought to represent early hemorrhage in the fragile portion of the plaque containing neovascularity. Plaques that are more heterogeneous, have irregular surfaces, and contain calcium are more difficult to characterize in a reproducible fashion. Their presence correlates with both patient symptoms and the presence of higher-grade stenoses of the internal carotid. They more likely represent plaques that have undergone more than one cycle of hemorrhage and repair. In general, the hemodynamically significant stenoses tend to be associated with large plaques that are heterogeneous in appearance and whose surface is irregular. This observation also lends support to the hypothesis that plaque growth combines episodes of rupture and subsequent repair.

DIAGNOSTIC CRITERIA (WALL THICKENING)

There has been increasing interest in the detection of early atherosclerotic lesions that could be monitored in a consistent fashion and used as a marker for either progression or regression of atherosclerotic disease. Recently, sonographic techniques have been used to measure the thickness of the intima-media complex. An increased thickness of this portion of the arterial wall has been shown to be associated with atherosclerotic change. Comparison between hypercholesterolemia and normal controls has shown a measurably increased thickness of the common carotid intima-media layer. Whether this thickening represents early atherosclerosis or a change that develops in association with the disease process is currently the subject of controversy. It is certain, however, that the thickness of this wall can be measured using sonographic approaches. The measurement is more accurate when performed on the far wall of the carotid artery where artifacts secondary to gain settings are less likely to obscure the interfaces. Thickening of the wall above 0.6 mm in a younger population is thought to represent evidence of early atherosclerosis. No studies have yet been performed to show that serial changes occur in response to either drug or dietary interventions.

INFLAMMATORY CHANGES

The atherosclerotic process affects mostly the intima and media layers of the vessel. Inflammatory processes such as Takayasu's arteritis or giant cell arteritis affect the media and adventitia (Fig. 4.39). The inflammatory process manifests itself as a diffuse thickening in the arterial wall that can be perceived on high resolution real-time sonography. This diffuse thickening has not been measured in any systematic fashion in patients with inflammatory arteritis. However, based on previous pathological studies, it is expected that the treatment of the arteritis should result in a response and in partial return to the normal appearance of the arterial wall with time.

DIAGNOSTIC ACCURACY (WALL THICKENING)

The validation of the in vivo measurements of carotid wall thickness have been mostly made by correlation with in vitro samples and pathology. Comparison between micrographs of arterial walls and sonograms have shown the clear delineation of the normal interfaces, which are the interfaces between the lumen and the intima, the media and the adventitia, and the adventitia and periadventitia. These interfaces are perceivable and can be imaged with ultrasound using carrier frequencies above 5 MHz.

The reproducibility of such measurements is currently being determined in multiple studies and the value of serial monitoring of wall thickness changes remains to be developed and shown over the next few years. Concern has been expressed as to the possibility that the lumina to intima interfaces perceived on sonography are artifactual in nature. Although in vitro experiments have, in part, shown that this is possible, the fact that the measurement actually correlates with atherosclerosis makes it likely that it will soon be an accepted tool.

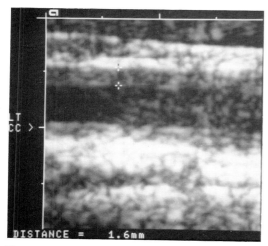

Figure 4.39. Diffuse thickening of the common carotid wall occurs as part of the aging process and can be seen in cases of more advanced atherosclerotic disease. In this 20-year-old, the sonogram of the mid common carotid artery shows a diffuse thickening of the arterial wall located between the cross-hairs. A normal thickness should be less than 0.8 mm. A diffuse vasculitis affecting the arterial wall and causing infiltration by inflammatory cells is responsible for the apparent thickening. This pathological process is more easily perceived by sonography than angiography, since the narrowing is often diffuse and affects long segments.

Masses and Aneurysms

The clinical finding of a palpable pulsatile neck mass often leads the patient to

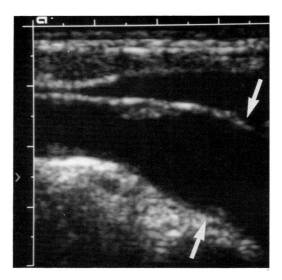

Figure 4.40. A true aneurysm of the innominate artery is rare. This marked dilatation of the innominate artery with a diameter greater than 2 cm is consistent with an aneurysm. We have occasionally seen extension of the aneurysm into the origin of the common carotid.

the noninvasive laboratory for further sonographic evaluation.

True aneurysms of the carotid arteries are very rare. They occur mostly secondary to a previous episode of trauma or as part of the more generalized tendency to develop aneurysmal arterial disease in the older patient (Fig. 4.40). The palpable mass is most often due to increased vessel tortuosity and ectasia secondary to atherosclerosis (Fig. 4.41).

A variety of neck masses will cause flow abnormalities that were often confused with stenoses in the era of CW Doppler evaluations. These include carotid body tumors (Fig. 4.42), or thyroid involvement by Graves' disease (Fig. 4.43) or adenomatous nodules (Fig. 4.44). Passive displacement of the carotid often creates the illusion that a large pulsatile mass is present (Fig. 4.45).

Vertebral Artery

The vertebral arteries on both sides normally arise from the subclavian artery distal to the thyrocervical trunk. These arteries course between the neural foramina from C2 through C6. They finally join at the base of the skull to form the basilar artery. On occasion, the left vertebral artery can originate directly from the aorta in 6% of patients.

Sonographic access to these arteries is basically over short segments that are visible between the segments of the cervical vertebral lamina (Fig. 4.46). The ability to evaluate flow and patency in this vessel has recently been shown to be above 71%. The presence of a normal direction of blood flow within the vertebral artery normally guarantees against occlusion. The inability to detect flow may represent occlusion or a technical limitation. A reversed pattern of flow suggests a pathological process such as subclavian artery occlusion and a syndrome referred to as the subclavian steal syndrome. Blood then flows from the opposite vertebral artery into the basilar artery and then in a retrograde fashion down the affected vertebral artery to supply the subclavian artery and the arm. More complex situations can show up because of the locations of stenoses or occlusions (Fig. 4.47) with the development of collateral flow through the carotid system and the circle of Willis. Lesions of intermediate severity can cause a loss in the unidirectional pattern of blood flow with reversal of blood flow occurring during diastole or may be unmasked by exercise or by changes in arm position.

There are no diagnostic criteria applicable for determining the severity of vertebral artery disease. Part of this limitation is the fact that clinical interventions are limited mostly to lesions affecting the origin of either the vertebral or the subclavian arteries themselves.

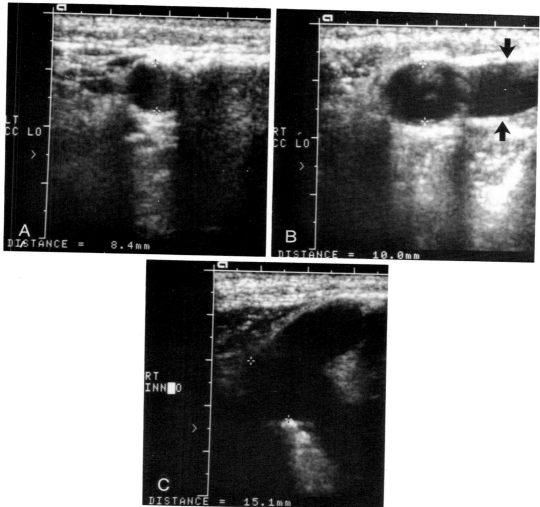

Figure 4.41. The patient presenting with a pulsatile neck mass is unlikely to have an aneurysm of the carotid artery. This entity is exceedingly uncommon. The newly felt pulsatile neck mass is often due to an ectatic arterial segment, to displacement of the carotid by another process such as an enlarged thyroid, or to a more diffuse increase in arterial caliber. **A,** The sonographic evaluation starts by imaging of the unaffected side. The normal common carotid measures 8.4 mm. **B,** On the affected side, the low common carotid appears to have a diameter of 10 mm. This apparent increase in size is in fact due to the position of the transducer. The walls of the innominate artery are inadvertently included in this measurement (*arrows*). **C,** The ectatic innominate has elongated, increased its diameter, and migrated upward in the neck, causing a pulsatile mass felt on clinical examination. Because of this displacement, the origin of the common carotid is easily seen. A repeat examination at 6 months to 1 year is recommended to ensure lack of progression of this asymptomatic enlargement.

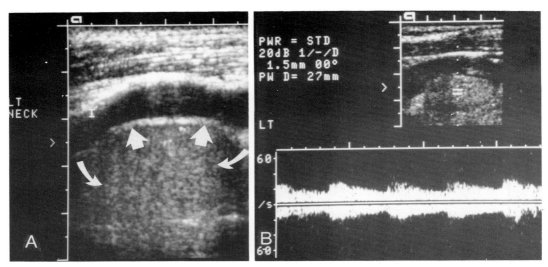

Figure 4.42. Masses involving the carotid bifurcation are rare. A lymph node may enlarge secondary to a localized head and neck malignancy. **A,** The more pathognomonic, albeit much rarer, entity is a carotid body tumor or paraganglioma. It appears as a well-circumscribed mass abutting the carotid bifurcation. It normally displaces the internal carotid (*arrows*) and is often intermixed with the external carotid branches. It has a somewhat heterogeneous appearance (*curved arrows*). The diagnosis is made by confirming the markedly vascular nature of the mass. **B,** The Doppler waveforms arising from within the mass show a consistent low-resistance pattern. This waveform is similar to that seen in a thyroid gland involved by Graves' disease. The location and position of the mass are sufficient to differentiate between these entities.

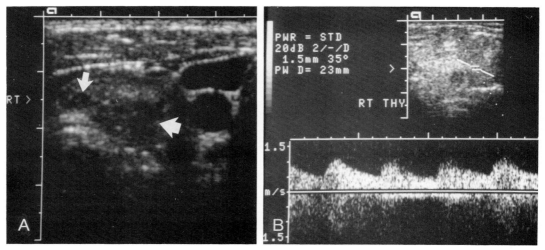

Figure 4.43. The common carotid artery runs in close proximity to the thyroid gland in the middle of the neck. There are three common manifestations of thyroid pathology that warrant mentioning. **A,** The first and most benign is the inadvertent detection of multiple sonolucent collections in the gland. These areas (*arrows*) correspond to cysts. This type of multinodular gland will normally contain at least two to three cysts. The presence of a solitary nodule, especially if it is solid and has an echogenic structure, warrants further investigation. **B,** On occasion, a CW pencil probe Doppler examination has been known to detect signals with high-frequency shifts despite the presence of a normal carotid bifurcation. The source of these high-frequency shift signals mimicking the presence of a stenosis is a diseased thyroid gland. These elevated velocity signals originate from the multiple arterial branches of a gland involved in Graves' disease. They can also be seen in cases of hypervascular adenomas.

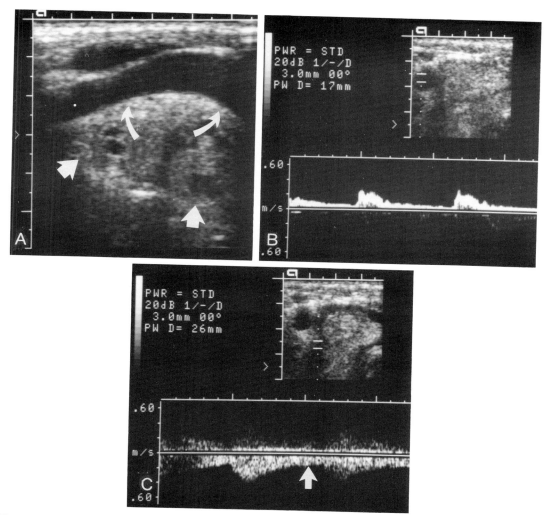

Figure 4.44. **A,** Adenomatous nodules are often the source of high-velocity signals within the common carotid. This two-dimensional image shows a large heterogeneous mass (*arrows*) displacing the common carotid artery superiorly (*curved arrows*). **B,** The location of the common carotid with respect to this mass is confirmed by using transverse Doppler imaging. The waveform sample within the common carotid shows a typical flow pattern. **C,** The Doppler gate is then displaced within the thyroid. The Doppler waveform obtained at this site shows a relatively low-resistance pattern (*arrow*) with a high diastolic flow component. Before duplex sonography, the presence of either thyrotoxicosis or autonomous hypervascular adenomas were the occasional source of high-velocity signals detected by CW Doppler. These were on occasion inadvertently diagnosed as high-grade carotid stenosis. This type of error is unlikely using duplex sonography.

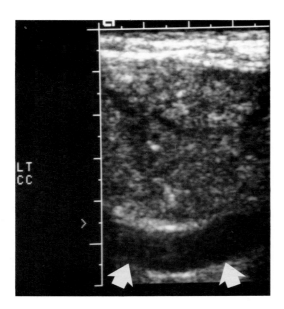

Figure 4.45. The presence of a palpable pulsatile mass in the neck is suspicious for the presence of an aneurysm. Besides the presence of ectasia, a markedly enlarged thyroid lobe may occasionally transmit pulsations from a low-lying common carotid (*arrows*).

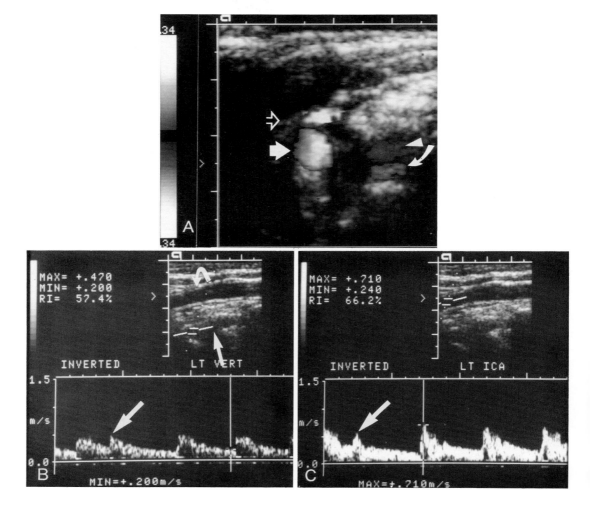

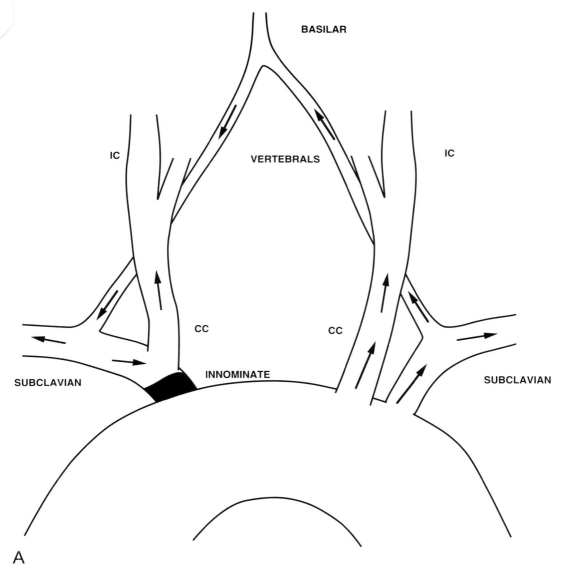

A

Figure 4.47. The subclavian steal syndrome is an example of the use of a collateral pathway to compensate for the effects of a proximal subclavian artery occlusion. Flow is redirected from either the opposite vertebral through the basilar artery or from the internal carotid through the circle of Willis to the subclavian artery distal to the occlusion. **A,** This example is a slightly more complex variant. The proximal occlusion involves the innominate artery. Blood flow is redirected from the

Figure 4.46. A (see color plate II), This transverse image of the lower neck shows the relative location of the common carotid artery (*arrow*) and the vertebral artery (*curved arrow*). The jugular vein (*arrowhead*) and the vertebral vein (*open arrow*) are located anterior to the corresponding arteries. **B,** The vertebral artery can be seen over a short segment in most patients. Although some authors suggest that a focal stenosis can be detected with some accuracy, we restrict our evaluation to detecting the presence of flow signals within this artery and determining their direction. In this case, the ipsilateral internal carotid (*curved arrow*) lies superior to the vertebral branch (*arrow*). **C,** The velocity signals arising from the internal or common carotid are also sampled to confirm the direction of blood flow. Both Doppler spectra contain an ectopic cardiac beat (*arrow*). The waveforms are also very similar in appearance, both showing a low-resistance pattern.

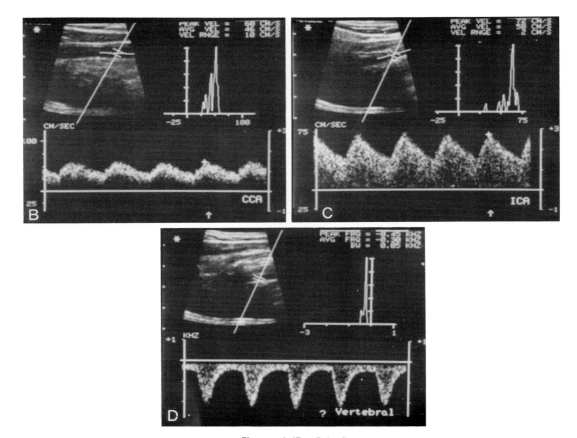

Figure 4.47. B to D.

opposite vertebral down the ipsilateral vertebral. The vertebral then goes on to supply not only the subclavian artery but also the ipsilateral common carotid and the internal carotid: Blood flow in both systems is markedly reduced. **B,** The presence of a low-resistance waveform within the right common carotid artery is suggestive of a proximal obstruction either at the level of the common carotid artery or within the right innominate artery. **C,** Determination of the peak systolic velocity in the internal carotid shows a markedly altered Doppler velocity waveform showing a low-resistance waveform and depressed velocities. **D,** Measurement of the direction of flow in the vertebral artery shows it to be reversed. This lesion is not typical of the subclavian steal syndrome, which is more common in the left subclavian artery and normally does not affect the velocity pattern within the common carotid. The lower resistance within the common carotid can be seen with a high-grade stenosis at the origin of the common carotid artery.

SUGGESTED READINGS

Blasberg DJ. Duplex sonography for carotid artery disease: an accurate technique. AJNR 1982;3:609–614.

Chambers BR, Norris JW. Outcome in patients with asymptomatic neck bruits. N Engl J Med 1986;315:860–865.

Colgan MP, Strode GR, Sommer JD, Gibbs JL, Sumner DS. Prevalence of asymptomatic carotid disease: results of duplex scanning in 348 unselected volunteers. J Vasc Surg 1988;8:674–678.

Erickson SJ, Mewissen MW, Foley WD, et al. Stenosis of the internal carotid artery: assessment using color Doppler imaging compared with angiography. AJR 1989;152:1299–1305.

Faggioli GL, Curl R, Ricotta JJ. The role of carotid screening before coronary artery bypass. J Vasc Surg 1990;12:724–731.

Fillinger MF, Reinitz ER, Schwartz RA, et al. Graft geometry and venous intimal-medial hyperplasia in arteriovenous loop grafts. J Vasc Surg 1990;11:556–566.

Grigg MJ, Papadakis K, Nicolaides AN, et al. The significance of cerebral infarction and atrophy in patients with amaurosis fugax and transient ischemic attacks in relation to internal carotid artery stenosis: a preliminary report. J Vasc Surg 1988;7:215–222.

Hatsukami TS, Healy DA, Primozich JF, Bergelin RO, Strandness DE Jr. Fate of the carotid artery contralateral to endarterectomy. J Vasc Surg 1990;11:244–251.

Moneta GL, Taylor DC, Zierler RE, Kazmers A, Beach K, Strandness DE Jr. Asymptomatic high-grade internal carotid artery stenosis: is stratification according to risk factors or duplex spectral analysis possible? J Vasc Surg 1989;10:475–483.

Polak JF, Dobkin GR, O'Leary DH, Wang A-M, Cutler SS. Internal carotid artery stenosis: accuracy and reproducibility of color-Doppler-assisted duplex imaging. Radiology 1989;173:793–798.

Poli A, Tremoli E, Colombo A, Sirtori M, Pignoli P, Paoletti R. Ultrasonographic measurement of the common carotid artery wall thickness in hypercholesterolemic patients. A new model for the quantitation and follow-up of preclinical atherosclerosis in living human beings. Atherosclerosis 1988;70:253–261.

Reilly LM, Okuhn SP, Rapp JH, et al. Recurrent carotid stenosis: a consequence of local or systemic factors? The influence of unrepaired technical defects. J Vasc Surg 1990;11:448–460.

Robinson ML, Sacks D, Perlmutter GS, Mannelli DL. Diagnostic criteria for carotid duplex sonography. AJR 1988;151:1045–1049.

Salonen R, Seppanen K, Rauramaa R, Salonen JT. Prevalence of carotid atherosclerosis and serum cholesterol levels in eastern Finland. Arteriosclerosis 1988;8:788–792.

Spadone DP, Barkmeier LD, Hodgson KJ, Ramsey DE, Sumner DS. Contralateral internal carotid artery stenosis or occlusion: pitfall of correct ipsilateral classification—a study performed with color-flow imaging. J Vasc Surg 1990;11:642–649.

Spencer MP, Reid JM. Quantification of carotid stenosis with continuous-wave (C-W) Doppler ultrasound. Stroke 1979;10:326–330.

Taylor LM Jr, Loboa L, Porter JM. The clinical course of carotid bifurcation stenosis as determined by duplex scanning. J Vasc Surg 1988;8:255:61.

Zierler RE, Kohler TR, Strandness DE Jr. Duplex scanning of normal or minimally diseased carotid arteries: correlation with arteriography and clinical outcome. J Vasc Surg 1990;12:447–455.

CHAPTER FIVE

Venous Thrombosis

Incidence and Clinical Importance

The incidence and prevalence of venous thrombosis can only be estimated, since most episodes are not detected clinically. Recent studies suggest that the prevalence of undetected pulmonary emboli in asymptomatic patients dying of unrelated causes in hospitals approaches 30%. The perioperative incidence of venous thrombi in high-risk populations can reach 30 to 50%. Since these emboli rarely cause symptoms, it has proven more difficult to determine the incidence of lower-extremity venous thrombosis than expected. Estimates made from the annual incidence of pulmonary embolism and lower-leg DVT suggest an approximately one-to-one concordance between episodes of pulmonary emboli and a likely source in the legs. In fact, it is believed that lower-extremity venous thrombosis is the source of the emboli in up to 95% of such episodes. Other less likely sources include the deep veins of the pelvis and the upper extremities. Conversely, not all lower-extremity thrombi need embolize. The incidence of symptomatic pulmonary embolism is thought to be 10 to 15% in patients with documented lower-leg DVT. More sensitive screening of patients with lower-leg DVT has shown an incidence of 35 to 50% of abnormalities consistent with asymptomatic pulmonary embolism.

Thrombi within the femoropopliteal veins (above the knee), and less often those limited to the calf veins (below the knee), are more likely to cause pulmonary emboli (Fig. 5.1). This puts the focus on performing careful sonographic examinations of this portion of the leg. Another factor to consider in patients who have a clinical suspicion of below-knee thrombosis is the use of serial ultrasound monitoring at the popliteal vein to document the spread of thrombus. Many experts believe that it is only when thrombus has spread into the popliteal vein that there is a clinical need to anticoagulate the patient. Proximal spread from thrombi residing in the calf veins is thought to occur in 20% of cases. This typical evolution of lower-leg DVT (i.e., origin in the calf vein and occasional spread into the more proximal popliteal vein) probably applies to most patients who present with lower-extremity DVT.

At least two patterns of clinical presentation are seen in patients with deep vein thrombosis. In the first, the thrombi are

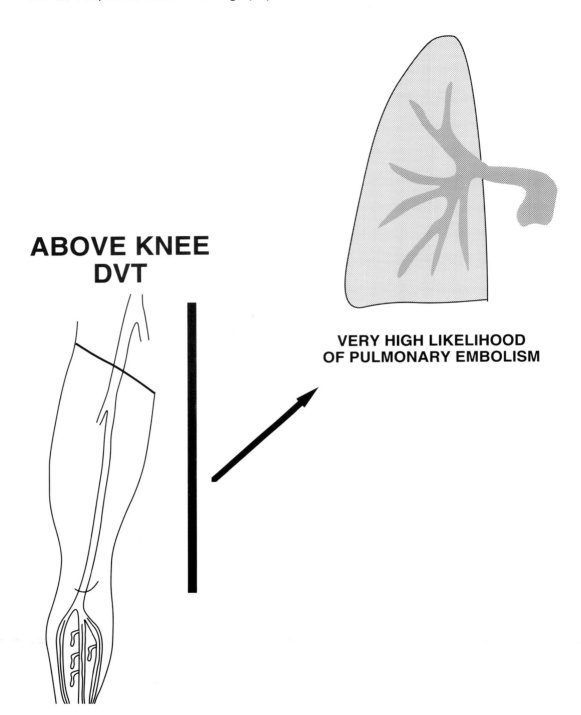

ABOVE KNEE DVT

VERY HIGH LIKELIHOOD OF PULMONARY EMBOLISM

Figure 5.1. Although sonography is capable of detecting calf vein thrombosis, the more clinically relevant thrombi are those that pose the greatest threat of causing pulmonary embolism. These are, in the vast majority, thrombi affecting the veins above the knee.

likely to have progressed above the knee at presentation. The majority of these thrombi tend to obstruct flow. The second applies to asymptomatic postoperative patients. These patients tend to have nonobstructing thrombi with a much larger proportion being located in the deep veins of the calf. The sonographic approach to these two types of patients is not the same. The pattern and natural history of both types of DVT are sufficiently different that the implications of a missed thrombosis will have distinctly different clinical implications.

Venous ultrasound of the lower extremity has emerged as a sensitive and accurate noninvasive test for confirming the presence of acute deep vein thrombosis. The high diagnostic accuracy, established in comparison with standard contrast phlebography in more than 2000 cases reported in the literature between 1980 and 1988, has caused it to replace contrast phlebography almost completely as the standard examination for the diagnosis of lower extremity DVT.

Lower Extremity

NORMAL ANATOMY

The general rule of deep venous anatomy of the leg is that every deep vein is accompanied by one artery that travels in close proximity to it.

The external iliac vein becomes the common femoral vein at the level of the inguinal ligament (Fig. 5.2). The common femo-

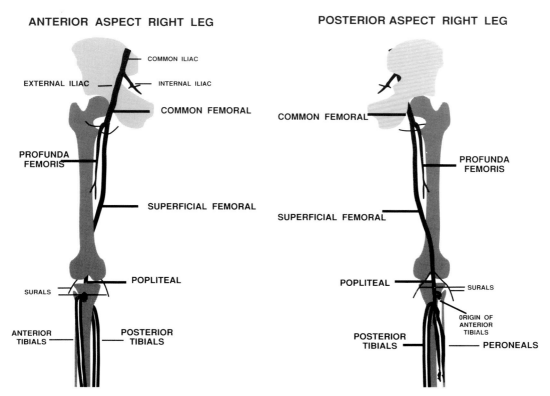

ANTERIOR ASPECT RIGHT LEG

COMMON ILIAC
EXTERNAL ILIAC
INTERNAL ILIAC
COMMON FEMORAL
PROFUNDA FEMORIS
SUPERFICIAL FEMORAL
POPLITEAL
SURALS
ANTERIOR TIBIALS
POSTERIOR TIBIALS

POSTERIOR ASPECT RIGHT LEG

COMMON FEMORAL
PROFUNDA FEMORIS
SUPERFICIAL FEMORAL
POPLITEAL
SURALS
ORIGIN OF ANTERIOR TIBIALS
POSTERIOR TIBIALS
PERONEALS

Figure 5.2. The anatomy of the deep veins of the lower extremity is subject to some variability. Most of this is accounted for by the instances of duplications of the femoral and popliteal veins.

ral vein lies medial and slightly deeper to the artery just below the groin crease. The first branch that arises from the common femoral vein is the greater saphenous vein, which courses medially and superficial to the fascia of the thigh and calf toward the foot. Within 1 to 2 cm, there is a major branching of the common femoral into the superficial and deep femoral veins (Fig. 5.3). The deep femoral (profunda femoris) vein drains the muscles of the thigh and courses more laterally and deep to the superficial femoral vein. When imaged from above, the deep (profunda) femoral vein lies on top of the deep femoral artery. The superficial femoral vein is the deep draining vein of the lower thigh and calf. It courses medial to the profunda femoral and stays deep to its accompanying artery. The superficial femoral vein lies deep or posterior to the femoral artery when imaged from the front of the thigh. Both the artery and vein enter the adductor (popliteal) canal when they cross beneath the adductor fascia in the lower third of the thigh. The vein still lies deep or posterior to the corresponding popliteal artery. Since the popliteal vein is normally imaged from the back of the leg rather than from the front, the popliteal vein will then be seen closer to the transducer than is the artery, i.e., superficial to the vein.

The lesser saphenous vein normally originates from the popliteal vein at or slightly above the mid knee and courses posteriorly and then laterally down the leg. It normally terminates just anterior to the lateral malleolus. The popliteal vein can often be followed to the proximal calf, where it separates into the anterior tibial vein and the tibioperoneal trunk. It is at this level that the veins are duplicated, i.e., for each accompanying artery, there are two veins (Fig. 5.4). Before this, the superficial femoral vein is duplicated over at least a short length in 15 to 20% of patients, while the popliteal is duplicated in up to 35% of patients. The duplicated seg-

ments of the superficial femoral vein vary in length and rejoin the main venous trunk (Fig. 5.5). The popliteal vein duplications tend to continue as separate duplicated segments. The anterior tibial veins can be from the front of the leg as they emerge after crossing the interosseous membrane. They are then lying on top of the membrane as they course down the leg. They cross the ankle as the dorsalis pedis veins. The tibioperoneal trunk is difficult to visualize in the upper third of the calf. The posterior tibial paired veins can be imaged as they migrate more superficially at the mid calf and then continue to the back of the medial malleolus. The paired peroneal veins lie deeper and closer to the fibula.

A typical examination of the lower leg veins should start with the patient lying on his or her back. This supine position will normally suffice for most patients. On occasion, it may be difficult to visualize the veins, even proximally in the thigh. This may be caused by cold, since the veins can constrict quite significantly. Another possibility is low blood volume. It may then be necessary to have the patient sit up slightly, increasing the pressure in the veins and causing them to distend. Normally transducer gel is generously applied to the skin of the thigh and behind the knee along the expected course of the superficial femoral and popliteal veins. This saves time when performing the sonographic examination.

Placing the transducer transverse, midway from a line drawn between the pubis and the iliac spine in the skin course, the common femoral vein is normally found easily with its accompanying artery lying to the side. The transducer is held such that the television screen shows an image corresponding to what an observer would see if he or she were looking at the patient from the foot of the bed. Duplex sonography and color Doppler mapping are used intermittently during the examination. When first learning to do the exami-

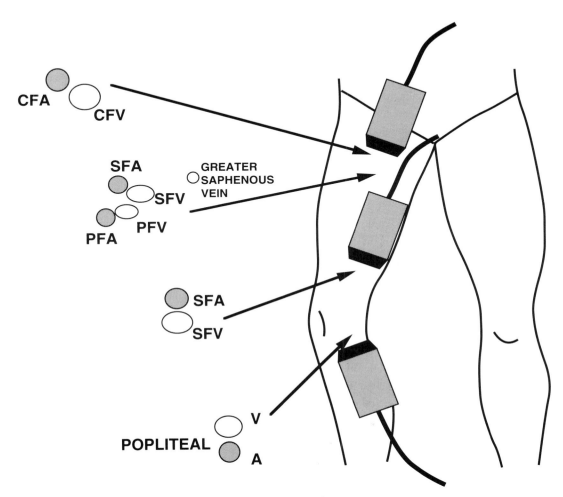

Figure 5.3. The venous ultrasound examination is performed with the subject supine. The transducer is held from the front and inner aspect of the thigh for imaging of the following deep veins: the common femoral (*CFV*), profunda femoral (*PFV*), and superficial femoral (*SFV*) veins. These are accompanied by the corresponding arteries. The common femoral artery bifurcates before the vein. The greater saphenous vein originates from the common femoral vein, just above the level of the bifurcation. At the level of the knee, the transducer is held from the back of the externally rotated and slightly bent leg. The popliteal artery now lies deep to the vein(s).

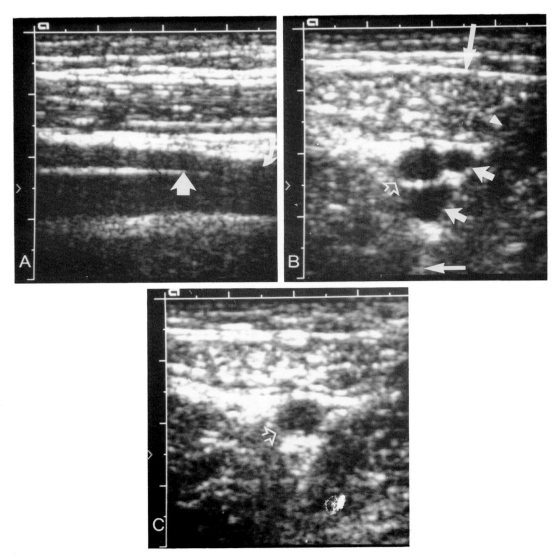

Figure 5.4. **A,** In this longitudinal image, a venous segment (*arrow*) is shown to join the superficial femoral vein (*curved arrow*). **B,** The first transverse image shows that there are two venous channels (*arrows*) lying on both sides of the superficial femoral artery (*open arrow*). The muscles of the thigh are also clearly shown with the sartorius located above (*long arrow*), the adductor magnus to the right (*arrowhead*), and the quadriceps to the left (*short arrow*). **C,** During compression, only the artery (*open arrow*) does not collapse. Duplicated portions of the superficial femoral veins can be seen in up to 30% of individuals. These tend to be small and normally rejoin the main vein after 5 to 15 cm.

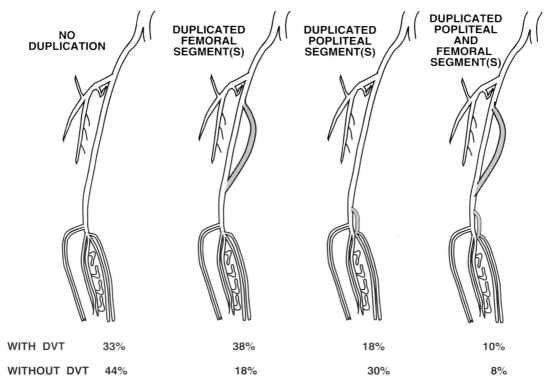

	NO DUPLICATION	DUPLICATED FEMORAL SEGMENT(S)	DUPLICATED POPLITEAL SEGMENT(S)	DUPLICATED POPLITEAL AND FEMORAL SEGMENT(S)
WITH DVT	33%	38%	18%	10%
WITHOUT DVT	44%	18%	30%	8%

Figure 5.5. The incidence of duplicated venous segments in the lower extremity is quite high. This diagram was created from information published by Liu et al. In general, there is a higher prevalence of duplicated femoral segments in patients with deep venous thrombosis. The commonly quoted incidence of 20% for duplicated femoral segments and of 30% for popliteal segments applies to normal venograms obtained in patients without deep vein thrombosis.

nation this is mostly to help in identifying and distinguishing vein from artery. With practice, the sonographer will use either modality to assess the blood flow pattern in the vein and deduce from this information the likelihood of either proximal or distal venous obstruction. Either modality may also be used to identify the presence of venous collaterals.

The examination often includes both sides even if only one limb is symptomatic. This is helpful in establishing "normal" anatomy in a given patient. Although the superficial veins are examined (Fig. 5.6), the focus of the examination is the deep venous system. The examination starts at the groin (Fig. 5.7). The origin of the greater saphenous vein is always identified. Within 2 to 4 cm distal to this point, the femoral artery branches into the superficial and deep branches. This occurs before the vein. One to two centimeters downstream, the common femoral vein also branches. The deep femoral vein migrates on top and medial to the artery, while the superficial femoral vein lies deep to the corresponding artery. The artery and vein are then normally followed easily to the junction of the mid and distal third of the thigh (Fig. 5.8). At this point, the vein and artery cross the adductor fascia and lie more deeply in the soft tissues. They become very difficult to visualize from the anterior and medial aspect of the

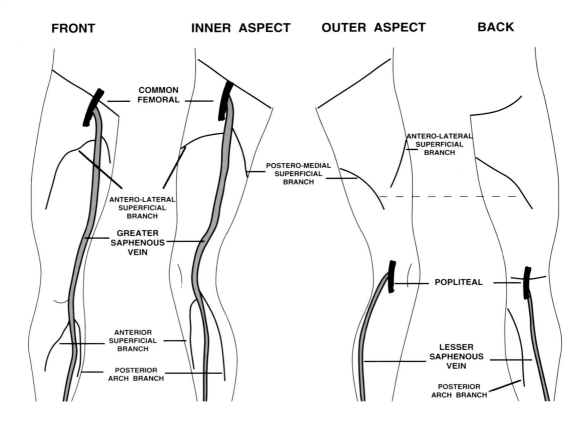

RIGHT LEG

Figure 5.6. The superficial veins of the leg form a complex network. The greater and lesser saphenous veins are consistent in their location for most individuals. The relative size and location of the various branches vary markedly from individual to individual.

thigh. One strategy for identifying and confirming patency of the vein is to use color Doppler mapping. Color Doppler imaging can penetrate more deeply into the thigh and show a patent venous segment because it uses a lower frequency than the gray-scale image. Another strategy is for the operator to use his or her free hand to grab the soft tissues along the inner back aspect of the thigh and lift them toward the transducer. This will bring both artery and vein closer to the transducer.

It may not be possible to image any lower in the thigh from the anterior scanning position. Some laboratories recommend that the patient then lie face down (prone) and that the examination continue in this position for both the popliteal veins and calf veins (Fig. 5.9). The knee should be held slightly flexed if this approach is used. We have come to favor another, simpler approach, which can be used even with patients who have undergone recent surgery. The leg is turned slightly outward while the knee is gently flexed. The transducer is then placed behind the knee. By moving it slowly upward, it is possible to reach the mid portion of the adductor canal. Sliding more inferiorly, the popliteal

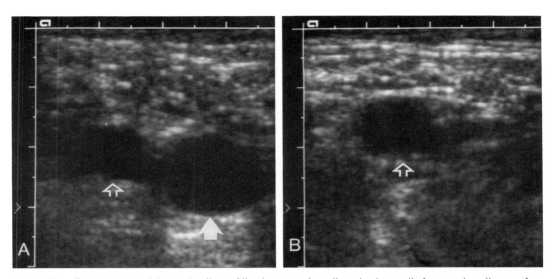

Figure 5.7. The sonographic evaluation of the lower-extremity veins is mostly focused on the performance of compression ultrasound along the full length of both the femoral and popliteal veins. Imaging is done with the transducer held transverse to the vein. The deep artery and accompanying vein(s) are identified. Pressure is applied on the skin. The vein collapses, creating the illusion of a "wink." **A,** At the level of the common femoral vein, the artery (*open arrow*) lies lateral and slightly superior to the vein (*arrow*). **B,** The vein collapses easily since it lies on top of the femoral head. The level of the femoral bifurcation is then evaluated, care being taken to well visualize the different arterial and venous branches. **C,** Transverse imaging then continues in the region of the thigh. The superficial femoral vein courses inferior (deeper) to the artery. The vein is often duplicated (20 to 30% of instances). **D,** A slight amount of pressure is normally sufficient to collapse the vein (*arrows*). It is often necessary to modify the imaging approach and the way in which pressure is applied to the skin once the region of the adductor canal is reached. **E** and **F,** The popliteal artery and vein are imaged with the transducer held behind the knee. This is more easily accomplished by having the subject slightly bend the knee and rotate it externally in a slight frogleg position. On transverse imaging, the artery (*open arrows*) now lies deeper to the vein (*arrow*). Duplication of part or all of the popliteal veins occurs in 30 to 35% of instances. During compression, the femur or tibia will often migrate into the image (*arrowhead*).

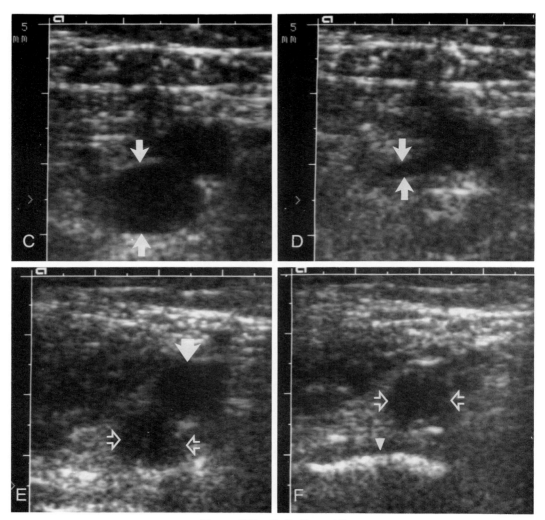

Figure 5.7. **C, D, E,** and **F.**

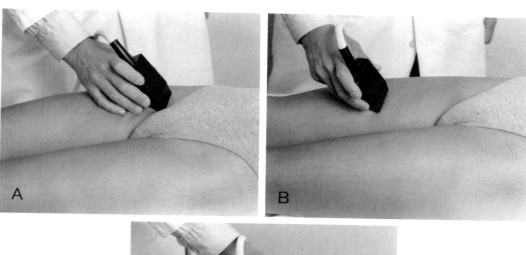

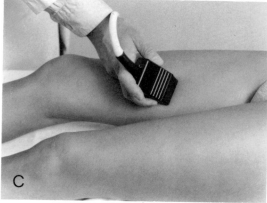

Figure 5.8. **A,** Imaging of the femoral and superficial femoral systems for the presence of acute deep vein thrombosis is normally done with the transducer held transverse to the vein. **B,** The transducer is displaced slowly along the anterior and medial aspect of the thigh. **C,** It may be necessary to reposition the transducer along the inner aspect of the leg to better apply compression.

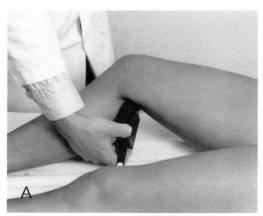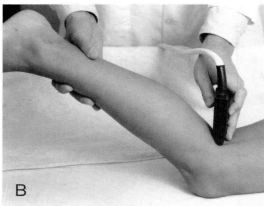

Figure 5.9. Evaluation of the popliteal vein can be performed in either of two standard positions. **A,** We prefer the more standard approach with the patient supine, the knee slightly flexed, and the leg rotated. The transducer then needs to be positioned at the posterior aspect of the leg. This frees the operator's hands for the performance of venous augmentation maneuvers. It is also more easily applicable to elderly patients or postoperative patients, who may be difficult to move. **B,** Imaging with the patient prone can be performed. If this is done, the knee may need to be slightly flexed to relieve potential extrinsic compression. The operator must also support the extremity to help relieve muscular contraction.

vein can be seen down to the level of the bifurcation of the popliteal vein into the anterior tibial and posterior tibial veins. There is then a relative blind spot since the tibioperoneal trunk lies deep to the gastrocnemius and soleus muscles. Bending the knee with the leg straight and holding the transducer posteriorly is often sufficient to permit visualization of this segment.

The calf veins (i.e., the muscular venous sinuses) normally are easily visualized with the knee bent (Fig. 5.10). The paired gastrocnemius veins are normally seen running parallel to the artery as they arise more proximally from the mid and lower popliteal vein (Fig. 5.11). The deeper located muscular venous sinuses communicate with either the peroneal or posterior tibial veins. The posterior tibial veins are easily seen with the leg lying flat on the bed and imaging from the medial aspect of the calf. The peroneal veins are also seen from this position. Color Doppler is often needed to help localize these veins (Fig. 5.10**D**). An alternate approach is to keep the leg flexed while imaging from the lateral posterior aspect of the calf. The peroneal veins can then be seen lying in close apposition to the fibula. The anterior tibial veins are seen lying on top of the interosseous membrane. They may be somewhat difficult to demonstrate, since they are often quite small and do not carry much blood flow.

On occasion, it may be necessary to have the patient sit up slightly to better distend the veins. Dangling the leg over the edge of the table is also a useful strategy for distending both the draining veins and the muscular venous plexus. Compression ultrasound is often difficult to perform in the latter position. Flow augmentation is also difficult to elicit.

DIAGNOSTIC CRITERIA

Venous ultrasound uses three important diagnostic criteria to determine the presence of acute deep vein thrombosis (Table 5.1). The first is direct visualization

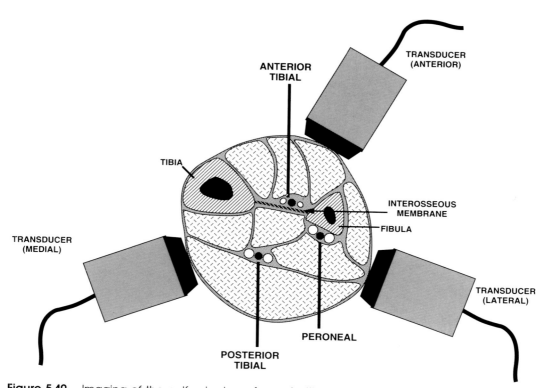

Figure 5.10. Imaging of the calf veins is performed with greater emphasis given to the posterior tibial and peroneal veins. The presence of anterior tibial venous thrombosis is quite rare and, on those rare occasions when detected in our laboratory, has tended to be in symptomatic patients who complained of pain at the anterior aspect of the calf. **A,** This diagram shows the relative position that can be used for calf vein imaging. The medial approach is always used. The lateral approach is best suited for the peroneals if they were not seen from the medial aspect. The anterior tibials are imaged from the anterior aspect. **B,** The posterior tibial veins are more easily seen from the medial aspect of the calf with the knee slightly flexed and the leg slightly rotated. They lie closer and more superficial to the transducer. **C,** Imaging of the more posteriorly located medial gastrocnemius muscle bundle and some of the soleus muscle can be achieved with the transducer placed slightly more posteriorly. The leg must be completely relaxed so that pressure can be transmitted through the thick muscles at this level. This imaging window can be used to evaluate the junction of the posterior tibial and peroneal veins. A lower-frequency transducer capable of better penetration is often necessary at this level. **D** (see color plate III), The paired deep veins of the calf are clearly seen with color Doppler imaging during venous augmentation. The transducer is located medially on the calf. The posterior tibial veins lie closer to the transducer (*arrows*) than the paired peroneal veins (*curved arrows*). **E,** If the compression maneuver cannot be performed directly at the level of the tibial peroneal trunk, the use of the longitudinal window and color Doppler to visualize flow within the vein can be used as an alternate means of excluding obstructive venous thrombosis. It is often necessary to apply a significant amount of pressure to visualize the tibial peroneal trunk at this level. **F,** On occasion it is necessary to position the transducer more laterally toward the fibula. The peroneal veins lie just inferior and posterior to the fibula. These veins can on occasion be better visualized with the patient dangling the leg over the edge of the bed. It is best to perform this maneuver at the end of a standard venous examination. Normal veins will distend and be difficult to compress when the patient is sitting due to the increased pressure. The partly obstructing venous thrombus in the calf veins will be better perceived, however, often appearing as a discrete echogenic structure located in the middle of a distended vein.

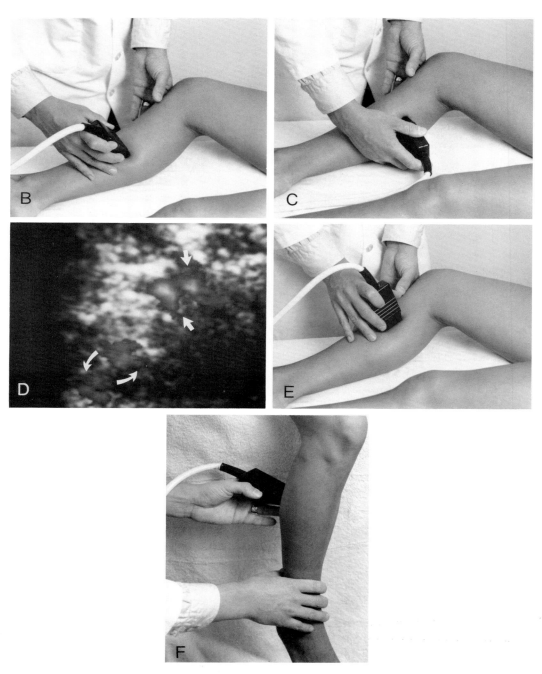

Figure 5.10. B to F.

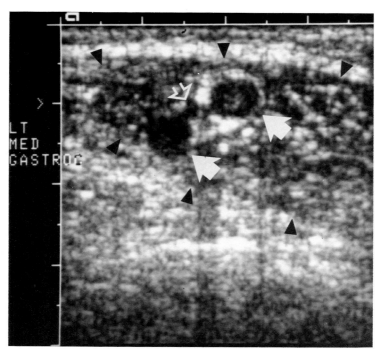

Figure 5.11. The sural veins drain the gastrocnemius muscle. They are duplicated and accompanied by an artery that lies in between (*open arrow*). These muscular veins are shown here distended by an acute thrombosis (*arrows*). Both contain echogenic material, facilitating the diagnosis of DVT. The medial head of the gastrocnemius is clearly discernible (*arrowheads*).

Table 5.1.
Diagnostic Features of Acute DVT

Thrombus characteristics
  Homogeneous
  Low echogenicity
  Leading edge often partly attached (nonobstructing)

Appearance of vein
  Distention
  Absence of flow
  Noncompressibility
  No collateral channels

of thrombus as an echogenic structure lying within the lumen of the vein. The second is measurement of the changes caused by the presence of thrombosis within the vein lumen. These indirect signs are passive distention of the vein by the acute thrombus and loss of normal venous compressibility when slight pressure is exerted on the skin overlying the vein. The third relies on detection of a change in the flow dynamics within the vein. In some cases there is total absence of flow, while in others a perturbed flow around a thrombus can be visualized.

Thrombus Visualization

Visualization of thrombus as an echogenic structure within the lumen of the vein is a very specific diagnostic criterion. When present, it is possible to unequivocally confirm the presence of acute venous thrombosis. There have been numerous attempts to determine the age of the thrombus as the echogenic structure of the blood clot evolves in time. Early on, echogenicity is thought to reflect red blood cell aggregation (Fig. 5.12). Within a day, the

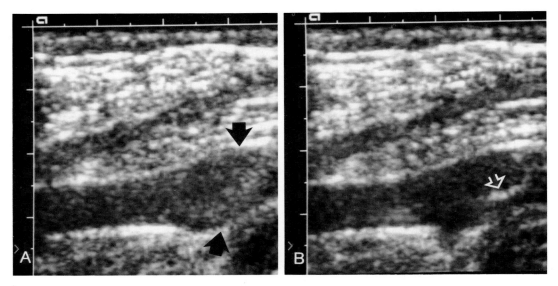

Figure 5.12. **A,** Slow-moving blood will commonly show zones of increased signal intensity corresponding to stagnation and layering of red blood cells. In this first image, relative stagnation of blood shows increased signals within a mildly dilated segment of the popliteal vein (*arrows*). **B,** This same level is imaged during the performance of a venous augmentation maneuver. Notice the valve leaflet, which is now open (*open arrow*). There is loss of the echogenic signals previously seen at the level of this valve.

cross-linking of fibrin and the development of internal zones of hemolysis are believed to be responsible for a relative loss of echogenicity. The thrombus is difficult to perceive. Within a few days, areas of increased echogenicity are intermixed with hypoechoic zones (Fig. 5.13). As the blood clot undergoes retraction and resorption over the ensuing weeks, the size of the vein decreases. If there is recanalization of the lumen, an isoechoic or slightly hyperechoic thickening of the vein wall will appear. Completely occluded veins that fail to recanalize show increasing echogenicity and a decrease in overall diameter. Attempts to age the thrombus by comparing in vitro observations to the in vivo situation have, unfortunately, given inconsistent results. This may be due to the fact that thrombus formation in vivo is a more dynamic process (Fig. 5.14). Two facts may explain the difficulties in determining the age of thrombus in a patient. The first is

that the process is not synchronous. Deep vein thrombus does not appear all at once in the full length of the involved vein. Rather, it grows slowly over the interval of days before it becomes symptomatic. The second is that there is, concurrent with a thrombotic process causing thrombus growth, a competitive fibrinolytic process that competes with thrombus formation and attempts to break apart and dissolve the forming fibrin matrix of the thrombus.

The major difficulty in using echogenicity as a diagnostic criterion is the need to accurately visualize all venous segments in the extremity. In an overweight patient or for a vein located deeply in the thigh, the overall noise due to scattering and other artifacts limits the quality of the sonogram. Adopting a lower-frequency transducer may solve the problem of penetrating to the location of the vein. Unfortunately, it is now well recognized that the blood clot that shows echogenicity at higher ultra-

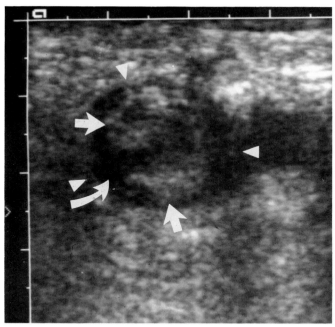

Figure 5.13. Acute thrombus will often contain areas of increased echogenicity and be identifiable as such on a gray-scale image. This sonogram shows a markedly distended common femoral vein (*arrowheads*), which contains intermixed echogenic (*straight arrows*) and nonechogenic (*curved arrow*) signals. This appearance is pathognomonic of acute DVT. The sensitivity of this finding is reported at 50%. We have found that it is often possible to find zones of increased echogenic signals in at least a small portion of veins affected by acute obstructing DVT. Similarly, nonobstructing DVT will often have a rim of increased signal at the interface between blood and thrombus. This is often better perceived on a longitudinal image, since the signal arising from the interface behaves as a specular reflector.

sound frequencies may be completely hypoechoic at lower ultrasound frequencies. This may therefore give a similar appearance to the thrombosed vein and the contiguously located artery.

Although very specific for the presence of acute vein thrombosis, visualization of an echogenic thrombus within a vein does not occur in every patient with DVT. It is the least sensitive sign for detecting the presence of acute thrombosis by sonography. It seems best for detecting nonobstructive DVT (Figs. 5.15 to 5.17). Estimates taken from the literature give this finding an approximate sensitivity of 50%. We believe that this can be as high as 75%.

Loss of Compressibility

The single most important criterion for making the diagnosis of acute deep vein thrombosis remains loss of compressibility of the vein (Fig. 5.18). The ultrasound examination is normally performed with a transducer held transverse to the lumen of the vein. The vein is identified as being either deep (femoral vein) (Fig. 5.19) or superficial (popliteal vein) (Fig. 5.20) to its accompanying artery. A slight amount of pressure is applied to the skin by pressing the transducer down. The pressure is released following apposition of the walls of the vein. This has the appearance of a

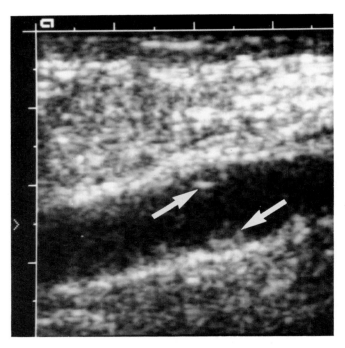

Figure 5.14. This longitudinal image is taken at the level of the popliteal vein valve (*arrows*). The popliteal vein at this level is noncompressible and contains thrombus. If gray-scale imaging alone had been used for the diagnosis of the presence of deep vein thrombosis, this examination would have been considered to be falsely negative.

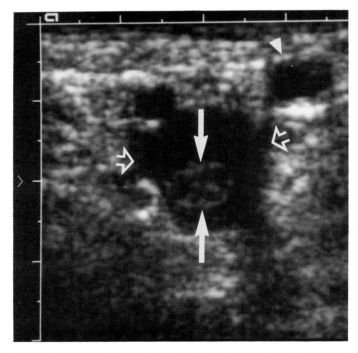

Figure 5.15. The standard sonographic evaluation of the deep veins of the leg starts at the level of the groin crease. Very extensive lower-extremity deep venous thrombosis is therefore likely to be detected early in the examination. This transverse image shows the more proximal tip of a large thrombus protruding into the middle common femoral vein. The thrombus (*arrows*) is clearly seen near the edge of the common femoral vein (*open arrows*). The greater saphenous vein is shown superiorly and to the right (*arrowhead*).

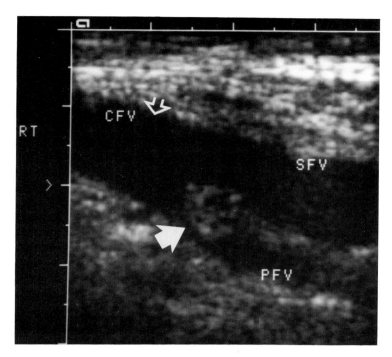

Figure 5.16. This longitudinal image shows an echogenic thrombus (*arrow*) within the profunda femoral vein and extending into the common femoral vein (*open arrow*). Isolated deep venous thrombosis of the profunda femoral vein is very uncommon. It is seen in patients following hip surgery or hip fractures. Local trauma related to the surgery or to the forces responsible for the fracture are transmitted to the endothelial lining of the vein. This local disruption of the endothelium then serves as a nidus for thrombus formation. Profunda femoral thrombosis can also be seen in patients with malignancies. In such cases it is rarely isolated but rather presents as one of many simultaneous sites of involvement. Patients in this category most likely develop these separate and multiple sites of venous thrombosis as part of their generalized thrombotic tendency.

wink during real-time imaging. The transducer is then moved 1 to 2 cm down the leg, and pressure is again reapplied. A normal response is complete collapse of the lumen of the vein before any distortion in the artery. Loss of venous compressibility or failure to appose the luminal surfaces of the walls of a vein is considered diagnostic of acute vein thrombosis (Fig. 5.21). This simple observation remains the most sensitive and most specific criterion for diagnosing acute obstructing and nonobstructing deep vein thrombosis of the femoral and popliteal venous segments (Table 5.2, Fig. 5.22). In some patients, the artery will occasionally compress before a

Table 5.2.
Sources of Error during Venous Compression Ultrasound

Occasional
Below-knee (infrapopliteal) thrombus
Segmental vein incompressibility (adductor canal)
Possible chronic DVT
Nonobstructing focal DVT
Vein duplication

Uncommon
Iliac vein thrombosis
Profunda femoris DVT

normal contiguous vein segment free of DVT. This has always turned out to be due to poor transmission of pressure down to

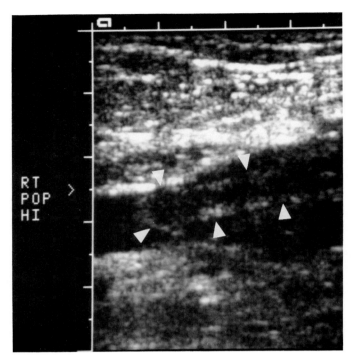

Figure 5.17. This nonobstructing thrombus in the popliteal vein is outlined by the *arrowheads*. This appearance is typical of this type of thrombus, which is also called "free-floating." These will typically move freely in the lumen of the vessel during real-time imaging.

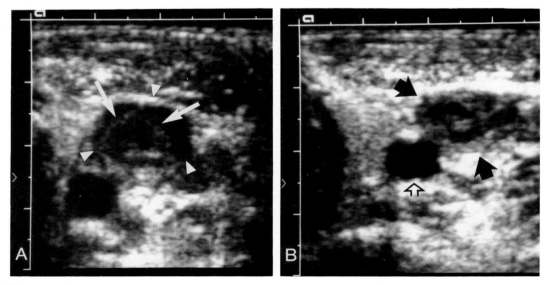

Figure 5.18. **A,** This transverse image shows that the popliteal vein has a slight amount of echogenic material within it (*arrows*). The vein itself is not distended (*arrowheads*). **B,** During compression, the lumen of the vein does not completely collapse (*arrows*). However, the artery is mildly deformed

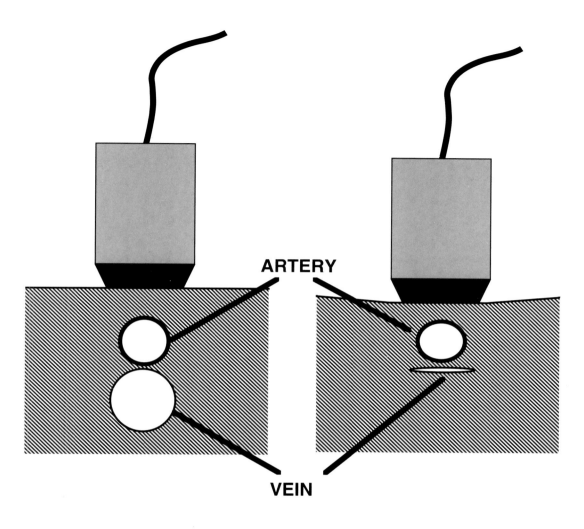

ARTERY

VEIN

BASELINE   **COMPRESSION**

Figure 5.19. The compression maneuver is performed with the transducer held transverse to the vein. Pressure is applied to the surface of the skin through the transducer. This is transmitted to the deeper structures and causes the vein walls to collapse. On real-time imaging, repeating this maneuver causes the vein to wink. The maneuver shown here is applied to the femoral vein, which lies deep to the artery. The artery should not deform before the vein. On rare occasions we have seen the artery collapse before the vein in patients with a prominent sartorius muscle. Reorienting the transducer more medially on the inside of the leg and repeating the compression maneuver then led to a normal response.

---

by the pressure applied on the skin (*open arrow*). This is the appearance of a partly obstructing thrombus. The possible causes of such a finding on sonography are partly obstructing acute DVT, chronic DVT, and an artifact due to patient positioning that causes poor transmission of the applied pressure to the level of the vein. The latter is the simplest to resolve by having the patient sit up or lie on his or her side. Differentiating acute from chronic DVT requires a more careful evaluation.

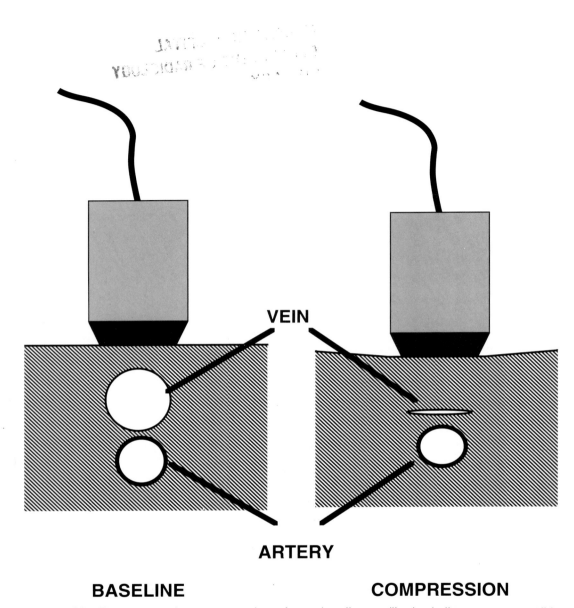

VEIN

ARTERY

BASELINE　　　　　　　　　　**COMPRESSION**

Figure 5.20. The compression maneuver is performed on the popliteal vein the same way as it is done for the femoral veins. The major difference is that the vein now lies closer to the transducer.

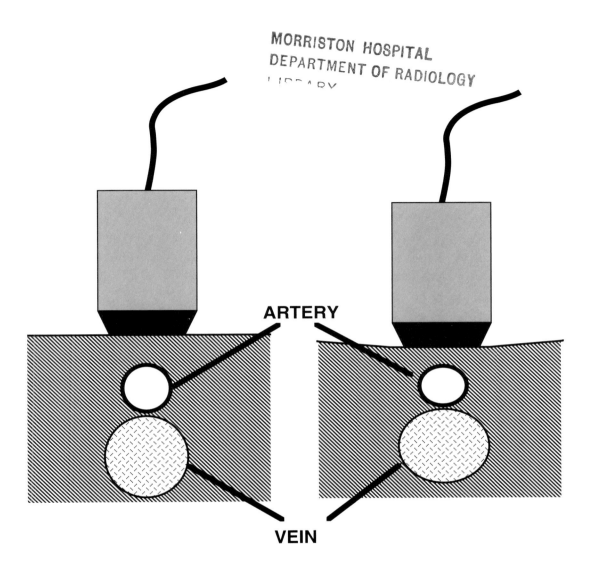

ARTERY

VEIN

BASELINE   **COMPRESSION**

Figure 5.21. An abnormal compression ultrasound is defined as a failure to appose the walls of the deep vein while pressure is applied onto the skin through the transducer. Sufficient pressure is exerted to the extent that the artery wall deforms slightly. An ancillary finding to the presence of DVT is distention of the vein. The additional presence of echogenic material in the vein lumen reinforces the diagnosis.

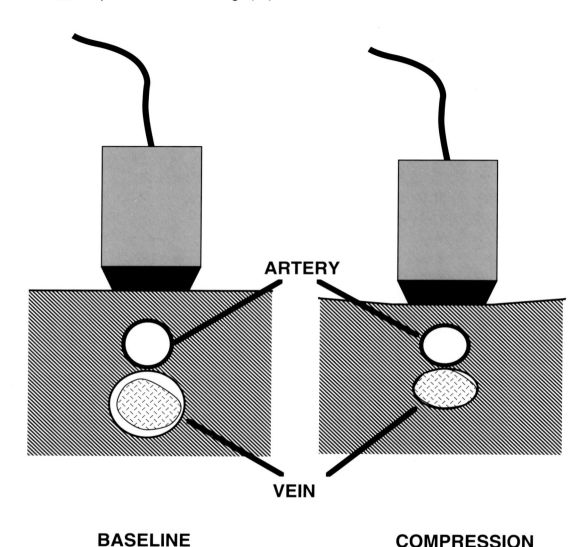

BASELINE   **COMPRESSION**

Figure 5.22. Compression ultrasound will also detect the presence of partly obstructing thrombus. There is failure of the walls of the vein to completely oppose during the compression maneuver. The vein is not distended. An echogenic structure need not be visualized in the vein lumen.

the vein partly because of patient anatomy (overlying muscle) or position. A slight change in patient position will normally correct the problem. The level of the adductor canal, just above the knee, is a difficult region to image by ultrasound (Fig. 5.23). Current strategies include imaging from the posterior aspect of the leg with pressure being applied either with the transducer, with a finger in close proxim-

ity to the transducer, or with a finger placed on the anterior aspect of the thigh. Another approach is to image from the anterior aspect of the thigh and to use the free hand to push the soft tissues and therefore the vein and artery toward the transducer. This thereby causes the vein to collapse. Imaging should be performed with the transducer transverse to the vessel and not parallel. If held parallel to the vein, it may be possible to miss a partly obstructing thrombus since the transducer may easily slip sideways during the compression maneuver. The nonobstructing thrombus may also be displaced while pressure is being applied (Fig. 5.24).

A consistent ancillary finding of acute obstructing vein thrombosis is distention of the vein lumen. This distention is thought to be secondary to the expansile forces generated by the fresh and expanding thrombus. This distending pressure is also the source of some of the pain that is experienced by the patient with acute thrombosis. Although expansion is seen, on occasion, with partly obstructing thrombus, it is more common when a fully obstructing thrombus is present. Partly ob-

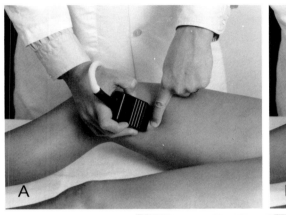
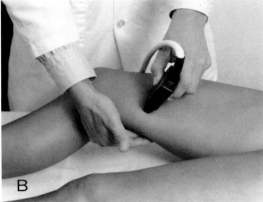
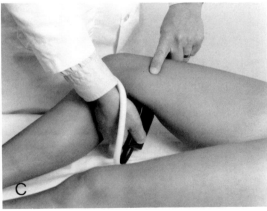

Figure 5.23. Difficulties in compressing and even visualizing the lower superficial and upper popliteal veins can be partly circumvented by additional maneuvers. **A,** The first useful maneuver is a means of compensating for poor transmission of pressure. The depth of the tissue attenuates the transmission of pressure from the transducer surface. The use of a finger placed on the skin beside the transducer often transmits pressure more efficaciously into the deeper soft tissues of the thigh and often compresses the vein where direct application of the pressure to the transducer has failed. **B,** The second approach to the problem is to position the free hand of the sonographer on the inferior aspect of the lower thigh and to lift the soft tissues toward the transducer. This will often cause real-time compression of the vein lumen. **C,** The last maneuver is to position the transducer posteriorly at the knee and to progressively move it up the back of the thigh to the highest level possible. If compression is not transmitted from the transducer, the opposite finger can be used to press on the anteromedial aspect of the thigh as shown here.

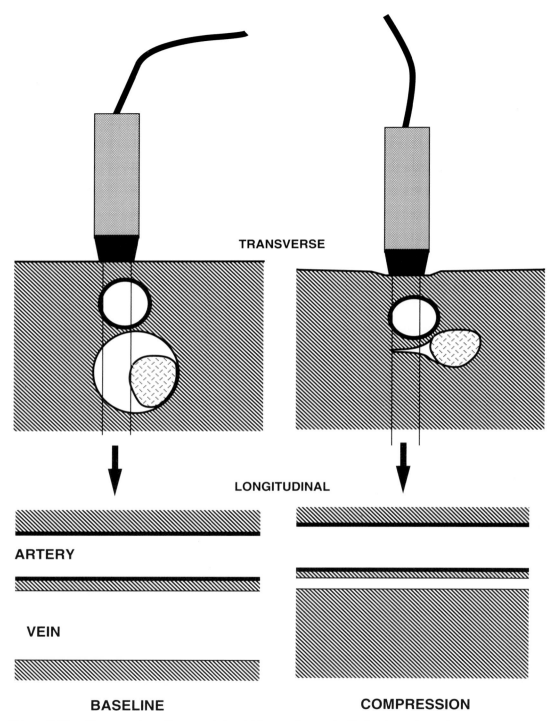

TRANSVERSE

LONGITUDINAL

ARTERY

VEIN

BASELINE

COMPRESSION

Figure 5.24. Compression ultrasound should be performed with the transducer held transverse to the vein. It is quite easy to miss venous thrombi while performing compression ultrasound with the transducer parallel to the vein. The field of view of the transducer can easily slide lateral to the vein. This creates the impression of a normal collapse of the vein walls. The longitudinal orientation of the transducer, however, is often useful in detecting echogenic structures in the suspected venous thrombus.

structive thrombosis can be perceived on the gray-scale image by virtue of visualizing an echogenic rim around the main body of the thrombus.

Altered Venous Flow

The last and largest category of changes that may be seen with acute venous thrombosis are detected as alterations to venous flow dynamics. The previous two criteria relied on accurate visualization of the vein with high-resolution sonographic imaging. Duplex sonography or color flow imaging are needed to evaluate the flow patterns within the venous lumen.

Normally, a cyclical respiratory variation should be seen superimposed on the more or less consistent flow within the major venous channels of the lower extremity (Fig. 5.25). On occasion, loss of this normal respiratory change may be due to patient positioning, low blood volume, or increased right-sided heart pressures. Loss of this respiratory variation may also be caused by an obstructing venous thrombus. An important ancillary maneuver has become an integral part of the sonographic examination; it consists of augmentation or accentuation of blood flow during compression of the calf (Fig. 5.26). This augmentation of the normal flow pattern within the vein is believed to be an accurate method for confirming the patency of the venous segments proximal and distal to the site where the Doppler signals are sampled (Fig. 5.27).

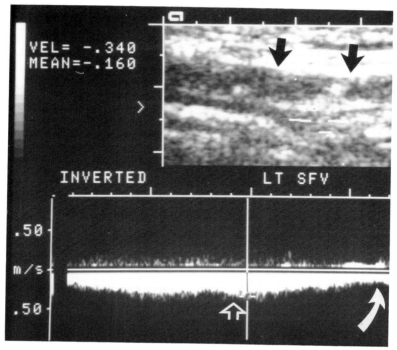

Figure 5.25. The Doppler gate in this image has been placed over the superficial femoral vein, which lies underneath the artery (*arrows*). The Doppler spectrum shows predominantly constant flow. Superimposed on this is a slight cyclical variation due to respiration. Flow increases when the patient is breathing out (*open arrow*) and decreases when the patient breathes in (*curved arrow*). In this image, the large markers on the time axis correspond to 1 second. The cyclical variation or phasicity corresponds to a respiratory rate of 20/min.

VENOUS AUGMENTATION
(NORMAL)

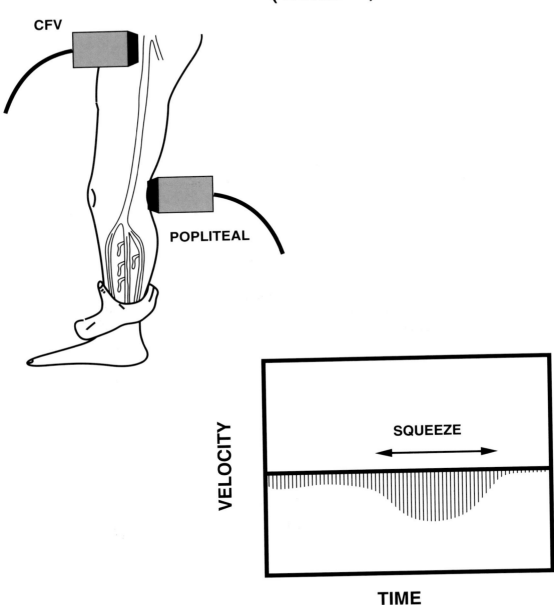

Figure 5.26. Venous flow augmentation is a standard maneuver used in Doppler ultrasound performed with a nonimaging probe and more recently using duplex sonography. The maneuver consists of squeezing blood from the calf veins, thereby increasing blood flow velocity in the proximal venous channels. The popliteal and common femoral veins are routinely sampled.

VENOUS AUGMENTATION
(DVT)

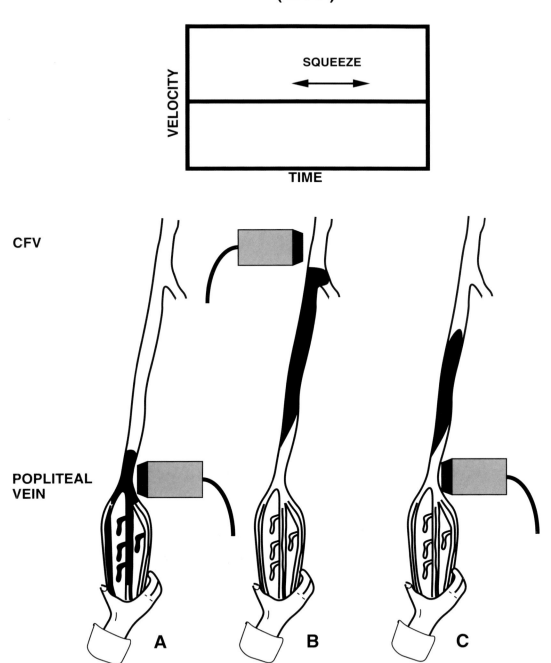

Figure 5.27. The absence of flow during venous augmentation is indicative of obstructing venous thrombosis. This can occur at the level of a thrombus (**A**) that fills and obstructs the normal lumen. This can also be seen downstream from the obstructive thrombosis (**B**), since the thrombus does not let any blood through the vein. Absence of flow can also be seen upstream from the obstruction (**C**). The latter is often seen at the level of the common femoral vein when there is iliac vein obstruction.

VENOUS AUGMENTATION
(DVT)

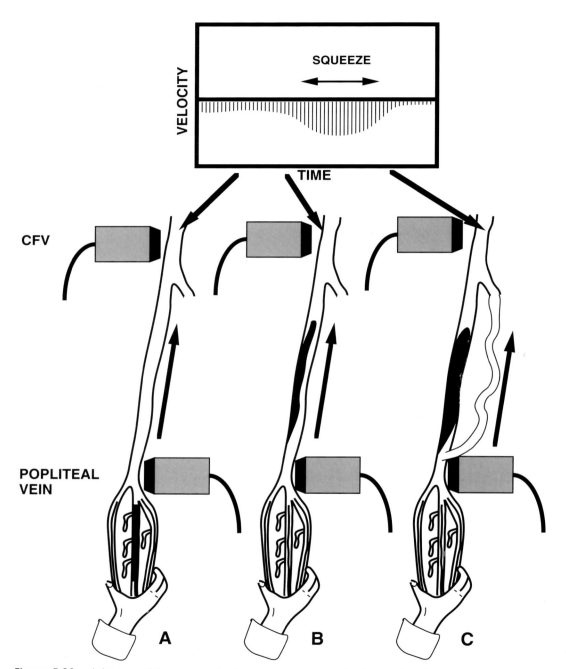

Figure 5.28. A few possible reasons for false negative examinations using Doppler sonography to detect venous thrombosis are shown here. The Doppler sampling is often performed only at certain locations on the leg since it would be time consuming to follow the full length of the veins. Failure to detect DVT is likely if the thrombosis is limited to the calf veins (**A**). Nonobstructing thrombosis is very likely to be missed either at points proximal and distal to the thrombus (**B**) as well as adjacent to the partly obstructing thrombus. This is less likely to be missed when color Doppler imaging is used. Obstructing thrombosis may also be missed (**C**) because of the development of large collaterals that bypass the obstruction.

Using the presence of flow as a means of excluding DVT, an accuracy of 90% has been reported. There are some limitations to this approach (Fig. 5.28). A partly obstructing thrombus, sparing a portion of the cross-sectional lumen of the vein, may not perturb venous flow. An obstructing thrombus involving only a part of the venous drainage of the leg but sparing important collateral channels may not have a significant effect on the flow pattern measured high up in the leg. This may hold

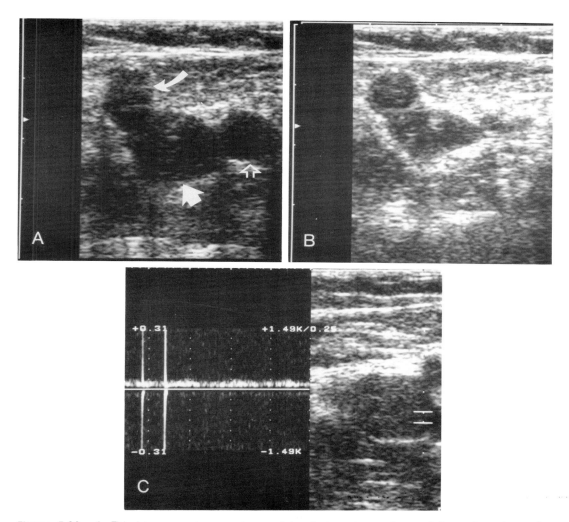

Figure 5.29. A, This transverse image shows distended common femoral (*arrow*) and greater saphenous veins (*curved arrow*). The artery is located laterally (*open arrow*). **B,** The compression view shows that the artery is partly collapsed while the veins are less affected. **C,** The last image shows a Doppler gate placed over the common femoral vein at the same level as **A** and **B**. A Doppler spectrum clearly shows flow around the thrombus despite the marked extent of the thrombus. The presence of flow signals in this case explains why standard duplex sonography or the use of hand-held CW probes can often miss the presence of thrombosis. Flow signals can persist despite an extensive thrombosis. Color Doppler mapping, however, does show the distribution of blood flow. In this case it demonstrated flow distributed at the periphery of the nonobstructing thrombus.

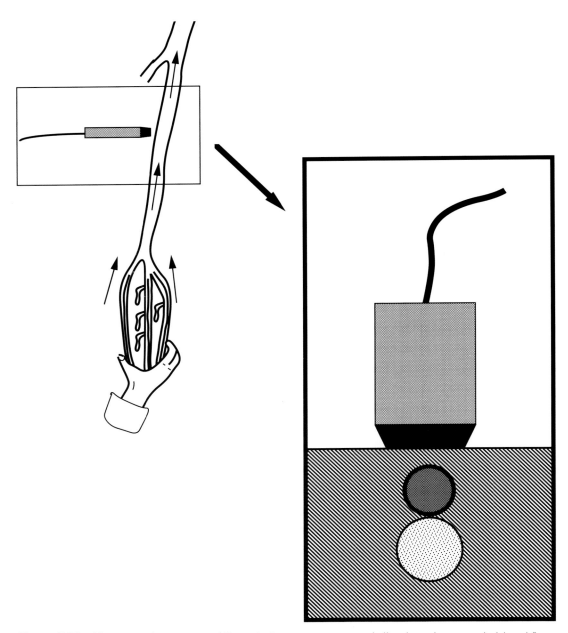

Figure 5.30. The normal response of the vein to venous augmentation is an increase in blood flow and flow velocity. This translates on the color Doppler image as a filling in of the visualized lumen of the vein. The vein lies deep to the artery.

true for thrombosis of the calf veins as well as those of the thigh. These thrombi can be missed if the examination is not performed over the full length of the vein.

Duplex sonography may miss partly obstructing thrombus since remaining flow around the thrombus appears normal (Fig. 5.29). Color Doppler flow imaging can easily display the flow patterns within the lumen of the vein (Figs. 5.30 and 5.31). Partly obstructing thrombus is normally outlined by the flowing blood. A rim of

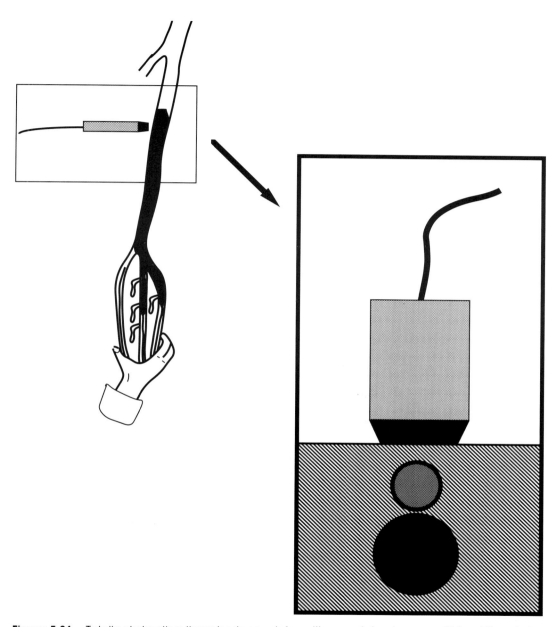

Figure 5.31. Totally obstructing thrombosis correlates with complete absence of blood flow during color Doppler imaging. On occasion, a duplicated vein may not be visualized. An occasional artifact may give the impression that some flow is present in the vein lumen. This is created by moving the transducer along the length of the vein. Depending on the color gain settings, color signals may show up in hypoechoic zones such as the thrombosed vein lumen. This artifact is due to the algorithm in the color devices that assigns color signals to areas without echoes instead of areas having echogenic structure.

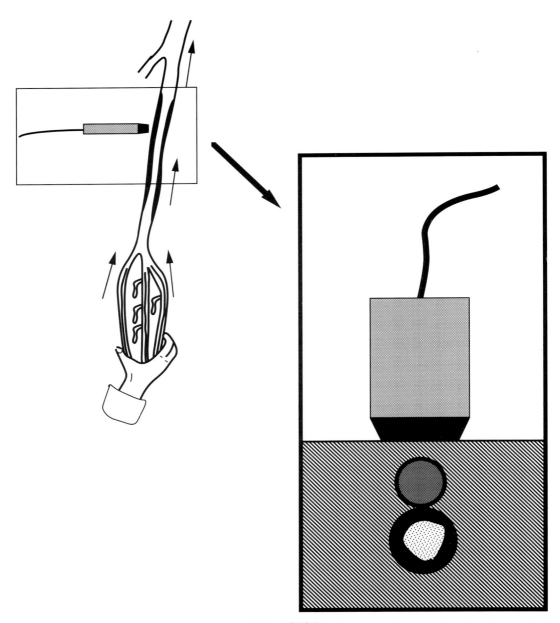

Figure 5.32. The identification of chronic DVT is facilitated by color Doppler imaging. Instead of flow directed to the periphery, as is the case in acute DVT, the color signals (*dotted pattern*) are seen in the center of the vein lumen.

increased flow signals is normally seen around the acute nonobstructing thrombus during venous flow augmentation (Figs. 5.32 and 5.33). There is, however, a major limitation to the approach. Loss of flow signals within a segment may be due to either complete involvement of the lumen of the veins by thrombus or either proximal or distal obstruction to flow (Fig. 5.34). This may lead the sonographer to overestimate the extent of the deep vein thrombosis.

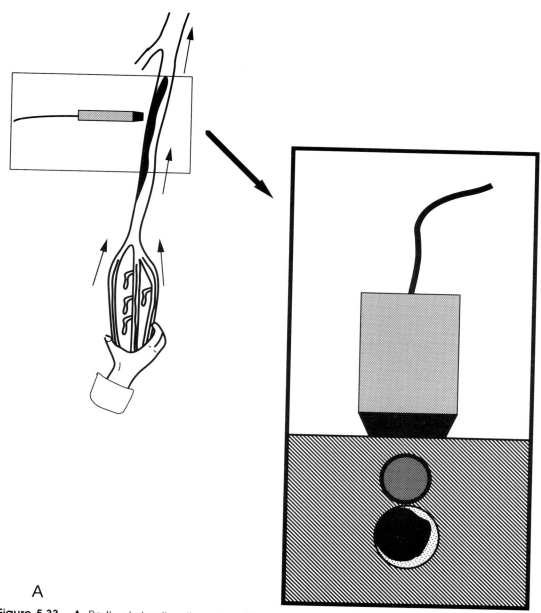

A

Figure 5.33. A, Partly obstructing thrombus still permits blood to flow around it both at rest and during venous flow augmentation. The thrombus (*black*) is outlined by the color signals (*dotted pattern*) when color Doppler imaging is done. This may help identify the extent of the thrombosis in large patients in whom compression ultrasound is difficult to apply. **B** (see color plate III), The presence of subtotal occlusive thrombosis within the popliteal vein is shown in this color Doppler image. The flow signals are seen at the periphery of the echogenic collection in the popliteal vein (*open arrows*). The artery lies deep to the vein (*curved arrow*). Artifacts related to the creation of the color image may overwhelm the smaller thrombi and give the impression of a normal color-filled lumen.

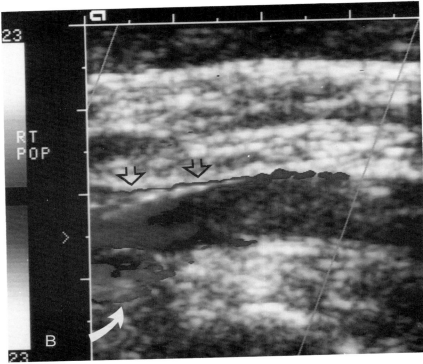

Figure 5.33. B.

The Valsalva maneuver is normally used to evaluate the patency of the iliac venous system or inferior vena cava at the level of the common femoral vein. A normal response consists of an increase in lumen diameter during the Valsalva maneuver. The diameter of the common femoral vein will normally increase by at least 15% from its baseline. Loss of this normal response may be secondary to either acute vein thrombosis or extrinsic obstruction of the iliac venous system. This maneuver, commonly used in most laboratories, may be difficult to elicit from a poorly cooperative patient. It may also be difficult to judge whether a 15 to 20% increase in diameter is in fact present. We have come to favor the use of flow measurements during the maneuver. Returning blood flow that ceases during the maneuver and then returns quickly is supportive evidence of an intact iliac vein (Fig. 5.35). Isolated iliac vein thrombosis is an uncommon clinical event often associated with a pelvic malignancy or pregnancy. Although the diagnosis might be suspected when poor flow and distention of the common femoral vein are seen (Fig. 5.36), it is hard to establish the extent of the thrombosis given that the iliac veins are difficult to visualize over their full length. Imaging using a sonographic window parallel to the iliac wing is possible. It is used on occasion to diagnose fully obstructing iliac vein thrombosis.

Diagnostic Accuracy
SYMPTOMATIC DVT

The accuracy of sonography for the diagnosis of acute thrombosis of either the femoral or popliteal venous segments (above the knee) is approximately 95%. Conglomerate data obtained from the literature suggest a sensitivity above 95% and a specificity greater than 97%. These data apply to both outpatients and hospitalized inpatients with symptomatic deep vein thrombosis. The diagnostic criterion on which the diagnosis has been based is loss of vein compressibility. Color flow Doppler imaging of the veins has recently been shown to help in visualizing partly obstructing thrombus within the lumen of the vein. It may also be useful in excluding venous obstruction as the pathological mechanism responsible for leg swelling. For example, in a patient presenting with marked thigh swelling, a normal flow pattern in the femoral vein is useful in excluding obstructing DVT as the source of the limb swelling. This does not exclude the possibility that nonobstructing thrombi are forming within the veins of the thigh, but it does exclude the presence of DVT as a cause for the clinical presentation.

Early reports on the accuracy of detecting symptomatic deep vein thromboses below the knee have estimated the sensitivity at about 20%. These data applied to situations where consistent attempts were not made to image the calf veins. Unfortunately, few studies have evaluated the accuracy of diagnostic sonography in the calf veins. The sensitivity is in fact above 80% in patients who manifest localized symptoms in the calf.

ASYMPTOMATIC DVT

Data on the evaluation of the postoperative or perioperative patient are sparser.

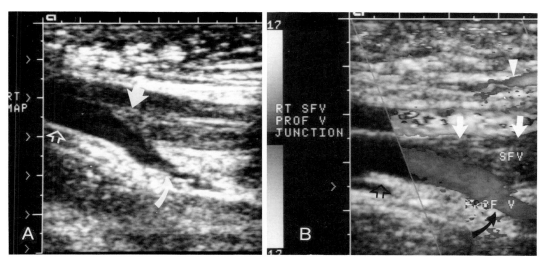

Figure 5.34. Involvement of the popliteal vein by deep vein thrombosis normally implies that the untreated thrombus will continue to spread more proximally. This will progress into the superficial femoral vein, ultimately reaching the level where the superficial femoral and profunda femoral veins join in the common femoral vein. In a given patient, it is difficult to predict which thrombi are more likely to spread into the more proximal veins. **A,** The trailing edge of such a thrombus (*arrow*) is shown protruding into the common femoral vein (*open arrow*) beyond the origin of the profunda femoral vein (*curved arrow*). In this case, collateral venous drainage of the lower leg has been established through the profunda femoral vein. **B** (see color plate III), Totally occlusive thrombus within the superficial femoral vein (*arrows*) is shown to extend into the common femoral vein (*open arrow*). Collateral flow is seen in the greater saphenous vein (*arrowhead*) and in the profunda femoral vein (*curved arrow*). The color Doppler signals were detected during venous augmentation of the calf veins. Increased flow in the profunda femoral vein is due to a large collateral communicating between the popliteal vein and the distal profunda femoral vein.

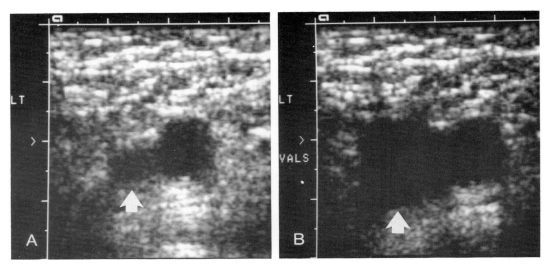

Figure 5.35. This series of images contrasts the normal response of the common femoral vein to the Valsalva maneuver to that seen when there is iliac vein obstruction. The Valsalva maneuver is a controlled elevation of intraabdominal pressure caused by bearing down against a closed glottis, similar to what is done while straining during childbirth or during a bowel movement. This effectively increases abdominal pressure, obstructs venous return, and distends the common femoral vein. The normal response is appreciated by comparing a transverse image of the normal common femoral vein at rest (**A**) to that of the vein during a Valsalva maneuver (**B**). The vein (*arrow*) distends dramatically. The effect on returning blood flow is shown in the Doppler waveform obtained during the maneuver (**C**). Venous flow has completely ceased and, in fact, has mildly reversed (*arrow*). This transient reversal is caused by the blood necessary to close the proximal femoral venous valve. With iliac vein obstruction, the Valsalva response is lost. The common femoral vein (*arrow*) is distended at rest (**D**) and shows no change during the maneuver (**E**). Common femoral venous flow is more dramatically affected (**F**). There is almost complete cessation of venous return at rest.

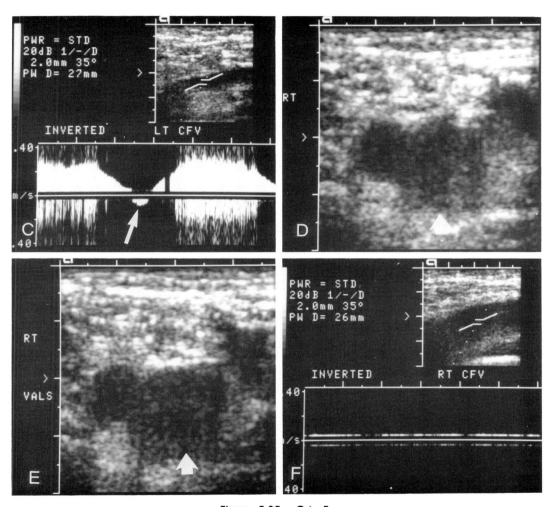

Figure 5.35. C to F.

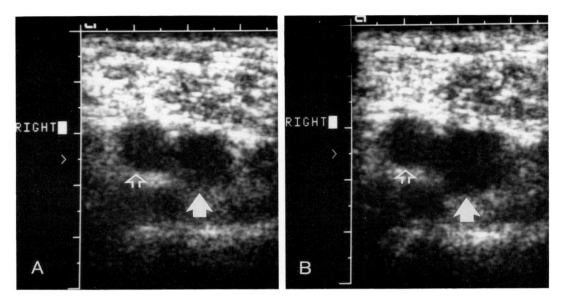

Figure 5.36. **A,** This first transverse sonogram shows the common femoral vein (*arrow*) and artery (*open arrow*). The vein is not abnormally distended. **B,** The second image was obtained during a Valsalva maneuver. The common femoral vein (*arrow*) does not show any significant change in diameter. An acute occlusion of the iliac vein will often cause distention of the femoral vein and loss of the Valsalva response. In a more chronic situation, the diameter of the vein will decrease, since collateral channels or partial recanalization of the iliac veins will help reestablish venous flow. The Valsalva response may remain absent for 3 to 6 months. After this, it may partly return as flow dynamics improve.

The diagnostic accuracy of sonography in asymptomatic deep vein thrombosis of the femoral and popliteal veins approaches that reported for the symptomatic population. However, care must be given to the way the examination is performed. The vein must be sampled more slowly, over its full extent, to exclude the smaller non-obstructing thrombi, which are the rule rather than the exception. The examination must also be performed on both extremities rather than directed to one limb. These patients also have a lower proportion of venous thrombi in the femoral popliteal system, with half the blood clots residing in the calf veins.

The diagnostic accuracy for deep vein thrombosis below the knee in this patient subset is less than for the femoral-popliteal veins. In fact, since the majority of thromboses in these asymptomatic patients are

nonobstructive, the sensitivity of the technique might lie in the 40% range. This may not be improved by the use of color Doppler sonography. The issue remains one for future investigation.

SERIAL SONOGRAPHIC STUDIES
Below-Knee DVT

Multiple studies using a radioisotope (iodinated fibrinogen) and phlebography have shown that up to 20% of calf vein thrombi will ultimately spread from their site of origin in the venous plexi of the muscles of the calf into the popliteal vein and then more proximally into the femoral venous system above the knee (Fig. 5.37). This has led to the current diagnostic strategy for suspected calf vein thrombosis: the serial follow-up of the lower extremity by compression ultrasound. The minority of thrombi that do spread to the popliteal vein and ultimately constitute the major risk for acute pulmonary embolism are diagnosed in the popliteal vein on repeat examination performed 1 to 3 days after the first baseline examination. This approach is made possible by the high accuracy of ultrasound for the diagnosis of DVT of the popliteal venous segments. Our own experience has shown that patients who present earlier in the evolution of DVT, when thrombus is still limited to the popli-

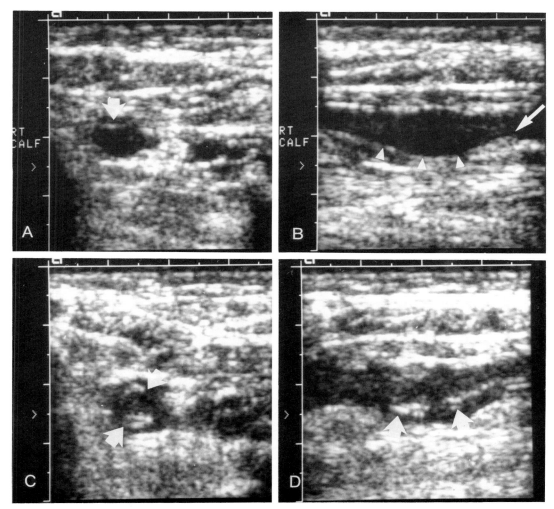

Figure 5.37. Thrombus tends to form in areas of stagnant or decreased venous blood flow. **A,** Early nonobstructing venous thrombosis has involved a portion of a mildly dilated segment of the tibial vein (*arrow*). **B,** The longitudinal image shows this thrombus just distal (*arrow*) to a small venous aneurysm (*arrowheads*). **C,** A repeat examination was performed 5 days later. On the transverse image, a larger nonobstructing thrombus is now better appreciated (*arrows*). **D,** The longitudinal image shows that this thrombus has also spread more proximally to involve the venous aneurysm (*arrows*). Venous aneurysms are rare and more often appreciated at the level of the popliteal vein. They are regions of poor blood flow. This in turn increases the tendency for thrombus deposition and spread. They can become symptomatic when their increased size exerts pressure on the surrounding soft tissues.

teal vein or below, are as likely to have the diagnosis made by ultrasound as those presenting with extensive femoral vein thrombosis. This is something of a trend. There used to be a clinical hesitation in performing venography in patients whose symptoms were minimal. Often, the patient presented with a markedly swollen leg and with a high probability of having femoral vein involvement. The dissemination of the sonographic methodology and its minimal associated risks has lowered the diagnostic threshold at which the examination is performed. It is now quite common to see patients presenting with only localized symptoms, often limited to the calf.

During the examination, the patient must identify the exact site of symptoms in the calf (Figs. 5.38 and 5.39). Imaging can then focus on this area of concern and help confirm the diagnosis of calf vein thrombus. Incidental diagnosis such as superficial phlebitis can often explain a patient's symptoms. The therapeutic strategies are, unfortunately, controversial, ranging from observation to full anticoagulation. This latter approach is based on the belief that calf vein thrombosis is a potential marker for a subset of the population at high risk for developing recurrent thrombophlebitis. Unfortunately, there are no published data validating a more integrated approach using the diagnostic capabilities of sonography to help guide the therapeutic strategy. An attempt to integrate the diagnostic approach to the therapeutic options is the use of serial monitoring at the popliteal vein. Anticoagulation is often withheld until spread is documented into the popliteal vein.

The type and extent of calf vein throm-

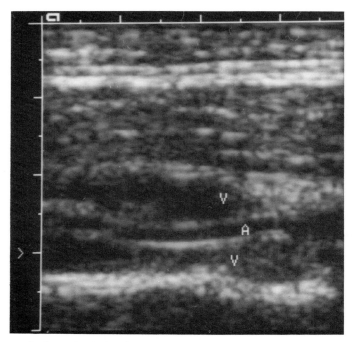

Figure 5.38. Deep vein thrombosis involving the paired draining vein is often diagnosed by compression ultrasound. In distinction to compression ultrasound performed in the thigh and behind the knee, compression can more easily be performed in the longitudinal plane, since the relationship between the artery and both veins can be kept during the compression maneuver.

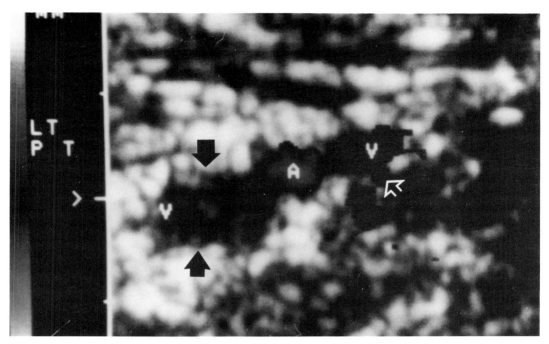

Figure 5.39. (see color plate III). Occlusive venous thrombosis of the posterior tibial veins has caused an absence of color Doppler signals in a distended vein (*arrows*). The artery is located between the thrombosed venous segment and the other patent posterior tibial vein (*open arrow*).

bosis should also be estimated. Thrombosis limited to the muscular veins probably warrants conservative treatment and simple monitoring for evidence of spread. Involvement of the paired tibioperoneal veins is more ominous and indicates the tendency of the thrombosis to spread. This is even more worrisome if the thrombus is obstructing. Over the last year, we have seen an increasing trend in the use of oral anticoagulation in patients with extensive obstructing deep vein thrombosis.

Calf vein thrombi, although believed to be the source of most of the deep venous thrombi, need not spread to all the calf veins before spreading to the popliteal vein and above. It is common to see sparing of at least one or two paired veins. The anterior tibials are rarely involved by deep vein thrombosis.

Above-Knee DVT

Nonobstructive DVT will tend either to resolve or to cause minimal changes in the wall of the vein (Fig. 5.40). Phlebographic studies have shown that above-knee obstructive venous thrombosis can have one of three major outcomes. Venous segments may become completely normal, recanalize in part, or show no significant change and remain completely thrombosed. These observations have recently been confirmed using sonography. Complete resolution of the occluding venous thrombus is seen in up to 53% of venous segments within the first 3 months following the acute thrombosis. Partial recanalization is the next most common outcome. It is normally associated with scarring and diminished caliber of the involved vein. If imaging is performed months or years af-

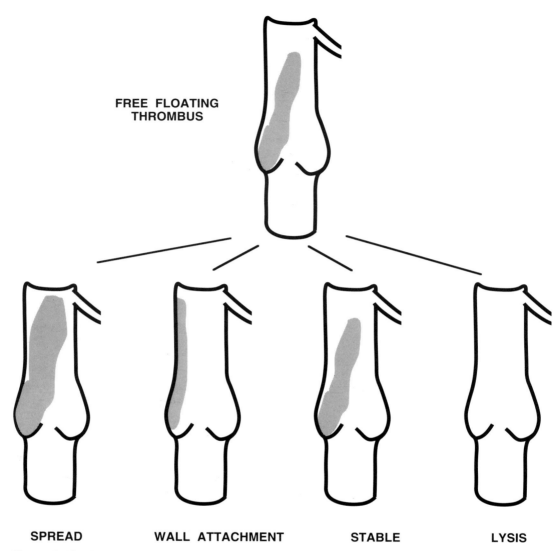

FREE FLOATING THROMBUS

SPREAD **WALL ATTACHMENT** **STABLE** **LYSIS**

Figure 5.40. The natural history of free-floating thrombi has been studied by performing serial venous ultrasound examinations. The majority show attachment to the wall by 7 to 10 days. Complete lysis occurs in a small percentage of cases within a week. Spread is also uncommon. The most common outcome is for wall attachment within a week and progressive lysis or incorporation over the next few months.

ter the acute DVT, many small channels are often seen. One of these multiple small channels is often the originally thrombosed segment. The other smaller collaterals develop either from the vena venorum of the vein or from new collateral branches that develop in response to the occlusion. The hyperplastic response of the endothelium of the vein wall is seen in venous segments whose thrombus is partly obstructing or that have almost completely recanalized. Following recanalization, valve function is often compromised and 25% of segments will show venous insufficiency 3 to 6 months following an episode of acute DVT.

A significant number of venous segments show persistent obstruction of the lumen. However, with time, the marked distention of the involved venous segment resolves. As the thrombus becomes organized and heals by fibrosis, the diameter of the vein decreases and it often cannot be perceived on repeat examination months later. Instead, smaller parallel channels are seen either above or below the artery.

Serial monitoring of these patients has also shown that many collateral pathways develop, often within the first day following diagnosis. These develop through the perforating veins into the superficial venous system or within partly duplicated venous segments, which are present in up to 25% of normal subjects. A very common collateral pathway joins the popliteal vein to the profunda femoris vein. This collateral is seen in 40 to 60% of patients. It is easily demonstrated by observing blood flow in the common femoral vein following venous augmentation of the calf veins. A normal response would consist of augmentation of flow in the superficial femoral vein, since blood reaches the common femoral vein mostly through this vein. If this large collateral is present, imaging over the junction of the profunda femoris and the superficial femoral vein will show that most of the blood flow reaches the common femoral vein from the profunda femoris vein (Fig. 5.34). This becomes more obvious if there is an obstructing thrombus in the superficial femoral vein. It is our standard practice to evaluate the blood flow pattern at the origin of the profunda femoris and superficial femoral veins. Whenever a preferential pattern of blood flow is seen at the profunda femoris vein, the possibility that there is or has been an episode of deep vein thrombosis affecting the superficial femoral vein is raised. The remainder of the examination is then performed more cautiously, by combining flow imaging with compression ultrasound with the expectation that an obstructive process involves the superficial femoral vein. If there is no acute thrombosis or evidence of chronic thrombosis (collaterals, wall thickening), the most likely explanation is the presence of an anatomic variant.

The patient presenting with a markedly swollen leg is a diagnostic dilemma. In most instances, the swelling in question is related to recent surgery or to a mass or obstructive process in the pelvis. The most difficult patient to deal with is the patient who also has such a large girth of the thigh that accurate visualization of all the veins cannot be successfully performed. Under these circumstances, a logical approach is to *exclude the presence of significant obstructive thrombosis responsible for the leg swelling*. This can be readily accomplished in almost all patients by performing an evaluation of the flow patterns in the common femoral and popliteal veins. Although this constitutes a limited examination, it can exclude the presence of obstructive thrombosis. This simple strategy is useless if the patient presents with a history of pulmonary embolism and the question asked is whether or not the legs are a source of the emboli. If there is obstruction to venous flow on one of the two sides, one may infer an obstructive thrombosis. A normal flow pattern seen in the common femoral and popliteal veins does not exclude the presence of smaller nonobstructive thrombi likely to be the source of pulmonary emboli.

The pattern of deep vein thrombosis favors the natural progression of thrombus from the calf upward to the femoral and iliac veins. A much less common pattern is that of iliac vein venous thrombosis that spreads downward to the femoral veins. This is more common in patients with pelvic malignancies such as prostate or testicular tumors in the male and ovarian or cervical neoplasms in the female. Bladder carcinoma can be seen in both. The presentation is often of unilateral painful leg swelling. Imaging may not necessarily show any thrombus or may show thrombus that involves the common femoral vein and a portion of the superficial femoral vein. When no thrombus is visualized at the iliofemoral junction, additional imaging can be performed using lower-frequency 3.5-MHz transducers. In general, these obstructive thrombi not only cause the response of the femoral vein to the Valsalva maneuver to be lost but also cause marked impairment to the normal respiratory variations and blunt the response to venous augmentation. A final diagnosis can be arrived at by direct femoral puncture and iliac venography. Computed tomography or serial monitoring for downward spread of the thrombus are alternative diagnostic approaches.

The pregnant patient may also present with a very similar unilateral leg swelling. This is most often on the left side. Iliac vein thrombosis is more commonly due to a combination of compression of the enlarging uterus and the propensity to stasis in the left iliac vein compressed by the overlying artery. In our limited experience, these thrombi normally spread downward within 2 to 3 days. If there is hesitation in performing a direct iliac venogram, serial monitoring can be done. However, it would be unwise to do so without attempting to image the iliac veins. The compressive effect of the uterus can often obstruct venous flow, blunting both the Valsalva response and the flow augmentation when the patient lies on her back. This relative obstruction is relieved by having the patient lie on her side. If this fails to relieve the venous obstruction, it should be assumed that an obstructive iliac thrombus is present.

The region of the adductor canal remains one of the most difficult areas to image. Strategies that rely on color flow mapping or duplex sonography are sufficient to exclude obstructive thrombosis but fail in excluding nonobstructing thrombus.

The latter may be more of a diagnostic problem for the postoperative patient, whereas the symptomatic patient is more likely to have obstructive thrombosis. However, it must be remembered that the use of venography is still recommended and available for these difficult cases.

Incidental Pathologies

The patient who presents with symptoms suggestive of deep vein thrombosis may in fact have other pathological entities responsible for the pain or leg swelling. Sonography can then be quite useful in sorting out the pathology responsible for the problem (Table 5.3).

In the case of marked swelling of the extremity, lymphedema due to obstruction of the lymphatics can be suspected whenever large marked lymph node masses are present in the groin yet the venous flow dynamics are normal.

Compression of the veins by an extrinsic process can also mimic deep vein thrombosis. Likely candidates include hematoma in the thigh and groin or tumor masses, as well as arterial aneurysms or pseudoaneurysms. These can be directly visualized by ultrasound. The compressive effect can easily affect the venous return and cause stasis and symptoms of leg

Table 5.3.
Miscellaneous Pathological Entities Detected in Patients Presenting with Suspected Acute DVT

Common
  Baker cyst (popliteal or synovial cyst)
  Hematoma

Uncommon
  Superficial phlebitis
  Cellulitis
  Pseudoaneurysm/aneurysm
  Lymph node masses/lymphatic obstruction
  Venous incompetence
  Pelvic masses
  Right-sided heart failure
  Venous varix

---

swelling. The two most dramatic cases of venous stasis we have seen were both caused by an expanding urinoma in patients following renal transplantation. The pelvic kidney and the urinoma compressed the adjacent vein to the point of almost total obstruction of lower-extremity venous return. Evacuation of the urinoma relieved the flow impediment (Fig. 5.41).

Other significant pathologic entities include Baker's cysts, also called popliteal or synovial cysts (Fig. 5.42). These can mimic the signs and symptoms of deep vein thrombosis to the point that the term pseudothrombophlebitis is often used to

describe this syndrome. It affects mostly patients with rheumatoid arthritis or osteoarthritis. These cysts have an oval shape and a heterogeneous structure that is mostly hypoechoic. It may mimic a large thrombus. Scanning up and down the leg shows this structure to be distinct from the vein and artery. The diagnosis of a ruptured cyst is more difficult, since a partly echogenic structure is not necessarily present in the popliteal fossa (Fig. 5.43). Often, a smaller collection has dissected downward in the muscular fascial planes of the calf muscles and can still be visualized. Most patients have an associated

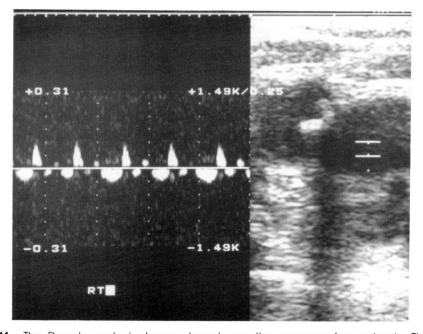

Figure 5.41. The Doppler gate is shown placed over the common femoral vein. The Doppler spectrum is abnormal and has a cyclical variation that mimics an arterial waveform. Such a pattern can occasionally be seen in patients with right-sided heart failure, in cases of AV fistula, and following renal transplantation. In cases of right heart failure, the presence of tricuspid regurgitation and vein distention due to increased blood volume are likely responsible for this waveform. Tricuspid regurgitation directly causes a change in blood flow with every cardiac beat. Vein distention causes it to appose closely against the artery, thereby helping to transmit the arterial waveform onto the vein. In a large AV fistula, the arterial waveform is transmitted directly into the vein. This is more likely to occur in larger chronic fistulas. The reason for this finding in patients following renal transplantation is unclear. This may be due to the presence of a shunt through the transplant. Volume overload and relative obstruction to venous return by a urinoma or lymphocele pressing against the iliac vein are other likely etiologies.

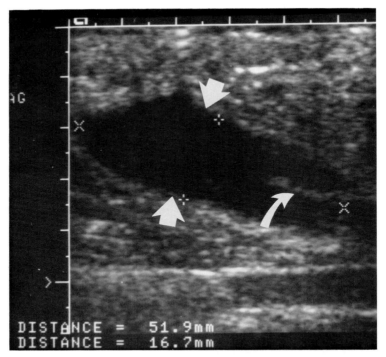

Figure 5.42. This well-circumscribed popliteal cyst (*arrows*) has a more complex architecture with some septation (*curved arrow*). The sonographic appearance of a more complex collection should suggest the possibility of an abscess. However, the sonographic appearance of popliteal cysts or of hematoma can vary tremendously, containing intermixed regions of increased and decreased echogenicity. The decision to perform an aspiration biopsy should be made on clinical grounds since the sonographic appearance of these entities shows such an overlap.

knee effusion, which can be better visualized as a collection in the suprapatellar pouch of the knee (Fig. 5.44).

Other causes of pain in the calf include a chronic evolving abscess (often associated with a cellulitis) and hematoma (often linked to muscle fiber rupture following vigorous exercise or blunt trauma) (Fig. 5.45). These show up as heterogeneous areas within a muscle or between muscle planes. They are too large to represent muscular veins. They are, however, similar to some of the localized muscle edema and reaction we have occasionally seen in association with deep vein thrombosis. At the very least, such cases warrant a repeat sonogram to confirm resorption of the process. The lack of any progression in the abnormality is reassuring even if it turns

out to have been a localized thrombosis. Damage to a muscle tendon can be confirmed by demonstrating edema at the site corresponding to the localized symptoms. Penetrating injuries to the calf and thigh can also cause hematoma, which compresses the venous system. Pseudoaneurysms will on occasion compress the adjacent vein and cause venous obstruction (Fig. 5.46). True venous aneurysms are rarely seen. These outpouchings of the veins are commonly the source of symptoms due to the localized pressure generated by their physical size. Their management tends to be conservative.

Two common pathological entities detected when screening patients are acute superficial phlebitis and venous insufficiency. Acute superficial thrombophlebitis is normally treated conservatively with leg elevation and compresses. It need not be viewed as always benign, however. A markedly dilated greater saphenous vein, distended with acute thrombus that protrudes into the common femoral vein, should not be brushed off. The extent of the thrombus and the caliber of the vein are important and should be reported. Anticoagulation has often been used to treat extensive superficial phlebitis in a large distended vein since it has a reasonable likelihood of spreading into the common femoral vein and causing pulmonary embolism. The presence of superficial phlebitis has also been linked with a high likelihood of coexistent deep vein thrombosis. These need not be symptomatic. Whenever detected, superficial phlebitis

should suggest the need for a more thorough examination of the deep veins.

Finally, the symptoms of venous insufficiency can mimic those of acute venous thrombosis. The presence of acute thrombus within dilated varicosities is also a likely source of symptoms localized to a small area of the leg. The identification of venous incompetence by sonography may often explain the patient's symptoms and the reason they presented for evaluation.

Upper Extremity
NORMAL ANATOMY

Venous imaging of the upper extremity is normally performed from the antecubital fossa to the medial head of the clavicle

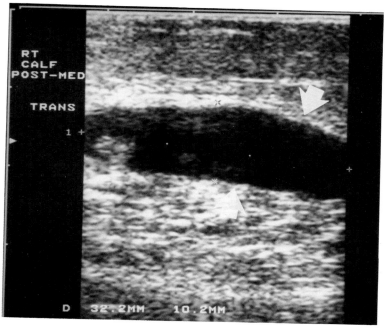

Figure 5.43. A popliteal cyst may cause acute symptoms when it ruptures or dissects into the soft tissues of the calf. This well-circumscribed, mostly echolucent collection (*arrows*) corresponds to the site of acute symptoms in the mid calf of this patient. It represents a popliteal cyst that has dissected downward into the calf. It is believed that the majority of popliteal cysts that rupture do not form discrete collections that can be seen by ultrasound. This belief has yet to be verified by a well-designed study using sonography. The differential diagnosis of the collection seen on this sonogram is that of hematoma or abscess.

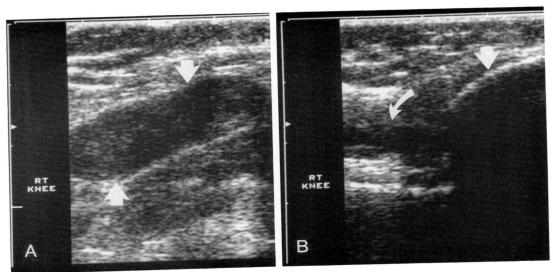

Figure 5.44. Patient referral to the noninvasive laboratory is made on the basis of symptoms suggestive of acute DVT. However, these may be the manifestations of a host of other pathologies. **A,** This longitudinal image shows a poorly echogenic mass (*arrows*) posterior to the knee. This represents a popliteal cyst. **B,** Imaging of the region of the suprapatellar bursa just above the knee cap shows a small knee effusion (*curved arrow*) just above the patella (*arrow*). Knee effusions may by themselves be the source of the patient's complaints. They are often associated with the presence of a popliteal cyst (whose synonyms include Baker's cyst and synovial cyst). Differentiating a popliteal cyst from a vein or other vascular abnormality is normally done by noting the absence of flow signals within the collection and by the lack of communication between the collection and either artery or vein.

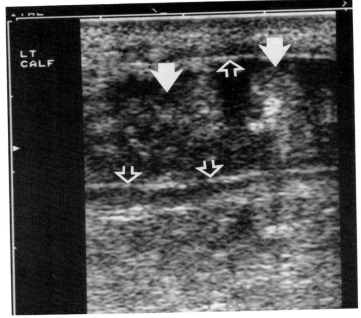

Figure 5.45. This large collection contains echogenic material (*arrows*). The circumference of the collection shows a rind of poor echogenicity (*open arrows*). No flow signals are detected within the collection. Subsequent aspiration biopsy and insertion of a drainage catheter confirmed the presence of an abscess.

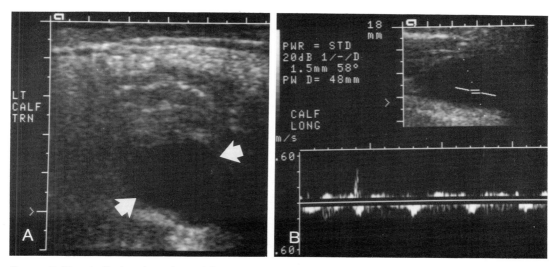

Figure 5.46. **A,** During imaging of the symptomatic calf of this patient, a large collection was appreciated to lie deep to the soleus muscle (*arrows*). **B,** Duplex ultrasound shows the presence of flow within this collection. This was subsequently proven to represent a pseudoaneurysm. The differential diagnosis of acute venous thrombosis includes Baker's cyst, pseudoaneurysm, abscess, or other masses.

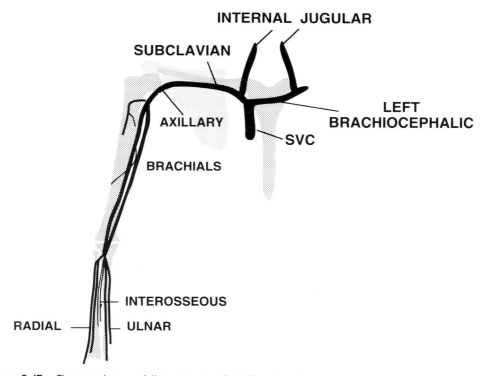

Figure 5.47. The anatomy of the upper-extremity veins shows a similar tendency for the more peripherally located veins—brachials and below—to be duplicated. The interconnections with the superficial venous system are also more variable.

(Fig. 5.47). The basilic vein is identified where it lies medially in the elbow (Fig. 5.48). It is followed upward until it often becomes duplicated and joins the brachial vein to form the axillary vein. The more laterally located cephalic vein courses laterally along the forearm, over the femoral head, and finally joins the axillary vein as it becomes the subclavian vein (Fig. 5.49). The brachial veins are duplicated and course parallel to the brachial artery until they anastomose with the basilic vein and continue as the axillary vein. Below the antecubital fossa, the veins course parallel to the artery and are difficult to visualize unless involved by thrombus. The subclavian vein can be imaged either from above or below the clavicle. From above, it lies deeper to the artery, while from below it lies more superficial to the artery (Fig. 5.50). The subclavian joins the internal jugular vein to form the brachiocephalic vein. Imaging is normally possible only to this level, with portions of the superior

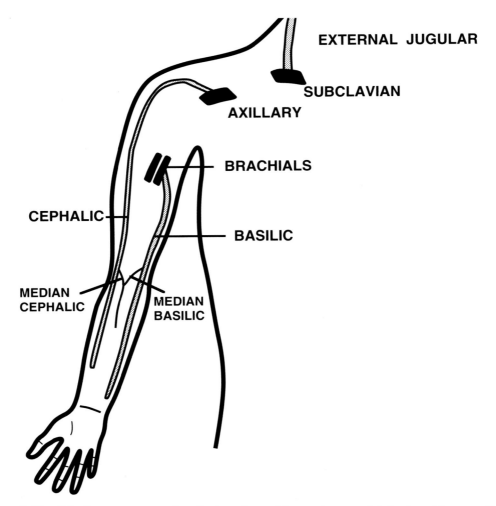

Figure 5.48. This diagram summarizes the locations of the major superficial veins of the arm. There is much more variability in the size and the location of the communications to the deep arm veins than the veins in the lower extremity.

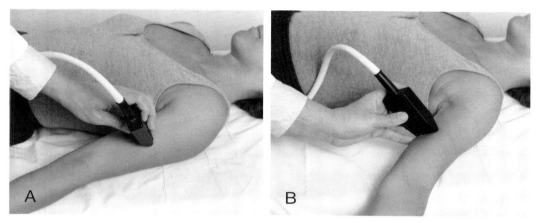

Figure 5.49. The superficial veins of the upper extremity can be quickly traced with the transducer. The patient should be perfectly supine or if possible in mild Trendelenberg position. **A,** The basilic vein can be followed from the medial aspect of the arm from the level of the elbow upward. It normally joins one of the two brachial veins at the mid arm level. **B,** The cephalic vein is normally evaluated with the transducer located more laterally. Care must be taken not to press on the skin, since the cephalic vein tends to be quite small and easily compressible.

vena cava only rarely being imaged. Imaging is normally performed with the head rotated away from the side being studied (Fig. 5.51). Better visualization of the brachiocephalic junction is occasionally achieved when the patient turns the head toward the side being imaged.

The internal jugular vein can be followed upward from the brachiocephalic vein. It runs superficial to the carotid artery and is easily followed to the carotid bifurcation. The external jugular vein joins the subclavian vein. It is so superficial that it is easily compressed by the slightest pressure on the skin.

DIAGNOSTIC CRITERIA

Exclusion of an obstructing process affecting the more central veins is accomplished by documenting the normal collapse of the subclavian vein in response to deep, rapid inspiration or sniffing (Fig. 5.52). As in the lower extremity, absence or loss of a normal response can be due to either intrinsic obstruction by thrombus or extrinsic compression of the vein by a mass or an infiltrative process due to tumor or inflammation (mediastinitis). Loss of compressibility remains the most reliable criterion for the diagnosis of venous thrombosis in the basilic, cephalic, brachial, and axillary veins (Fig. 5.53). Either absence of flow or loss of compressibility is needed to make the diagnosis of thrombosis within the subclavian vein. In the distal third, the vein is accessible to direct visualization and can be compressed. The mid portion is often obscured by the clavicle and only total obstruction of this vein segment can be excluded by demonstrating good flow signals within the segments on both sides corresponding to the distal and proximal thirds of the clavicle. In the proximal third, the presence of an echogenic nidus (Fig. 5.54) and loss of flow signals (Fig. 5.55) within the vein can be used as diagnostic criteria. The accuracy of the examination is higher in the jugular vein since it is easily compressible along its full length (Fig. 5.56).

Despite the difficulties discussed above, the diagnostic accuracy of this examination is quite high. Reported series are either too

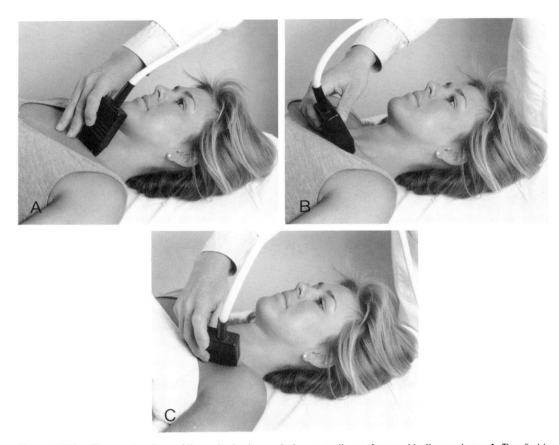

Figure 5.50. The evaluation of the subclavian vein is normally performed in three steps. **A,** The first is the use of a supraclavicular window to identify the origin of the subclavian vein as it communicates with the brachiocephalic vein. This window is also useful in evaluating the proximal subclavian artery. **B,** An infraclavicular approach is needed for the evaluation of the mid portion of the subclavian artery and vein as they emerge from underneath the clavicle. **C,** The transducer is then displaced laterally along this infraclavicular window for further evaluation of the subclavian vein and artery as they migrate more laterally and become the axillary vein and artery, respectively.

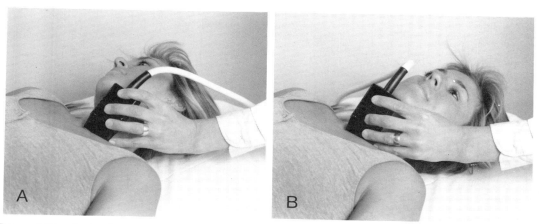

Figure 5.51. Evaluation of the junction of the proximal brachiocephalic vein can be quite difficult. **A,** The standard imaging position is shown here with the transducer in the supraclavicular window pointing toward the feet, almost parallel to the body. The head is slightly rotated away from the transducer. **B,** A slightly more difficult position for the patient to adopt is with the head turned slightly toward the transducer. This helps better visualize the origin of the brachiocephalic and the junction with both the internal jugular and the subclavian vein.

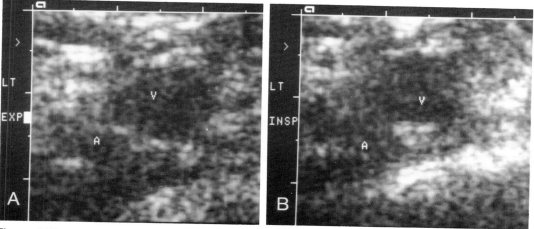

Figure 5.52. **A,** The normal response of the subclavian vein to deep inspiration is collapse of the wall. This image taken from the infraclavicular projection shows a normal resting of the vein (V). Notice that the vein lies superficial to the artery (A). **B,** During the inspiration there is no significant change in the diameter of the vein (V). The loss of this response is suggestive of a proximal obstruction within either the subclavian vein, the brachiocephalic vein, or the superior vena cava.

small or did not use a sufficient number of gold standard examinations (most often venography) to permit an accurate estimate of the sensitivity or specificity of the technique (Table 5.4). The accuracy of the technique is quite high in cases of sponta-

neous effort thrombosis and in instances where indwelling catheters are in place (Fig. 5.57). Concurrent obstruction due to a mediastinal process may sufficiently depress blood flow that the signals are difficult to detect by either color flow mapping

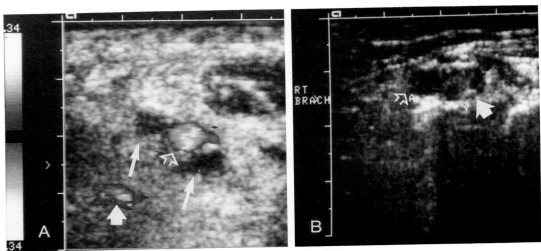

Figure 5.53. **A** (see color plate III), This transverse color Doppler image of the arm shows duplicated brachial veins lying to both sides (*arrows*) of the brachial artery (*open arrow*). Both veins are involved by acute venous thrombosis. Color signals are seen within the more medially located basilic vein (*large arrow*). **B,** This transverse image shows echogenic material within one of the two brachial veins (*arrow*). The other brachial vein has collapsed normally in response to the compression maneuver, whereas the artery (*open arrow*) is still clearly seen. Spontaneous thrombosis of the brachial vein is extremely rare. It is normally, as in this case, associated with the percutaneous placement of a venous catheter or intravenous line. It may also be due to the peripheral extension of a more central axillary or subclavian vein thrombosis.

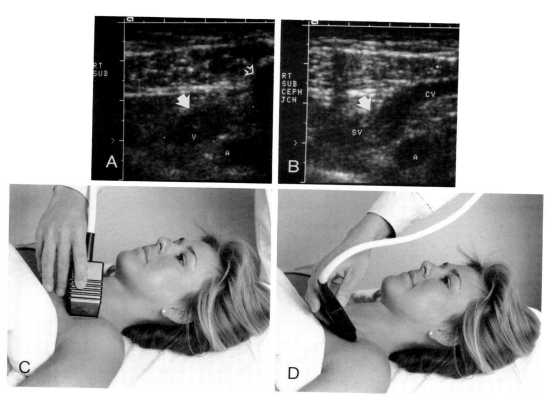

Figure 5.54.   The presence of deep vein thrombosis in the subclavian vein can also be ascertained using the compression maneuver. **A,** In this first image, a transverse projection taken from an infraclavicular projection shows the subclavian vein superficial to the artery. The edge of the clavicle is indicated by the *open arrow*. There is faintly echogenic noncompressible material within the vein. **B,** A longitudinal image taken at the same level shows the cephalic vein (*CV*) joining the axillary vein to become the subclavian vein (*SV*). Echogenic material is again seen within the vein (*arrow*). **C** and **D,** The corresponding projections were acquired in both the transverse (**C**) and the longitudinal (**D**) planes.

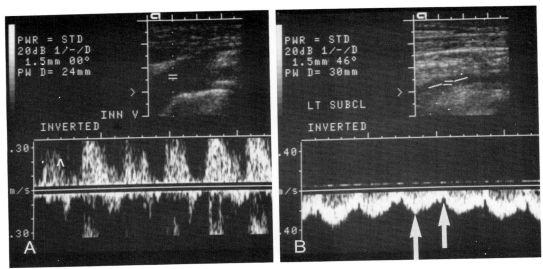

Figure 5.55. The flow signals transmitted within the brachiocephalic (**A**) and subclavian (**B**) veins reflect mostly changes in blood volumes secondary to cardiac activity (*arrows*). These are due to atrial contraction and a small amount of reflux during atrial contraction. The transmission of these signals can occur in most individuals into the subclavian vein system. Loss of these signals is suggestive of proximal obstructive process.

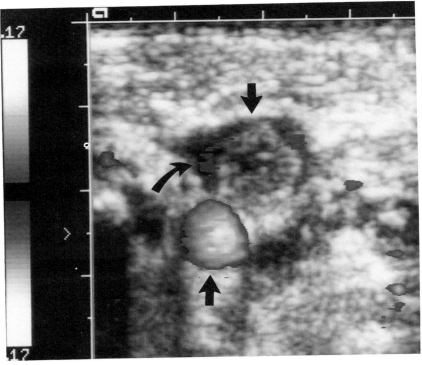

Figure 5.56. (see color plate III). Transverse images taken of the lower neck show a partly obstructing echogenic collection (*top arrow*) within the internal jugular vein. Faint signals are seen at the periphery of this subtotally occlusive thrombus (*curved arrow*). The common carotid artery lies deeper (*bottom arrow*).

Table 5.4.
Causes of Deep Venous Thrombosis of the Upper Extremity

Traumatic
Indwelling venous catheters
Intravenous irritants (radiographic contrast material, chemotherapeutic agents)
Clavicular or first rib fractures
Postoperative (chest wall, orthopedic, lymph node dissection)
Effort thrombosis
Thoracic outlet syndrome

Nontraumatic
Malignancy
Congestive heart failure
Extrinsic mediastinal venous obstruction
Idiopathic

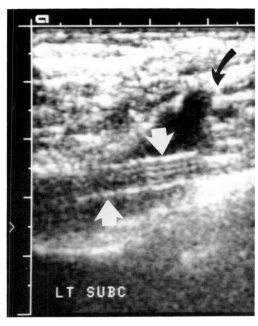

Figure 5.57. The sonographic appearance of the multiple-lumen Hickman catheter is shown in this oblique sonogram. The catheter is normally inserted in the subclavian vein just inferior to the clavicle and along the outer third of the vein. It is then advanced so that the tip lies in the superior vena cava. It consists of two parallel catheters, one shorter than the other. This geometry generates a reverberation artifact with multiple parallel lines (*arrows*) seen on the image. The catheter has been inserted at the level of the cephalic vein (*curved arrow*).

or duplex sonography. The sonographic examination can then easily overestimate the presence or extent of concurrent venous thrombosis within the proximal two-thirds of the subclavian.

SUGGESTED READINGS

Baldridge ED, Martin MA, Welling RE. Clinical significance of free-floating venous thrombi. J Vasc Surg 1990;11:62–69.

Barnes RW, Nix ML, Barnes CL, et al. Perioperative asymptomatic venous thrombosis: Role of duplex scanning versus venography. J Vasc Surg 1989;9:251–260.

Cheely R, McCartney WH, Perry JR, et al. The role of noninvasive tests versus pulmonary angiography in the diagnosis of pulmonary embolism. Am J Med 1981;70:17–22.

Comerota AJ, Katz ML, Greenwald LL, et al. Venous duplex imaging: should it replace hemodynamic tests for deep venous thrombosis? J Vasc Surg 1990;11:53–61.

Comerota AJ, Katz ML, Grossi RJ, et al. The comparative value of noninvasive testing for diagnosis and surveillance of deep vein thrombosis. J Vasc Surg 1988;7:40–49.

Cronan JJ, Leen V. Recurrent deep venous thrombosis: limitations of US. Radiology 1989;170:739–742.

Dismuke SE, Wagner EH. Pulmonary embolism as a cause of death. The changing mortality in hospitalized patients. JAMA 1986;255:2039–2042.

Dorfman GS, Cronan JJ, Tupper TB, Messersmith RN, Denny DF, Lee CH. Occult pulmonary embolism: a common occurrence in deep venous thrombosis. AJR 1987;148:263–266.

Foley WD, Middleton WD, Lawson TL, Erickson S, Quiroz FA, Macrander S. Color Doppler ultrasound imaging of lower-extremity venous disease. AJR 1989;152:371–376.

Husni EA, Williams WA. Superficial thrombophlebitis of lower limbs. Surgery 1982;91:70–74.

Kakkar VV, Howe CT, Flanc C, Clarke MB. Natural history of postoperative deep-vein thrombosis. Lancet 1969;2:230–232.

Krupski WC, Bass A, Dilley RB, Bernstein EF, Otis SM. Propagation of deep venous thrombosis identified by duplex ultrasonography. J Vasc Surg 1990;12:467–475.

Lagerstedt CI, Olsson CG, Fagher BO, Oqvist BW, Albrechtsson. Need for long-term anticoagulant treatment in symptomatic calf-vein thrombosis. Lancet 1985;2:515–518.

Liu GC, Ferris EJ, Reifsteck JR, Baker ME. Effect of anatomic variations on deep venous thrombosis of the lower extremity. AJR 1986;146:845–848.

Loring W. Venous thrombosis in the upper extremities as a complication of myocardial failure. Am J Med 1952;397–410.

Moser KM, LeMoine JR. Is embolic risk conditioned by location of deep venous thrombosis? Ann Intern Med 1981;94:439–444.

Prescott SM, Tikoff G. Deep venous thrombosis of the upper extremity: a reappraisal. Circulation 1979;59:350–355.

Sevitt S, Gallagher N. Venous thrombosis and pulmonary embolism: a clinico-pathological study in injured and burned patients. Br J Surg 1961;48:475–489.

Skillman JJ, Kent KC, Porter DH, Kim D. Simultaneous occurrence of superficial and deep thrombophlebitis in the lower extremity. J Vasc Surg 1990;11:818–824.

Thomas ML, O'Dwyer JA. Site of origin of deep vein thrombus in the calf. Acta Radiol Diagn 1977;18:418–424.

Wright DJ, Shepard AD, McPharlin M, Ernst CB. Pitfalls in lower extremity venous duplex scanning. J Vasc Surg 1990;11:675–679.

CHAPTER SIX

Chronic Venous Thrombosis and Venous Insufficiency

Chronic Deep Venous Thrombosis

The prevalence of chronic deep vein thrombosis is largely unknown. It is likely that the vast majority of patients who have had symptomatic deep vein thrombosis have some form of residual damage to the vein wall or to the venous valves. Significant numbers of these patients are likely to return to the noninvasive laboratory. They present with chronic complaints such as leg swelling and also with clinically suspected DVT, since one of the greatest risk factors for deep vein thrombosis is a previous episode of deep vein thrombosis. The changes in both vein anatomy and function caused by the previous episode of DVT can be quite confusing. The time required to perform the sonographic examination is often increased. Patients with a previous episode of asymptomatic deep vein thrombosis are less likely to show any evidence of chronic changes in the deep and superficial veins. This is presumably due to the contained nature of the nonobstructive thrombosis that has occurred in the vast majority of these cases. In addition to anatomic changes, there are significant functional changes that develop sub-sequent to an episode of acute DVT leading to valvar incompetence and venous insufficiency (Fig. 6.1). This topic is discussed in the second section of this chapter.

The major concern for the sonographer is the possible confusion between the changes due to a current acute episode of deep venous thrombosis and the more chronic changes secondary to the healing process that has occurred following a previous episode. Differentiating between the two is often not possible in one session. In case of doubt, venography can be used to give supplemental information. In general, however, the findings of the venographic examination need to be combined with the results of the sonographic examination. Another approach is to perform a repeat examination, since chronic DVT is unlikely to change over a few days.

ANATOMY

The healing process that affects the deep vein does so in a diffuse fashion. Even if complete lysis of the venous thrombus is achieved, residual trauma to the endothelial cells of the vein wall may cause a hyperplastic response. This thickening is similar to the intimal hyperplastic

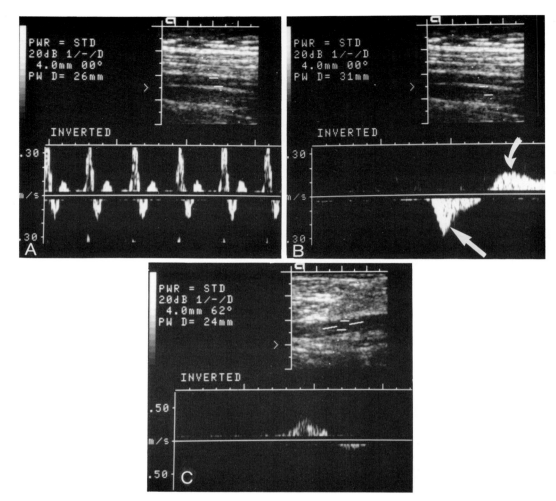

Figure 6.1. The deep veins can be evaluated for the presence of incompetence in the same way as the superficial system. **A,** The Doppler gate is first positioned over the artery accompanying the deep vein. This documents the location of the vein and confirms the direction of blood flow. **B,** The gate is then moved over the vein. Reflux is diagnosed whenever reverse flow (*curved arrow*) follows venous augmentation (*arrow*). **C,** The superficial system (greater and lesser saphenous veins) is also evaluated. This step is taken since venous incompetence of the deep veins will often lead to compromised function of the perforators and then of the superficial veins. In this case, the greater saphenous vein was competent.

response seen following arterial wall injury. In general, however, the proliferation is manifested as a diffuse thickening of the vein wall extending into the lumen at the site of previous thrombus deposition (Fig. 6.2). Sonographic imaging cannot easily be used to differentiate between the early phase of resorbing thrombus and the later development of a true hyperplastic response. The echogenicity is often similar to that of an acute thrombus, although the fibrous nature of the resorbing thrombus does cause some increased echogenicity (Fig. 6.3). Thrombus resorption takes place due to two major physiological mechanisms. The first is actual lysis of the throm-

ACUTE DVT

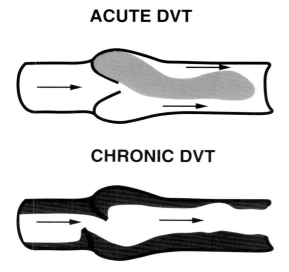

CHRONIC DVT

Figure 6.2. Differentiation of a segment affected by chronic DVT from one with acute DVT is aided by images taken parallel to the affected vein. The nonobstructing thrombus will tend to adhere to one wall and to have blood flow around it. Chronic DVT tends to affect the walls of the vein in an almost circumferential fashion. Blood flow takes place in the center of the lumen. It is very difficult to distinguish these two entities on the basis of one examination only. A repeat examination a few days later can be used to confirm significant acute DVT, since the latter is likely to have spread.

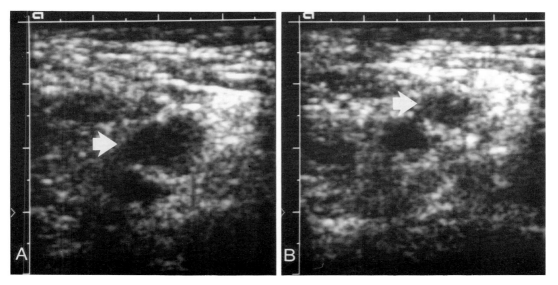

Figure 6.3. The diffuse neointima that forms in venous segments previously involved by acute DVT may cause diagnostic difficulties. **A,** In this first transverse image a normal-caliber popliteal vein (*arrow*) is clearly seen beside the artery. The vein has a slight amount of echogenic structure within it. **B,** The second transverse image obtained during compression shows that the vein (*arrow*) fails to collapse. The differential diagnosis should include a nonobstructing acute deep vein thrombosis or evidence of chronic deep vein thrombosis—a healed episode of DVT. Differentiating between the two can be quite difficult. The use of phlebography may help clarify the diagnosis. Serial sonographic examinations performed over the next few days will likely show spread if the finding corresponds to an acutely evolving DVT. Color Doppler may help verify the chronic nature of these changes in the vein wall, since combined longitudinal and transverse images may clearly show their circumferential distribution. A possible limitation to this approach is the possibility of acute DVT in a vein with chronic changes. For this reason we favor the use of repeat sonographic examinations repeated once, and on occasion twice, at 2- to 3-day intervals.

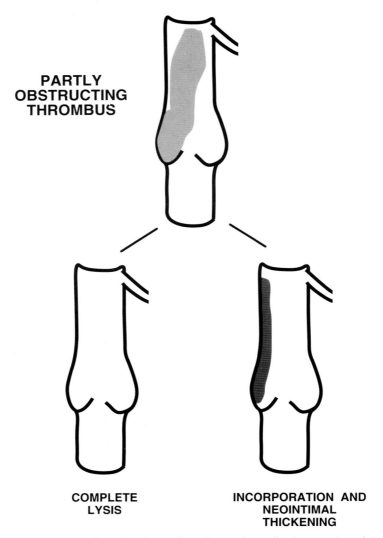

Figure 6.4. Partly obstructing thrombosis has less damaging effects on valvar function than obstructing DVT. In general, the thrombus will either be completely resorbed or will be incorporated into the vein wall. Most patients have a combination of obstructive and nonobstructive thrombi in different venous segments. As such, they are likely to have some residual changes in some of the involved venous segments.

bus. This is the most important factor affecting the ultimate appearance of the residual thrombus (Fig. 6.4). The size of the thrombus, its obstructive or nonobstructive nature, and the amount of regional blood flow affect the rate of lysis. Nonobstructing thrombus in a high-flow venous channel is more likely to resorb quickly. Fully obstructing thrombus in a

duplicated superficial femoral vein is likely to persist for a much longer amount of time. The rate of lysis is a function of the exposure of local lytic agents such as plasmin with the elements of the clot matrix. The larger the surface area of exposure, the faster the lytic process takes place. The second mechanism responsible for clot resorption is a fibroelastic response similar

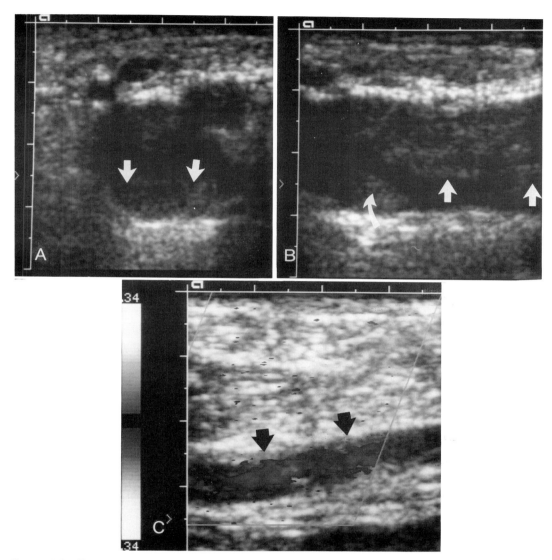

Figure 6.5. The chronic thickening of the vein wall is sometimes difficult to clearly visualize in the smaller-caliber veins of the leg. **A,** This transverse image of the common femoral vein of a patient with a previous episode of DVT shows a diffuse thickening of the vein wall (*arrows*). The appearance, although suggestive of chronic DVT, might still represent acute DVT. **B,** The longitudinal image shows that the vein wall is affected on both sides (*arrows*), while the lumen is free of obstruction. A valve has been incorporated (*curved arrow*) in this diffuse process. **C** (see color plate IV), The more typical appearance of chronic deep vein thrombosis during augmented flow is preferential distribution of color signals to the center of the lumen (*arrows*). Both walls of the popliteal vein are thickened consistent with the presence of neointima formation secondary to the previous episode of acute deep vein thrombosis.

to scarring. The earliest manifestation of this process is the early adherence of the partly obstructing thrombus to the wall of the veins. This attachment is normally achieved by seven days. Following this, there is a neovascular response arising in the vein wall and a fibrous transformation of the adherent thrombus. This process continues for months. It accounts for the increased echogenic appearance of the thrombus. Superimposed on this process is return of the endothelium to the surface occupied by the thrombus (Fig. 6.5).

PATTERNS AND DIAGNOSTIC CRITERIA

The presence of very small venous channels in the expected location of a vein is a common finding following an episode of obstructive DVT (Fig. 6.6). These correspond either to partially reopened native venous segments, to small channels of the vena venorum of the affected vein that have enlarged in time, or to small parallel collateral channels that have developed in response to the adjacent obstruction (Fig. 6.7). These channels may be hard to visualize with the patient supine. Having him or her sit up will distend them slightly more and make them easier to perceive. The native vein often has developed such scarring that it may not even be visualized.

Another typical presentation is that of a small vein whose diameter is less than expected (Fig. 6.8). A parallel collateral is often seen. The small vein often has evidence of wall thickening, which is more easily perceived while imaging parallel to the axis of the vein. The thickening most

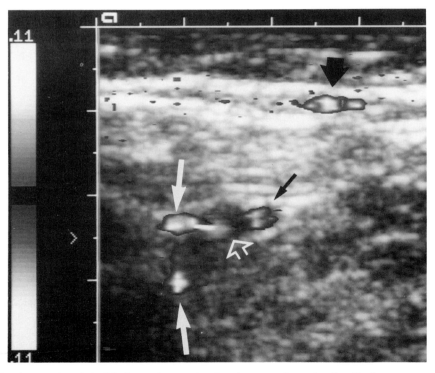

Figure 6.6. (see color plate IV). A previous episode of venous thrombosis will often cause a change in the pattern and distribution of flow within the deep and superficial venous system. The greater saphenous vein has increased flow signals within it (*arrow*). There are multiple collaterals (*long arrows*) around the superficial femoral artery (*open arrow*).

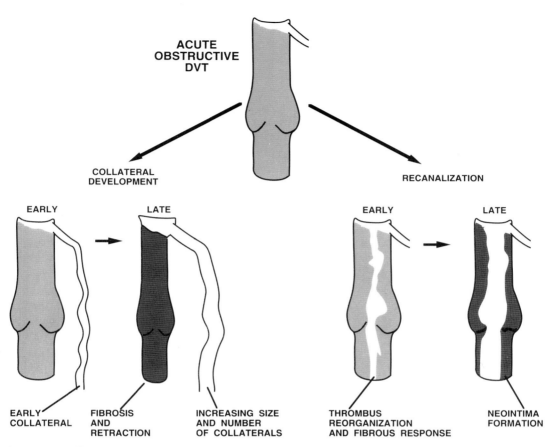

Figure 6.7. The outcome of obstructive deep vein thrombosis varies from individual to individual and is difficult to predict. One scenario is the development of collaterals capable of taking up most of the blood flow returning from the leg. The thrombosed segment is then likely to scar down and heal by fibrosis rather than recanalize. Another scenario is the early recanalization of the obstructed lumen. In the later stages, this leads to a thickened neointima in the vein wall. Valve function is likely to remain compromised. Complete recanalization is seen in up to 50% of affected segments. This is more likely if the original thrombus was partly obstructing.

likely represents a mixture of a hyperplastic response of the endothelium and some residual thrombus that is becoming incorporated into the wall during the scarring (fibroblastic) response.

Finally, an almost normal-appearing vein can be seen by sonography. The presence of a previous episode of DVT can then be suspected only if adjacent venous segments show the changes described above or if there has been good documentation of a previous episode of acute thrombosis.

Differentiation between acute and chronic DVT is difficult. There are, however, some simple rules that help make this distinction in the majority of cases. For example, an acute obstructing DVT normally distends the vein, while in chronic DVT, the vein lumen is small. In acute nonobstructing DVT, flow of blood is normally around the thrombus. The thrombus is also often eccentric, with a larger portion anchoring it to one of the vein walls. In chronic DVT, flow of blood is directed toward the center of the lumen since the

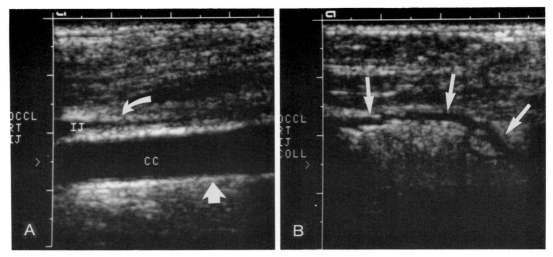

Figure 6.8. The vein affected by an episode of acute DVT does not always recanalize. **A,** In this longitudinal image, the mid common carotid artery (*arrow*) lies beneath an internal jugular vein that tapers abruptly (*curved arrow*). **B,** Farther down, at the level of the distal common carotid and internal jugular vein, only small venous collateral branches are seen (*arrows*). This patient had a previous catheter-related thrombosis of the internal jugular vein. Instead of completely or partially recanalizing, the vein remained occluded and small collateral branches developed. In our experience, upper-extremity venous thromboses are more likely to cause a permanent occlusion of the vein, while recanalization is more common in the lower extremity.

INCIDENCE OF POST-PHLEBITIC SYMPTOMS

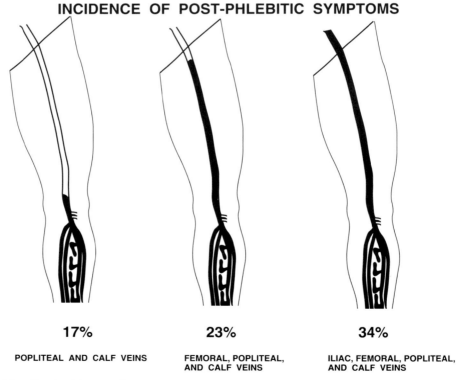

17%

POPLITEAL AND CALF VEINS

23%

FEMORAL, POPLITEAL, AND CALF VEINS

34%

ILIAC, FEMORAL, POPLITEAL, AND CALF VEINS

Figure 6.9. The incidence of post-phlebitic symptoms is related to the extent of previous episodes of deep vein thrombosis. These symptoms become manifest a few years following the acute inciting episode. The more extensive involvement of the iliac and femoral veins shows a higher incidence of chronic symptoms of leg swelling and skin discoloration. This decreases somewhat when only the

thickened mildly echogenic material of the hyperplastic intima often involves the circumference of the vessel.

DIAGNOSTIC STRATEGY

In cases where ultrasound cannot definitely confirm that acute DVT is present, phlebography remains an important additional investigation. This additional step may be necessary when patients present acutely and more aggressive intervention is being considered. This is likely in a patient who is thought to be sending pulmonary emboli from a source in the leg but who also has a contraindication to anticoagulation.

If there is no need for acute intervention, serial monitoring of the extremity may help differentiate between acute and chronic DVT. Repeat ultrasound by day 3 following the first examination often helps differentiate between an acute process and evidence of previous DVT. Acute DVT will normally show change and spread, especially if anticoagulation has been withheld. Chronic DVT should show no change. Even if an acute thrombus is misclassified as a chronic one, the fact that the thrombus remains stable over the next 3 days suggests that is unlikely to spread.

RECOMMENDATIONS

Changes in the sonographic appearance of the vein can persist in up to to 50% of patients 2 years after the acute event. Repeat ultrasound can help document the baseline appearance of the veins and may prove quite useful, given that a high proportion of patients with a previous episode of DVT go on to have another episode.

Longitudinal and transaxial imaging should be used to study the appearance of the veins. If needed, a venographic study is often useful in differentiating between acute and chronic DVT. Finally, serial sonography in selected cases may help to confirm that the changes seen are stable and are not due to developing thrombus.

Venous Insufficiency
INCIDENCE AND CLINICAL IMPORTANCE

The incidence of venous insufficiency is even more difficult to estimate than that of deep vein thrombosis or pulmonary embolism. The symptoms are often insidious and chronic and manifest as leg swelling, pain, and skin changes. The prevalence of the problem in the general population is close to 3%. In the lower extremity, venous insufficiency may be secondary to a defect in vein valve function or evolve as a sequela of deep venous thrombosis (Fig. 6.9). Venous insufficiency ultimately leads to chronic elevations of the interstitial pressures in the lower leg. The basic malfunction is an inability of the venous system to clear blood volume from the veins of the lower leg, specifically from the calf, and for blood to pool in the veins. Although it is standard practice to consider superficial vein insufficiency and deep vein insufficiency as separate entities, both often coexist. Pooling of blood in the superficial veins causes distention and exacerbates the effect of faulty valves. It also impairs clearance of blood and decreases the efficiency of the calf pump (Fig. 6.10), exposing the soft tissues to chronic elevations of pressure (Fig. 6.11).

---

femoral veins have been involved. The relationship with calf vein DVT is not as clear cut. Patients who are examined for suspected calf vein DVT but who are shown to have a negative phlebographic examination still have close to a 10% incidence of post-phlebitic symptoms. It is unclear what the etiology of this problem is. There is an estimated doubling in the likelihood that symptoms will appear if there is a documented episode of calf vein DVT.

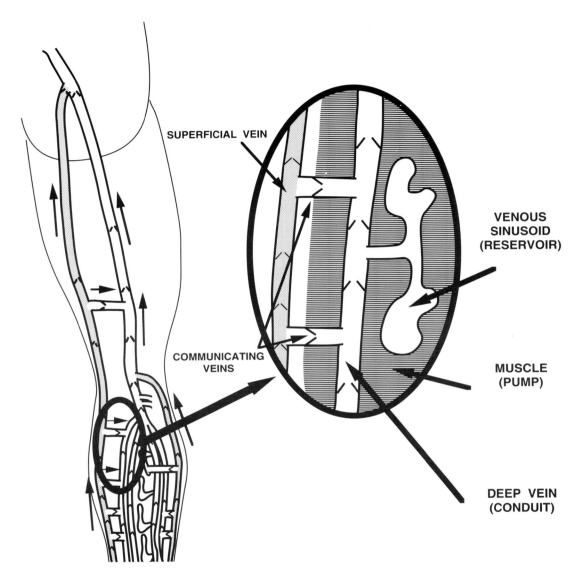

Figure 6.10. The communicating or perforating veins permit blood flow from the superficial veins into the deep veins. A series of valves acts as an anti-reflux mechanism to prevent flow from the deep into the superficial system. The muscular venous sinus, the deep veins, and a portion of the perforators are located within the deep compartment of the calf. This constitutes the calf pump mechanism.

Superficial venous insufficiency often comes to the attention of the patient or physician when distended superficial venous channels dilate. These varicose veins are normally treated for cosmetic reasons. However, there is another important reason for detecting and treating them early.

The passive distention of the superficial venous channels and the development of varicosities where large volumes of blood can pool will ultimately lead to a malfunction of the deep vein system through persistently elevated pressures and distention at the level of the perforating veins that communicate between the deep and superficial venous system (Fig. 6.12). Once this occurs, the deep system becomes subjected to chronic and persistent elevations in pressure. This then leads to distention and the increased likelihood of additional damage to the venous valve mechanism by distention of the supporting valve ring.

Valves fail to function normally and local reflux increases. This can progress and, by involvement of a larger number of venous segments, worsen the severity and extent of the symptoms.

Deep venous insufficiency is often caused by a previous episode of deep vein thrombosis (Fig. 6.13). At most, 60% of patients

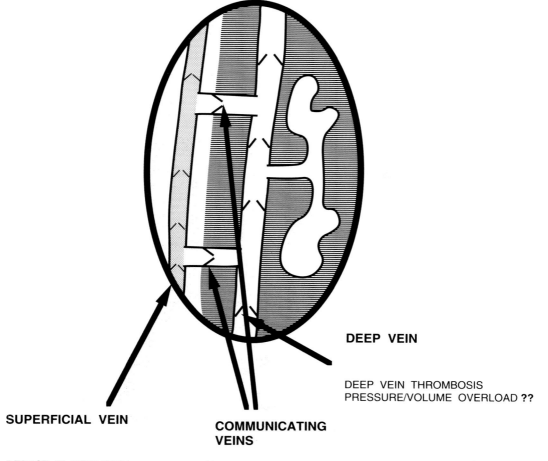

DEEP VEIN

DEEP VEIN THROMBOSIS
PRESSURE/VOLUME OVERLOAD **??**

SUPERFICIAL VEIN

COMMUNICATING VEINS

DEFECT IN VEIN WALL
PRESSURE/VOLUME OVERLOAD
TRAUMA
SUPERFICIAL PHLEBITIS

PRESSURE/VOLUME OVERLOAD
DEEP VEIN THROMBOSIS

Figure 6.11. The various mechanisms thought to be responsible for venous insufficiency are summarized in this diagram. The deep and perforating veins are more likely to have been damaged following an episode of acute DVT, while an inherent weakness in the superficial vein wall accounts for most cases of superficial vein insufficiency. We have occasionally seen cases of combined superficial and perforator vein insufficiency with sparing of the deep veins. This suggests that superficial insufficiency may lead to perforator valve dysfunction, at least in the more chronic cases.

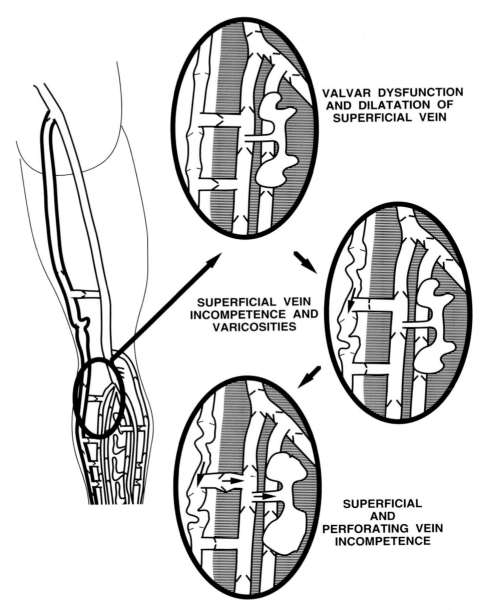

**VALVAR DYSFUNCTION
AND DILATATION OF
SUPERFICIAL VEIN**

**SUPERFICIAL VEIN
INCOMPETENCE AND
VARICOSITIES**

**SUPERFICIAL
AND
PERFORATING VEIN
INCOMPETENCE**

Figure 6.12. This diagram summarizes a potential pathway for combined superficial and perforator vein dysfunction. Superficial venous insufficiency develops because of an inherent weakness in the vein wall leading to vein valve dysfunction. With time, the chronic elevations in volume cause increased distention of the perforators and some dysfunction of their valves. This need not cause dysfunction of the deep draining veins. Instead, the perforator vein permits the exchange of blood with the muscular venous sinusoid, which is devoid of any valve. This is the source of additional symptoms and exacerbates the superficial venous insufficiency. It is unclear whether this situation can progress to affect valve function of the deep draining veins.

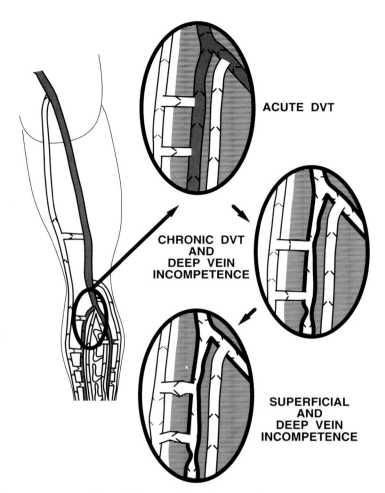

Figure 6.13. The common pathway in the evolution to a combined pattern of superficial and deep vein insufficiency is shown here. A previous episode of deep vein thrombosis compromises deep venous valve function. Either the perforating vein valves are involved in the original episode of DVT or they become incompetent following chronic exposure to elevated distending pressures. The dysfunction of the perforators leads to chronic volume overload of the superficial veins, causing wall distention and ultimately valve dysfunction.

with obvious clinical venous insufficiency give a history of previous deep vein thrombosis. The reflux that then occurs is most likely due to direct damage to the valvar mechanism following the episode of DVT. Five to six years following an acute episode of DVT with extensive involvement of the femoral and popliteal veins, up to 75% of patients will have symptoms of venous insufficiency. Patients whose thrombosis affected only the calf veins

have a 20% chance of developing symptoms. During the healing phase of an acute vein thrombosis, there is an early transient interval of 1 to 2 months when up to 50% of venous segments show valve dysfunction. Valve function can remain compromised with 25% of segments showing venous reflux 3 to 6 months following the acute episode of DVT.

It is clear that the common mechanism responsible for the presence of venous insufficiency is vein valve dysfunction. An inherent weakness of the valve mechanism may cause failure of the bicuspid leaflets to coapt. Chronic elevation of intraabdominal pressures during pregnancy may cause transient dysfunction of the superficial venous system. Redistribution of blood flow in response to vein obstruction that has been only partly relieved by the development of collaterals following deep vein thrombosis is also an inciting factor for deep valve dysfunction. Scarring of the valve leaflets is the likely explanation for deep vein insufficiency following acute DVT. The co-existence of superficial and deep vein insufficiency is likely due to the development of valve dysfunction in the communicating channels between the superficial and deep veins. Venous insufficiency of the deep veins can, with time, cause the perforating veins to become incompetent. This will transmit increased volume to the superficial system and start a process of vein distention and the development of varicosities and cause dysfunction of the valve mechanism. Conversely, chronic dysfunction of the superficial system can only affect the deep veins once the integrity of perforating vein valves has been compromised. The increased pressure and blood volume cause the vein valves in these perforators to malfunction. Reflux then occurs back and forth into the deep system of the calf, compromising calf pump function.

ANATOMY

Deep Venous Valves

The number and distribution of the venous valves within the iliac, femoral, and popliteal veins vary from individual to individual. In the iliac vein, there may be one valve in the external iliac in up to 33% of cases. There is a common femoral vein valve in up to 75% of patients. There is almost always a valve in the superficial femoral vein just beyond the origin of the

profunda femoris vein and one in the upper third of the popliteal vein just below the distal end of the adductor canal. The number in the superficial femoral vein can vary from one to four. The popliteal has, in general, two valves near the knee joint. The tibial and peroneal veins have, considering their length, a much greater density of valves. There is in general a valve every 1 to 3 cm. The draining veins that communicate with the soleal and gastrocnemius venous plexi have valves as well. However, the muscular veins themselves are without valves.

Superficial Veins

The greater saphenous is the major draining vein running from the common femoral to the medial malleolus of the ankle. It normally splits into two major trunks proximally in the thigh: the anterolateral and the posteromedial branches.

The lesser saphenous runs from the popliteal posteriorly in the calf to the lateral malleolus.

Perforating Veins

There exist communicating veins between the superficial venous system (e.g., the greater and lesser saphenous veins) and the deep veins of the leg (e.g., the superficial femoral, the popliteal, and the tibioperoneal veins) (Fig. 6.14). They contain valves that are arranged so that blood flows from the superficial system into the deep system. These perforating veins are seen at specific levels in the thigh and calf. There is normally one in the mid thigh. It penetrates through the fascia around the sartorius muscle (Hunter's canal) and joins the greater saphenous to the superficial femoral veins. In the calf, there are two major groups of perforating veins. The first group is located medially. A vein communicates between the greater saphenous and the posterior tibial vein approximately 10 cm below the knee. Lower down, a

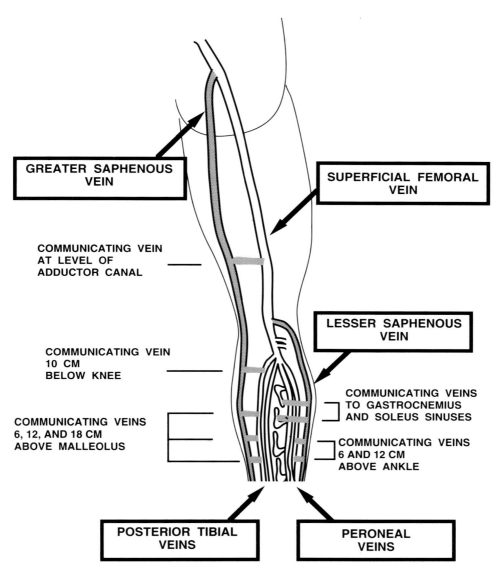

Figure 6.14. The anatomic connection between the deep and superficial venous systems is ensured by a series of communicating veins, also called perforators. The approximate number and location of these veins is shown here, from a posterior view of a right lower extremity.

grouping of three veins is normally located 5 to 6 cm above the medial malleolus. They communicate between the posterior tibial veins and a more posterior arch branch of the greater saphenous vein. A second set of veins is located on the lateral aspect of the leg. A lateral communicating vein nor- mally connects the peroneal vein to the lesser saphenous in the lower third of the calf. At the same level, two more posteriorly located veins often join the lesser saphenous to the peroneal veins either directly or through side branches to the soleal or gastrocnemius veins.

Function

The valves of the veins arise from a collagen ring and are themselves composed of collagen. They are bicuspid. Congenital absence of the venous valves is very rare. These patients will have chronic venous insufficiency.

The mechanism most often responsible for valve dysfunction is passive dilatation of the valve ring. This can occur in response to prolonged elevations of venous pressures. The vein wall, which dilates in response to pressure elevation and the increased volume of blood, pulls on the valve ring that is anchored to it. The valve leaflets then lose the ability to coapt their surfaces and to prevent reflux. This mechanism is likely to affect the superficial veins. These are not supported by the surrounding subcutaneous tissues and are more likely to distend in response to elevated pressures. The deep veins are surrounded by muscles and a matrix of organized fascia and are less likely to distend. Valvar dysfunction need not be permanent. During pregnancy, the combination of chronic elevation of intraabdominal pressure and the release of hormones, which causes loss of strength of the collagen matrix, often causes transient superficial vein insufficiency. These changes will reverse at least in part following delivery.

The deep veins are surrounded by muscles and supporting fascia. These supporting structures limit the veins' ability to distend. The amount of pressure necessary to cause reflux of these valves is much greater than for the superficial system. A likely explanation for the development of deep vein insufficiency is direct damage to the valve following an episode of DVT. The valve cusps are damaged in one of two ways. Either they are incorporated into the recanalization process or they become part of the fibrointimal thickening of the vein wall. Even if there is complete lysis of thrombus, the leaflets may remain thickened and contracted due to scarring. The leaflets then lose their ability to coapt.

The valves within the perforating veins permit blood flow only from the superficial system into the deeper veins. This simple physiological fact explains the coexistence

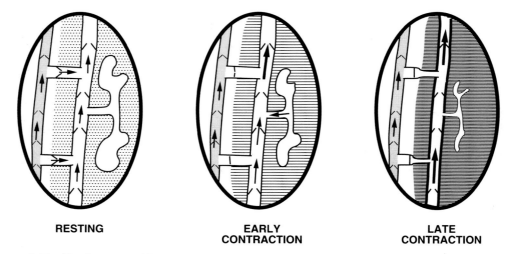

RESTING **EARLY CONTRACTION** **LATE CONTRACTION**

Figure 6.15. The integrity of the perforating veins ensures proper function of the calf pump. Drainage of the superficial venous blood takes place at rest during the relaxation phase. The anti-reflux mechanism of the perforator vein valves prevents blood from being expulsed from the high-pressure deep calf venous blood into the superficial low-pressure system.

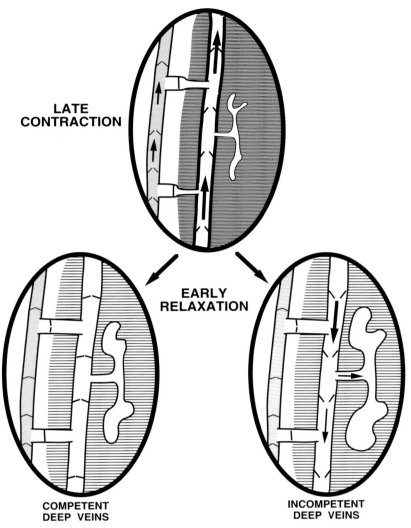

LATE CONTRACTION

EARLY RELAXATION

COMPETENT DEEP VEINS

INCOMPETENT DEEP VEINS

Figure 6.16. The action of the calf pump is to promote venous return from veins within the muscles of the calf as well as from the veins draining the skin. Under normal circumstances, contraction of the calf pump empties both systems. With competent deep veins, the blood volume slowly increases through continued antegrade arterial inflow. If the deep veins are incompetent, there will be reflux of blood and continued congestion of the calf veins.

of superficial and deep vein insufficiency. The valves of the deep venous system act as a series of locks that prevent reflux of blood down the leg (Fig. 6.15). If the patient stays immobile, flow is consistently going through from the artery, arterioles, capillaries, venules, and veins. Pressures are equal and the valves are open. It is following forced emptying of a portion of

the blood volume within the calf veins that the function of the deep venous valve becomes apparent (Fig. 6.16). Use of the calf muscles (or muscle pump) causes, during contraction, emptying of a good part of the venous blood pool. Following this, there is a decrease in pressure in the vein lumen—in fact, almost a suction effect. This draws blood from the superficial system and aids

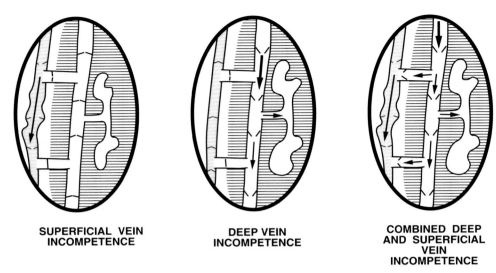

SUPERFICIAL VEIN INCOMPETENCE   DEEP VEIN INCOMPETENCE   COMBINED DEEP AND SUPERFICIAL VEIN INCOMPETENCE

Figure 6.17. Venous insufficiency can be caused by one of the mechanisms shown here. The first depicts reflux limited to the superficial venous system alone. This is normally associated with superficial varicosities. The perforators are competent. The second is isolated deep vein reflux. This is most often the sequela of a previous episode of acute DVT. The deep venous valves are damaged during the healing phase. The superficial and perforator vein valves remain intact. The third is a combination of both superficial and deep vein insufficiency. This is likely the end result of a previous episode of DVT that involved both the deep and the perforator vein valves.

forward flow from the capillaries and venules. This helps to reduce the interstitial pressure in the lower leg. If this mechanism fails due to a persistently distended vein or to reflux downward from the more proximal incompetent segments of the vein, the flow of blood within the superficial system (which drains the skin and subcutaneous tissues) and the deep venules is decreased. There is no temporary decrease in the venous pressure (Fig. 6.17). This chronic pressure elevation causes a buildup of fluid in the interstitial tissues of the lower leg. This can then progress to more chronic changes, skin pigmentation, skin atrophy, and actual ulceration.

PATTERNS AND DIAGNOSTIC CRITERIA

Our normal screening procedure for evaluating a patient with venous insufficiency is performed as follows (Fig. 6.18): The deep system is first imaged with the patient supine or partly sitting to evaluate the presence and extent of changes due to previous episodes of venous thrombosis. The greater saphenous vein is then followed with the transducer held transverse and rotating the leg outward. The patient may be asked to bend the knee so that the proximal lesser saphenous vein, which arises from the mid or distal popliteal vein, can be evaluated (Fig. 6.19). The patient is asked to perform a Valsalva maneuver and the sonographer squeezes the thigh proximal to the site of Doppler measurements. Flow down the leg is considered abnormal. Color may be used with the transducer held perpendicular or parallel to the vein. Duplex sonography is performed parallel to the vein (Fig. 6.19).

For more elaborate evaluations of the pattern and possible sites of reflux, the examination is performed with the patient standing and putting most of his or her weight on the leg not being examined. The Doppler gate is positioned over the same

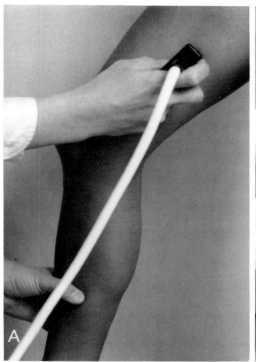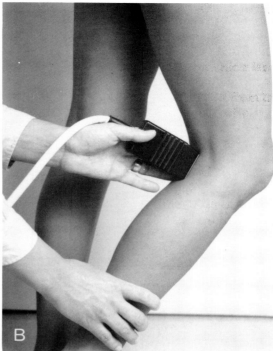

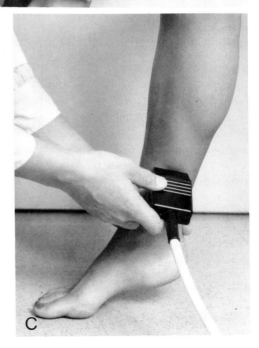

Figure 6.18. The deep venous system is normally evaluated for the presence of either acute or chronic deep vein thrombosis using standard imaging approaches. An assessment is then made of valvar function. The evaluation of the superficial as well as the deeper veins for venous insufficiency is best performed with the patient standing and instructed not to put weight on the extremity being examined. **A,** The course of the greater saphenous vein is then followed with the ultrasound transducer. Either color Doppler or a Doppler gate placed over the greater saphenous vein is used to sample velocity signals during the performance of venous augmentation by squeezing the lower calf. **B,** Evaluation of the lesser saphenous vein is performed with the transducer positioned posteriorly from its origin in the popliteal vein all the way down its course as it slowly migrates laterally to lie anterior to the lateral malleolus of the ankle. **C,** Transverse imaging is often useful for the evaluation of the perforating veins. These are searched for at their typical locations at the inner and outer aspects of the lower calf and at the inner aspect of the thigh. The free hand is used to perform the venous augmentation maneuver by squeezing either distal or proximal to the location of the transducer.

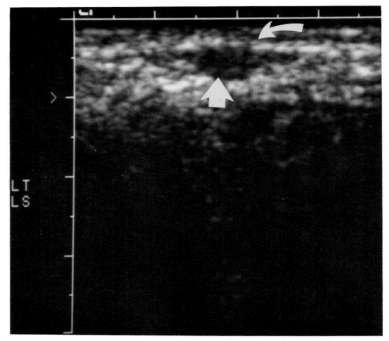

Figure 6.19.   The lesser saphenous vein (*arrow*) is difficult to follow. It can easily be confused with a sural vein at its origin from the popliteal vein. It then courses deep to the fascia (*curved arrow*) for a variable distance down the calf. In the majority of patients it has emerged from the fascia and lies quite superficial at the level of the mid calf. It courses more laterally and can then be easily lost from the gray-scale image since it is easily collapsed by the transducer during imaging. Two sets of perforators communicate with it in the lower calf.

sites mentioned above. This time, the free hand of the operator squeezes the calf. Following venous augmentation, there should not be any significant reflux of blood. A short reflux of blood is often noted (Fig. 6.20). This is normally due to the smaller amount associated with closure of the venous valve and filling of venous channels that do not contain valves (Fig. 6.21). Persistent reflux for more than 1 second is considered to be abnormal. The level of the reflux can then be mapped out.

Sonography is easily used to confirm the diagnosis of superficial venous insufficiency (Fig. 6.22). Although the presence of varicosities is often manifested clinically, sonographic real-time imaging can help document the size and extent of the

dilated venous channels (Fig. 6.23). Duplex sonography and color Doppler imaging can then be used to document the pattern of flow. The presence of a congenital AV fistula is part of the differential diagnosis of distended venous channels. However, these will contain high-velocity flow signals, whereas varicose veins contain relatively stagnant blood. Reflux is documented in the superficial system by using the same maneuvers used for the deep system. Although an examination of the superficial venous system is of interest by itself, the most important contribution of sonography is in documenting the extent of the reflux and in confirming the absence of coexistent deep vein reflux and perforating vein dysfunction (Fig. 6.24).

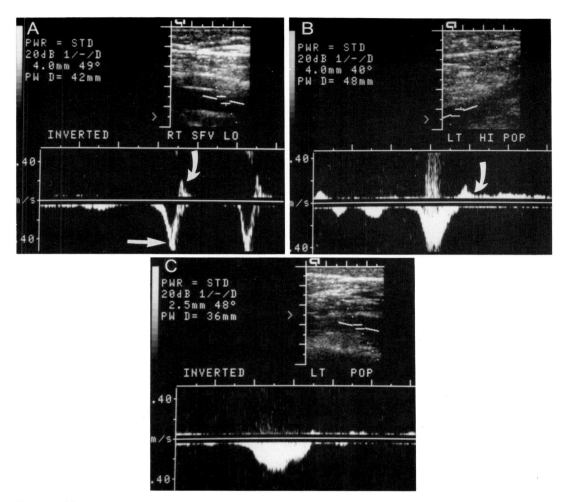

Figure 6.20. A normal amount of reflux is normally present in the larger-caliber superficial femoral vein and can also be seen in the proximal popliteal vein. **A,** The Doppler gate has been positioned over the distal superficial femoral–proximal popliteal vein. Following augmentation (*arrow*), there is a very brief period of reflux (*curved arrow*). This is believed to be caused by the amount of blood necessary to close the open venous valves. This effect can be very pronounced in the common femoral or proximal superficial femoral veins of certain individuals. The greater the distance between the venous valves and the greater the caliber of the vein, the more pronounced the transient reflux. **B,** The Doppler gate is now positioned over the proximal popliteal vein. Here again, a small amount of reflux is seen but it persists a bit longer (*curved arrow*). The blood that has been evacuated during venous augmentation is now refilling the muscular veins proximal to a venous valve. This effect has been accentuated since the patient has voluntarily stopped contracting the calf muscles. **C,** The lower popliteal vein communicates distally with the paired draining veins of the calf. They have innumerable valves, which are closely spaced. The physiological reflux necessary for valve closure is barely perceived on the Doppler spectrum.

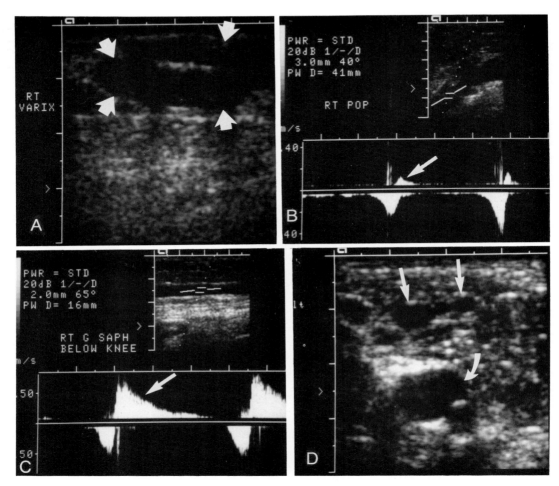

Figure 6.21. Doppler sonography can be used to comprehensively evaluate the venous system of patients with suspected venous insufficiency. **A,** A varix can easily be distended by having the patient stand upright. This patient had a localized varix (*arrows*) that was easily seen on a gray-scale image of the calf. **B,** The proximal popliteal vein was evaluated for the presence of reflux. The valvar mechanism is intact with only a small amount of physiological reflux being present (*arrow*). **C,** Evaluation of the greater saphenous vein showed pathological reflux (*arrow*). **D,** The sural veins (*arrows*) communicate directly with the popliteal vein (*curved arrow*). A small amount of blood will normally reflux into them from the popliteal vein following the venous augmentation maneuver and is partly responsible for the physiological reflux shown in **B**.

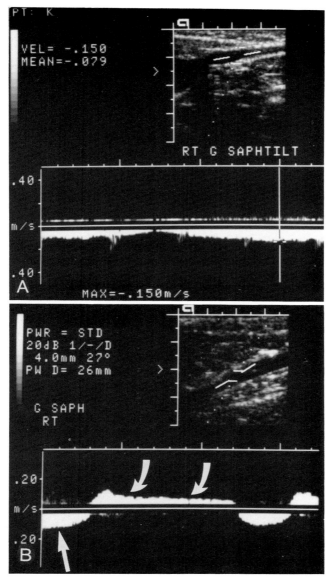

Figure 6.22. **A,** The normal flow pattern in the greater saphenous vein is quite variable. In this patient, blood flow velocity is of lower amplitude but similar to that seen in the femoral veins. The normal respiratory phasicity is clearly superimposed on the constant low-velocity waveform. In many individuals, blood flow will often be barely detectable. **B,** The normal response to an augmentation maneuver with the patient upright is to see an increased amplitude in the velocity coincident with the squeezing of blood from the muscular venous sinuses. In this patient with superficial venous insufficiency, the squeezing of blood from the leg veins has caused a greater amplitude in the velocity of returning blood (*arrow*) in the greater saphenous vein. This should be followed by either absent or low-velocity signals due to a decrease in the amount of returning blood. In this patient, flow reverses (*curved arrow*) for a period of 2 seconds. This is diagnostic of superficial vein reflux (insufficiency).

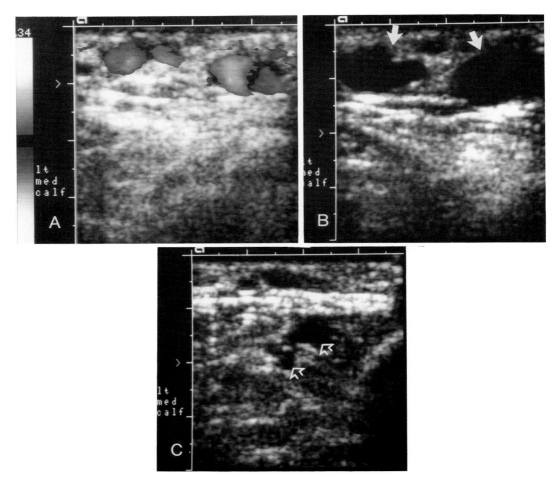

Figure 6.23. Dilated perforating veins are commonly associated with superficial varicosities. **A** (see color plate IV), Color flow mapping shows these moderately distended varicosities to have a heterogeneous pattern of blood flow during venous augmentation. The flow velocities are of low amplitude. **B,** This transverse image of the calf shows a moderately dilated varicosity (*arrows*) in the lower portion of the greater saphenous vein. **C** and **D,** The next two images were taken just inferior to this point. They show a very tortuous channel (*curved arrows*) winding from the varix to the more deeply located posterior tibial veins (*open arrows*). **E,** The incompetence of the superficial veins is documented in the last image where a Doppler gate has been placed over the varix. Augmented flow (*arrow*) is followed by a longer period of reversed flow (*curved arrow*), indicative of reflux.

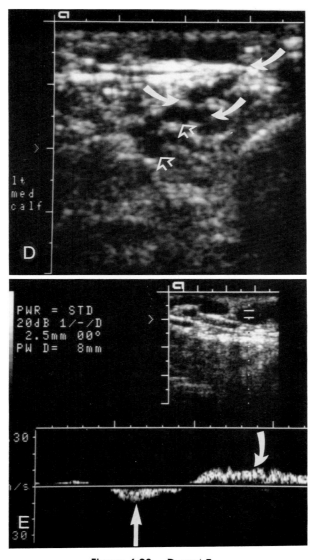

Figure 6.23. **D** and **E.**

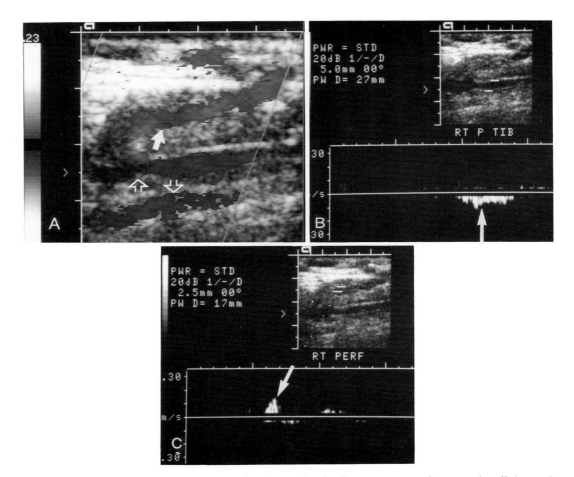

Figure 6.24. The evaluation of the perforating veins for the presence of venous insufficiency is difficult using duplex sonography alone. The Doppler signals are of small amplitude, since only small amounts of blood are moving back and forth. The perforators may also be difficult to visualize on the gray-scale image because of their small size and tortuous course. They are often easily perceived with color Doppler mapping. **A** (see color plate IV), Reversal of the flow direction is clearly shown in a lower-calf perforator (*arrow*). The normal direction of flow in the posterior tibial veins (*open arrows*) is encoded in blue and directed toward the upper portion of the extremity. Flow in the perforating vein is encoded in red and is abnormally directed outward from the deep venous system toward the superficial venous system. **B,** This longitudinal image of the posterior tibial veins in the lower third of the calf shows a normal albeit small-amplitude response to venous augmentation (*arrow*). **C,** This same longitudinal image now shows the Doppler gate positioned over the incompetent perforating vein. The Doppler signals show flow directed away from the deep system and into the superficial system (*arrow*). This is contrary to the normal direction of flow from the superficial to the deep veins. This therefore represents evidence of venous insufficiency.

SPECIFIC MANEUVERS

The diagnosis of deep venous insufficiency is made by confirming the presence of reflux in the deep veins during maneuvers using either duplex sonography or color Doppler imaging.

With duplex sonography, reflux in the greater saphenous vein can be shown during the Valsalva maneuver. This same maneuver can be used for the proximal superficial femoral and profunda femoral veins (Fig. 6.25). It is less reliable at the level of the popliteal vein. An alternate approach is compression of the thigh muscle to demonstrate reverse augmentation of blood at the level of the popliteal vein (Fig. 6.26). The popliteal vein valves are the critical sites to assess if deep vein valve reconstructive surgery is being considered.

Newer methods of quantifying reflux with Doppler sonography have recently been proposed. One group has shown that a standardized compression cuff at the thigh can be used to estimate reflux. The thigh is compressed with the patient on a

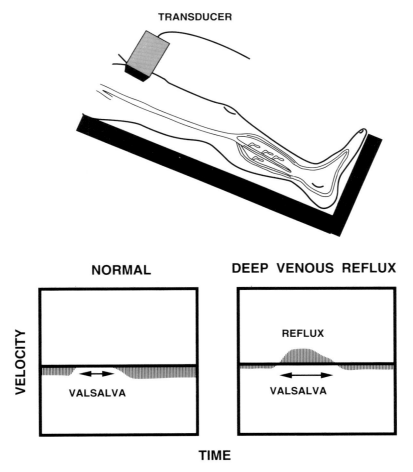

Figure 6.25. An alternate means of detecting the presence of venous insufficiency is to have the patient perform a Valsalva maneuver. The normal response is cessation of returning blood flow. The response in the incompetent vein is reversed blood flow. This examination is more easily performed with the patient lying approximately 15° from the horizontal.

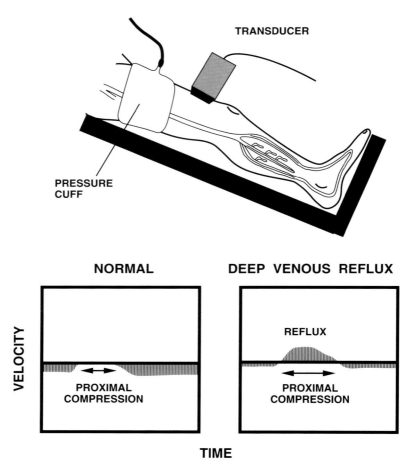

Figure 6.26. The use of a cuff placed over the proximal thigh has been used as a substitute for the Valsalva maneuver. A short inflation to a standardized pressure is performed. The amount and duration of reflux is measured. A simpler variant of this approach is to manually squeeze the patient's thigh and to look for any reversal of flow on the Doppler waveform. This examination is best done with the patient tilted upward by approximately 15°.

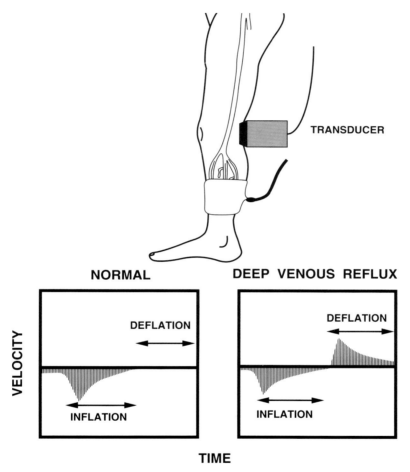

Figure 6.27. The amount of venous reflux can be semi-quantified by using a cuff placed over the calf as a means of delivering a controlled inflation. The height of the venous reflux can then be measured.

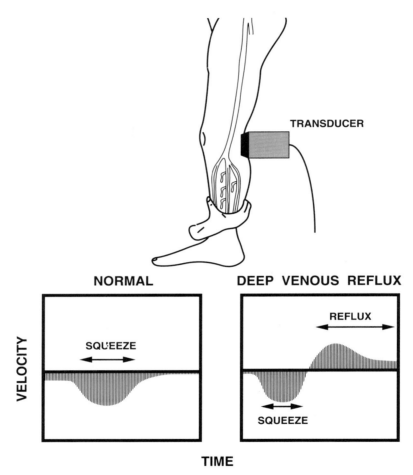

Figure 6.28. The presence of venous insufficiency is easily detected by observing the Doppler waveform. The incompetent vein will show a large amount of reversed flow following venous augmentation. This is not seen in the normal vein with competent valves. This examination is normally performed with the patient standing while putting most of their weight on the leg which is not being examined.

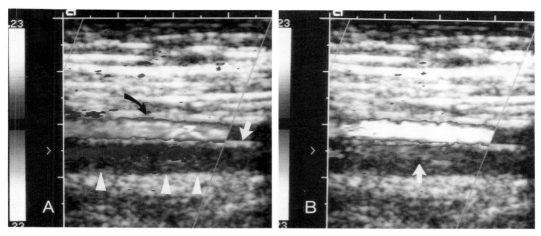

Figure 6.29. **A** (see color plate IV), The presence of chronic venous thrombosis in this extremity is manifested by the presence of heterogeneous material within the superficial femoral vein (*arrow*) lying deep to the artery (*curved arrow*). This diffuse wall thickening of the vein is suggestive of a previous episode of thrombosis (*arrowheads*). There is no abnormal distention of this channel. The augmented flow signals in blue are located in the center of the vein. **B** (see color plate IV), This reversal of color Doppler signals (*arrow*) in red signifies retrograde flow down the incompetent vein, which has previously been involved by deep vein thrombosis.

tilt table, and the velocity duration or reflux is measured. Another group has proposed the use of distal compression with a standard inflation of a calf pressure cuff (Fig. 6.27). The appearance of delayed reflux following augmentation is then quantitated. Both examinations are performed with the subject upright or semi-upright with weight bearing on the opposite leg so that the calf muscles are relaxed.

We have further simplified this technique by measuring the amount of reflux following compression of the calf and partial emptying of the blood volume in the calf with the free hand of the sonographer (Fig. 6.28). The patient is asked to stand, putting most of his or her weight on the leg not being examined. The calf is then squeezed and the amount of reflux is measured at different locations in the leg (Fig. 6.29). This latter approach is closer to the normal physiology of reflux, which tends to have its effect when patients are standing. However, it can be quite awkward for the sonographer, who must often bend down or squat while going through the maneuvers.

SUGGESTED READINGS

Browse NL, Burnand KG, Lea Thomas M. Diseases of the veins. Pathology, diagnosis and treatment. London: Edward Arnold, 1988.

Jay R, Hull R, Carter C, et al. Outcome of abnormal impedance plethysmography results in patients with proximal-vein thrombosis: frequency of return to normal. Thromb Res 1984;36:259–263.

Killewich LA, Bedford GR, Beach KW, Strandness DE Jr. Spontaneous lysis of deep venous thrombi: rate and outcome. J Vasc Surg 1989;9:89–97.

Marder VJ, Soulen RL, Atichartakarn V, et al. Quantitative venographic assessment of deep vein thrombosis in the evaluation of streptokinase and heparin therapy. J Lab Clin Med 1977;89:1018–1029.

Robertson BR, Nilsson IM, Nylander G. Thrombolytic effect of streptokinase as evaluated by phlebography of deep venous thrombi of the leg. Acta Chir Scand 1970;136:173–180.

Rosch J, Dotter CT, Seaman AJ, Porter JM, Common HH. Healing of deep venous thrombosis: venographic findings in a randomized study comparing streptokinase and heparin. AJR 1976;127:553–558.

Schulman S, Lockner D, Granquist S, Bratt G, Paul C, Nyman D. A comparative randomized trial of low-dose versus high-dose streptokinase in deep vein thrombosis of the thigh. Thromb Haemost 1984; 51:261–265.

Vasdekis SN, Clarke GH, Nicolaides AN. Quantification of venous reflux by means of duplex scanning. J Vasc Surg 1989;10:670–677.

Widmer LK, Zemp E, Widmer MT, et al. Late results in deep vein thrombosis of the lower extremity. Vasa 1985;14:264–268.

CHAPTER SEVEN

Peripheral Arterial Diseases

The role of sonography in the diagnosis of peripheral arterial disease is changing. The imaging tasks currently performed in the noninvasive laboratory can be grouped into two broad categories. The first comprises the more traditional diagnostic tasks, which consist of evaluating the nature of masses in close proximity to a vessel and of determining whether an iatrogenic injury has caused a pseudoaneurysm, hematoma, or AV fistula. Once the nature of the perivascular collection has been determined by sonography, the localized nature of the process often leads to surgical intervention without preoperative angiography. Absence of blood flow in a perivascular collection is a reassuring finding. The nonvascular nature of the mass makes it likely that an aspiration biopsy can be safely performed. A more conservative approach with clinical observation and optional follow-up by repeat sonography can be adopted whenever a hematoma is thought to be present. The second category is increasing in importance. It comprises a broader application of Doppler sonography to the detection of stenoses or occlusions in the peripheral arteries and in bypass grafts. This application is similar in nature to the use of sonography for making the diagnosis of significant stenoses of the carotid arteries. The major difference between both tasks is a function of the length of the arteries that must be imaged. In the leg, the sonographic transducer must cover distances 5 to 10 times greater than those covered in the neck. A more effective imaging strategy that relies on color Doppler mapping is the only practical way of performing this type of study within reasonable imaging times. Although it can be used to detect the presence and location of significant arterial lesions in the lower extremities, duplex sonography requires 60 to 120 minutes. Color Doppler imaging of the leg arteries is more effective and can be achieved with imaging times of 15 to 30 minutes.

Incidence and Clinical Importance

PSEUDOANEURYSMS

A peripheral arterial mass that develops acutely rarely occurs without a history of previous trauma or surgical intervention (Fig. 7.1). The presence of a pseudoaneurysm is suspected following arterial catheterization or in association with an arterial catheter that has been in place for a

SYSTOLE

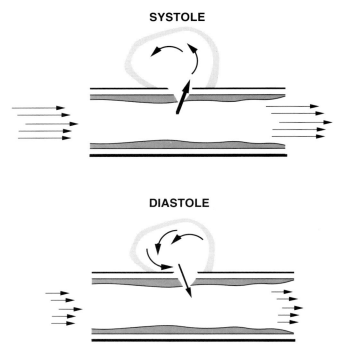

DIASTOLE

Figure 7.1. A false aneurysm is a contained rupture through all three layers of the arterial wall (intima, media, and adventitia). A persistent communication between the site of rupture and the arterial lumen permits entry and egress of blood from the "collection." The pattern of blood flow within the collection is "swirling" in nature, showing a mixture of colors corresponding to this circular motion of blood. Color Doppler mapping or duplex sonography is essential in making this diagnosis. False aneurysms are at risk of expanding and causing local symptoms due to compression of adjacent nerves or vessels. They may also go on to rupture.

few days. The incidence of this complication is close to 0.5 to 1% following catheterization. The site of catheterization is almost always the common femoral artery. The pseudoaneurysm lies in close proximity to the entry site into the arterial lumen. It is, on occasion, distant by a few centimeters. It is, however, connected to the lumen by a channel of variable width and length. Arterial punctures that enter above the inguinal ligament are more likely to have this complication. The full extent of the collection may be difficult to evaluate, since it often extends into the pelvis. Pseudoaneurysms localized below the inguinal ligament are often caused by poor compression following the removal of the arterial catheter. Risk factors for their develop-

ment include deeply lying arteries due to body habitus, the use of anticoagulants, and the use of larger-diameter catheters (7Fr or above; 3Fr catheters are 1 mm in diameter). Localized pseudoaneurysms also occur at brachial artery arteriotomy sites following cardiac catheterization. Pseudoaneurysms that arise in association with vascular surgical procedures are discussed in Chapter 8. More slowly enlarging masses can develop following arterial injuries that have been missed. The mass slowly enlarges with time, often shows thrombus deposition, and remains at risk for possible rupture.

AV fistulas are also quite common following the percutaneous insertion of catheters. These are often caused when an arterial puncture has been performed too low, below the junction of the profunda and superficial femoral arteries. The incidence of an AV fistula is also estimated at 0.5% following arterial catheterization. Risk factors include the use of anticoagulants and poor technique during the catheterization. Congenital AV fistulas are rare and are often detected early in life. A missed AV fistula can often cause significant shunting, artificially causing an increase in cardiac output as it progressively enlarges.

ANEURYSMS

Aneurysmal disease of the artery is commonly categorized as a form of atherosclerosis. However, although aneurysmal and peripheral arterial disease coexist in most instances, isolated aneurysm formation without significant atherosclerotic involvement is not uncommon (Fig. 7.2). Primary aneurysmal disease is now thought to represent a pathological entity in which the primary defect lies in a weakness of the components of the arterial wall itself. This is supported by the genetic association seen in certain families with primary aneurysmal disease. This hypothesis is supported by the observation that popliteal artery aneurysms are often bilateral—35 to 50% of the time. Similarly, there is often a coexistent aneurysm of the aorta—20 to 35% of the time. There are also more diffuse forms of aneurysmal disease with diffuse enlargement of the peripheral artery being present on one side, both sides, or

SYSTOLE

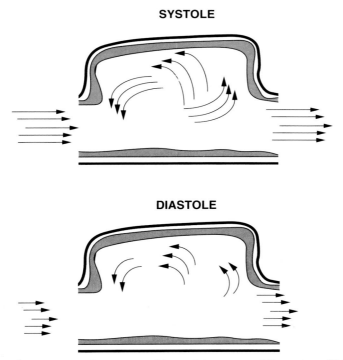

DIASTOLE

Figure 7.2. A saccular aneurysm is an eccentric protuberance of the artery. All three layers of the wall remain intact. The marked eccentricity of the collection makes it possible for the same type of swirling motion to be set up. This motion is more commonly perceived during a portion of the cardiac cycle. The presence of a saccular aneurysm should suggest the possibility of an infectious agent such as *Salmonella*. Most saccular aneurysms are atherosclerotic in nature.

limited to the proximal arteries. These are referred to as cases of primary arteriomegaly. The presence of atherosclerosis with plaque deposition and occlusions is associative and not causative. The occlusions occurring with aneurysmal disease are more abrupt and are due to embolization of the thrombus that forms along the wall of the aneurysm (Fig. 7.3).

PERIPHERAL ARTERIAL STENOSIS

Symptomatic peripheral arterial disease is estimated to have a prevalence of 5 to 10% in the population above 70 years of age. Many patients suffer from peripheral vascular disease for years before seeking medical assistance. This is a reflection of the normal development of collateral channels, which are often sufficient to maintain sufficient perfusion to the extremity in the older patient as long as he or she does not exercise or ambulate too vigorously. In general these patients adapt by decreasing their levels of activity as their disease progresses. Despite this, subjective worsening in symptoms occurs in 28 to 60% of patients over 2 to 5 years. Amputation

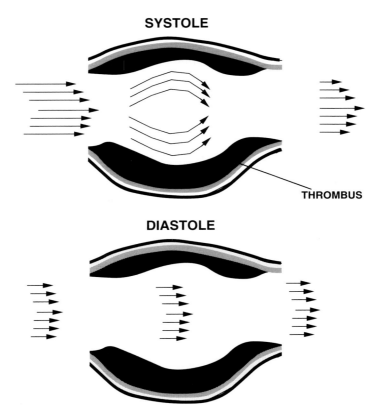

Figure 7.3. The traditional arterial aneurysm is a more or less symmetrical expansion of the arterial walls. All three layers are involved. They have a strong tendency to have thrombus deposit against the intima and to somewhat smooth out the divergent walls. The appearance and flow patterns within the lumen are variable and depend on the extent of filling in of the lumen by thrombus. The diagnosis is made on gray-scale imaging, with Doppler analysis giving some supplemental information. The major complications are continued growth and rupture of the aneurysm, occlusion due to thrombosis, and episodes of peripheral embolization of some of the thrombus deposited in the aneurysm.

rates in these nontreated patients vary between 2 and 6% over a 2.5- to 8-year interval.

The estimated yearly mortality rate in these patients with peripheral arterial disease is greater than 5% and does not depend on whether or not a revascularization procedure has been performed. The coexistent atherosclerotic involvement of the carotid and coronary circulation accounts for the high mortality of this patient cohort. Of patients presenting for peripheral revascularization, the prevalence of concurrent severe coronary artery disease is 28%. Myocardial infarction is the primary cause of death in patients with peripheral arterial disease.

The important clinical events that prompt the patient to seek medical assistance are the development of chronic skin and soft tissue changes reflecting arterial insufficiency and the presence of poor wound healing. Another presentation is the development of acute embolic events originating from a more proximal arterial lesion such as an ulcerated plaque.

The high success rate of revascularization procedures has diminished the likelihood that peripheral arterial lesions will progress to the point of amputation during the lifetime of the patient. The high mortality rate in this patient group due to age and coronary events increases the chance that a revascularization procedure will remain successful (i.e., maintaining a patent arterial bypass graft) at the time of death.

The two noninvasive screening tests widely used for screening for the presence of peripheral arterial lesions are segmental pressure measurements and pulse volume recordings. Both noninvasive tests can confirm the presence of significant stenotic lesions in the femoropopliteal or aortoiliac arteries. However, they are unable to accurately identify the severity or extent of arterial involvement. They are therefore poorly predictive in identifying patients who might have arterial lesions amenable

to limited interventions such as angioplasty or atherectomy rather than more extensive revascularization surgery.

Lower Extremity
NORMAL ANATOMY

The patient is normally imaged supine. The femoral and popliteal arteries of the leg travel with an accompanying vein, while the lateral descending branch of the profunda femoral artery and all of the arteries in the calf are accompanied by two veins.

The common iliac arteries originate from the aorta and are most often seen with the transducer (2.5 to 3.5 MHz) placed over the umbilicus. The bifurcation is more obvious on transverse images than on longitudinal images. Successful visualization of the full extent of the iliac artery is possible 40 to 50% of the time at frequencies above 5.0 MHz but is more easily achieved at 2.5 to 3.5 MHz. The optimal window is one with the transducer placed just medial to the anterior iliac spine and oriented parallel to the iliac wing. At the bifurcation of the common iliac artery, the internal iliac most often lies deep to the external iliac. The more distal portion of the external iliac artery can often be seen with a 5.0-MHz transducer. The vein lies deep to the artery and can be easily identified by using the venous augmentation maneuver during scanning.

The common femoral artery starts at the level of the inguinal ligament and continues for 4 to 6 cm until it branches into the superficial and deep femoral arteries (Fig. 7.4). Imaging is performed with the transducer placed either anteriorly or slightly toward the medial aspect of the thigh. The early bifurcation of the artery before that of the common femoral vein is best appreciated on transverse scans (Fig. 7.5). Below this, the transducer is kept longitudinal (Fig. 7.6). The deep femoral ar-

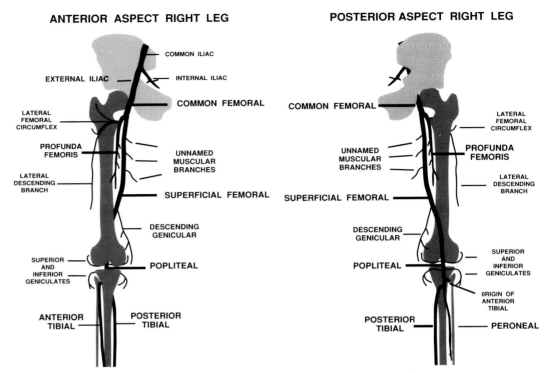

Figure 7.4. The major arteries of the leg include the profunda femoris, which supplies the muscles of the thigh; the superficial femoral artery, which acts mostly as a conduit but sends off a few branches to supply the mid and lower thigh muscles; the popliteal artery, which crosses the knee joint before bifurcating into the tibioperoneal branches that feed the muscles of the calf. Claudication manifests itself mostly as a cramping sensation in the calf brought on by exercise. A narrowing or occlusion in any portion of the superficial femoral, popliteal, or tibioperoneal branches is therefore likely to be the source of this problem.

tery lies lateral to the superficial femoral artery and quickly branches to supply the region of the femoral head and the deep muscles of the thigh (Fig. 7.7). A medial origin of the profunda femoris occurs in 2 to 5% of patients. The presence of peripheral arterial disease is normally associated with collateral pathways, which tend to develop from the branches of the deep femoral artery and from the lower portion of the superficial femoral artery. The superficial femoral artery continues along the medial aspect of the thigh at a depth of 3 to 8 cm until it reaches the adductor canal near the junction of the middle and lower thirds of the thigh. The vein lies below it as

it courses in the medial thigh. In cases of suspected occlusion and absent arterial flow signals, venous Doppler flow signals should be used to confirm correct placement of the transducer and to determine whether imaging is being performed over the expected location of the artery. The artery dips deep to the upper boundary of the adductor canal formed by the fascia arising from the adductor magnus muscle and continues as the popliteal artery. Imaging may not be possible with the leg held in a neutral position, partly due to the marked depth of the vessel and partly because of the poor penetration of the ultrasound beam through the fascia. The leg is

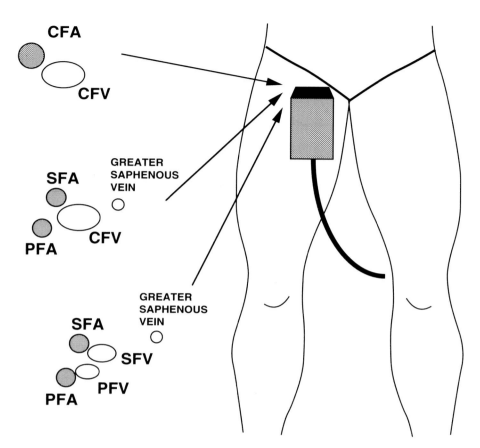

Figure 7.5. The region of the groin is a very difficult area to sort out. The easiest way to gain an understanding of the different relationships between the branching arteries and veins is to move the transducer down in the transverse plane. When using color Doppler mapping, the arteries and veins are easily distinguished from each other. If no color option is available, the Doppler gate can be used to sequentially interrogate the different arteries and veins. Once the different vessels have been identified, it is relatively easy to turn the transducer in a longitudinal plane and to evaluate that portion of the artery.

therefore externally rotated and the knee slightly bent in a frog leg position (Fig. 7.8). If the transducer is held on the anterior aspect of the lower thigh, the free hand can sometimes be used to pull the soft tissues closer to the transducer. This may help visualize the artery and vein to the level of the patella. Both artery and vein can then be followed from a posterior approach. The transducer is placed posteriorly at the level of the knee joint. The popliteal artery and vein are identified and

followed as they slowly move more medially within the adductor canal. The tendon of the semimembranosus muscle sometimes makes it difficult to keep the transducer in a transverse orientation. A longitudinal position is then often necessary if Doppler signals are to be taken. This is also helpful in evaluating the diameter of the artery in cases of suspected aneurysms. Using this posterior approach and moving downward, the artery continues to lie deep to the vein. At the level of the

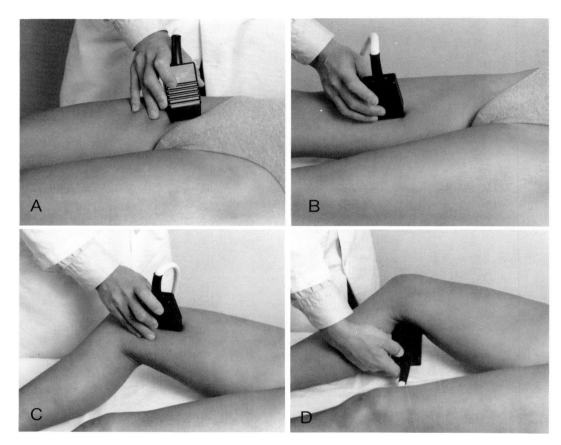

Figure 7.6. The evaluation of the lower-extremity arteries can be done by serially displacing the longitudinally oriented transducer along the course of the femoral and then the popliteal arteries. **A,** The examination normally starts at the level of the groin crease. **B,** The transducer is slid along the inner aspect of the thigh while color Doppler flow signals are obtained of the artery lumen. **C,** At the level of the lower thigh, the knee is slightly flexed and the leg externally rotated. The transducer can then be pressed in the soft tissues at the palpable interface between the more anteriorly located vastus medialis muscle and the more medially located sartorius muscle. **D,** Finally, the transducer is positioned posteriorly for imaging of the popliteal artery. The leg remains in an externally rotated position with the knee slightly flexed. Imaging from the posterior projection with the patient prone is sometimes necessary. Under these circumstances, the knee is slightly flexed. This position is also useful when evaluating for the presence of popliteal artery entrapment.

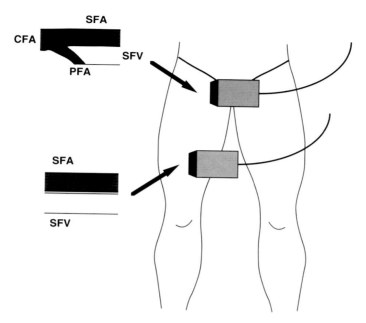

Figure 7.7. Imaging of the superficial femoral artery is done from the anterior aspect of the thigh. The bifurcation of the common femoral artery (*CFA*) into the profunda femoris artery (*PFA*) and the superficial femoral artery (*SFA*) must be identified in every patient. Imaging is more easily performed in the longitudinal plane. Although duplex sonography can be used to image the artery and evaluate flow patterns, we rely almost exclusively on the color Doppler map to follow the artery and detect sites of increased frequency shifts. These are then evaluated with the aid of Doppler wave-form analysis.

knee joint it sends off small geniculate branches. Approximately 6 to 8 cm from the knee joint it branches into the anterior tibial artery and the tibioperoneal trunk. The tibioperoneal arteries are accompanied by two veins. The anterior tibial artery courses into the anterior compartment of the lower leg after crossing through the proximal portion of the interosseous membrane. It lies on top of the membrane until it finally crosses the ankle joint as the dorsalis pedis artery. The two accompanying veins are often difficult to visualize. The tibioperoneal trunk gives off the posterior tibial and the peroneal arteries, which supply most of the calf muscles (Fig. 7.9). The posterior tibial lies more superficially and can be imaged from the medial aspect of the calf. It is accompanied by two veins,

which can be followed down to the medial malleolus. The peroneal artery lies deep to the posterior tibial artery when imaged from the medial aspect of the calf. It lies in close apposition to the fibula. This can be taken to advantage by imaging from the lateral aspect of the calf. It is often necessary to bend the knee to better visualize it. The peroneal artery terminates as small branches that cross the ankle joint. It serves as an important collateral pathway. In some laboratories, the prone position is adopted for imaging of the popliteal and tibioperoneal arteries. We use this approach in cases of suspected aneurysms whenever a satisfactory sonographic window cannot be obtained by flexing the knee and externally rotating the leg. Whenever the diagnosis of popliteal artery

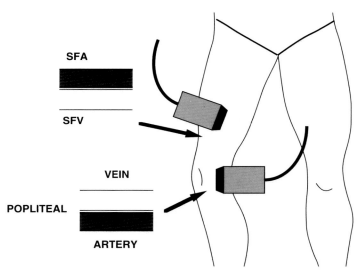

Figure 7.8. The region of the adductor canal is a difficult one to evaluate. Most of the errors in detecting stenoses of the femoropopliteal arteries occur at this level. It is normally evaluated with the leg slightly bent at the knee and the leg turned outward. As the transducer progresses downward over the lower thigh, it is placed halfway between the back and the front of the thigh. By exerting a moderate amount of pressure, the transducer will often slide between the sartorius and the vastus medialis muscles in a window that shows the artery. From the back of the knee, the transducer is slid upward and medially to follow the artery until the tendon of the semimembranosus muscle gets in the way. Both these approaches used in combination normally permit the evaluation of the popliteal artery lying in the adductor canal.

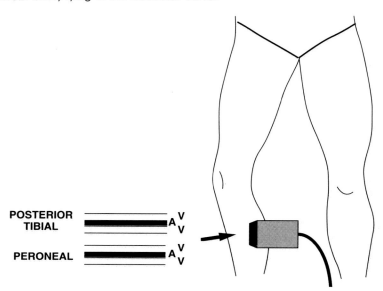

Figure 7.9. The tibioperoneal arteries are normally best seen with the transducer held midway between the front and back of the calf. The posterior tibial arteries should be seen in almost all individuals. The more deeply located peroneal artery is accessible in most patients from this approach. In those few in whom there is a problem, the transducer should be placed just to the side and behind the fibula. The artery will then be easily identified. The anterior tibial artery is normally best seen from the front, lying on top of the interosseous membrane. Both the anterior tibial and the posterior tibial arteries continue down to cross the ankle. The posterior tibial does so behind the medial malleolus. The anterior tibial becomes the dorsalis pedis artery as it crosses the anterior ankle joint. The peroneal ends 4 cm above the ankle joint.

entrapment is suspected, we perform imaging in both the prone and upright positions.

NORMAL FLOW PATTERNS

The flow pattern in all of these branches is typically triphasic (Fig. 7.10). There is an early systolic acceleration in velocity followed by a brief period of low amplitude flow reversal before returning to antegrade diastolic flow of lower velocity. There is more of a pulsatile pattern in the profunda femoris artery. The amount of flow reversal decreases in the arterial branches below the knee. The response to either exercise or ischemia is a loss of this triphasic pattern and the development of a more monophasic pattern with a loss of the period of flow reversal and a persistent antegrade flow during diastole. Published ranges of normal velocities for the different arterial segments depend on the method used to acquire the Doppler spectra. The values derived from older Doppler probes will be much lower, since the mean velocity is being measured (Fig. 7.11).

As mentioned earlier, flow velocity through the accompanying veins has values of 0.1 to 0.2 m/sec. It normally shows respiratory variation, which can be detected at the lower scale settings of the Doppler velocity displays. Flow augmentation following compression of the calf veins is an important maneuver useful in confirming proper positioning of the ultrasound transducer. It is useful in guaranteeing that the Doppler gain is properly set and that Doppler signals are detectable at the level of the accompanying artery. Absent or low-amplitude Doppler spectra sampled in the artery are then accepted as being accurate representations of arterial lesions.

ABNORMAL FLOW PATTERNS
Vascular Masses

Avascular masses do not generally contain any flow signals detectable by either color Doppler mapping or duplex sonography. If the mass lies in close proximity to an artery, however, pulsations from the artery can be transmitted to the mass. These show up as low-amplitude signals, which can be falsely believed to represent evidence of flow within the mass. A simple way to correct this problem is to decrease the color sensitivity of the device so that there are no color or Doppler signals generated around the artery itself when imaging slightly above or below the location of the mass.

Hypoechoic masses may often show an accentuated transmission of color signals through their substance. This artifact is due to the relative sensitivity adjustments made in the algorithm used to superimpose color flow information on the gray-scale images. Regions with echogenic signals are more likely not to represent vascular channels. Manufacturers will therefore decrease the likelihood that color signals will be superimposed on any area that contains strong gray-scale echoes. Conversely, they increase the amount of color signals that will be mapped over an area that does not have many gray-scale echoes, since moving blood is relatively anechoic. This difference accounts for the transmission of arterial pulsations as color signals into any poorly echogenic periarterial collection such as a hematoma. Similarly, it accounts for the presence of color signals in any region of the image with low-amplitude gray-scale signals. Finally, the relative motion of the transducer due to transmitted pulsations causes the transducer to move with respect to the collection. This can also cause color signals to be mapped onto the anechoic collection.

Pseudoaneurysms remain the most important category of perivascular masses requiring accurate diagnosis. These are caused by a rupture in the arterial wall. The resultant collection of blood is retained within the soft tissues and possesses a communication to the artery. This creates a typical pattern of blood flow

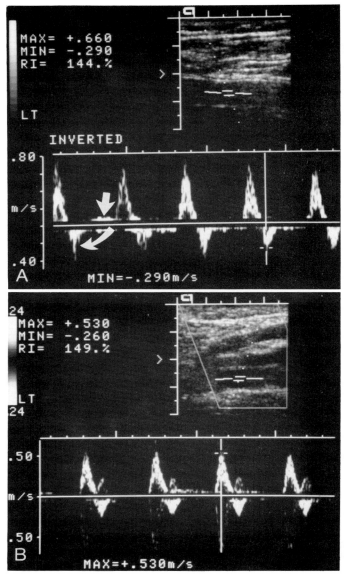

Figure 7.10. The typical Doppler waveform of the lower extremity artery consists of three parts. The first is a period of forward flow during systole. This is followed by a brief period of flow reversal. Finally, a low-amplitude component of forward flow can often be detected during diastole. This idealized triphasic waveform is not necessarily present in all normal individuals. **A,** A Doppler velocity waveform taken in the distal superficial femoral artery of this patient shows a strong forward velocity component (0.66 m/sec) and a significant amount of flow reversal (−0.29 m/sec). Flow is reversed (*curved arrow*) during early diastole and then forward (*arrow*). Both are of low amplitude and may be difficult to see on the Doppler waveform tracing. **B,** The Doppler velocity waveform from a normal popliteal artery shows both the forward (0.53 m/sec) and the reverse components of blood flow (−0.26 m/sec). In this case, the presence of flow during diastole is either absent or lower than the wall filter or lower-velocity threshold of the device. The arterial waveform sampled lower in the leg appears more pulsatile (i.e., having a higher relative amount of reversed flow with respect to the forward flow).

**PROCESSED USING
ZERO-CROSSING DETECTOR** **AVERAGE OF INSTANTANEOUS
FREQUENCIES (VELOCITIES)**

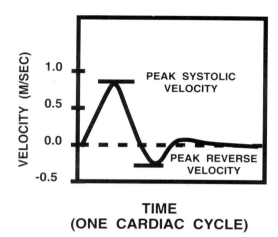

	PEAK SYSTOLIC VELOCITY	PEAK REVERSE VELOCITY
FEMORAL ARTERY	0.30-0.50 M/SEC	0.06-0.12 M/SEC
POPLITEAL ARTERY	0.25-0.30 M/SEC	0.08-0.12 M/SEC

Figure 7.11. **A,** The velocity values for the leg arteries often quoted in the literature have been obtained from older-generation Doppler devices. However, the peak velocity measured from such a tracing is in fact the maximum of the *mean* velocity and not the maximal velocity. This is roughly half of what is measured on a Doppler spectral waveform. **B,** The range of normal velocities obtained in the leg arteries by Doppler spectral analysis varies between 0.5 and 1.4 m/sec. More distally, the velocity decreases paradoxically as the arterial diameter decreases. The arteries are not acting as simple conduits. If they were, a decrease in diameter would correspond to an increase in velocity. These arteries send off smaller branches that shunt blood flow away from the main arterial conduit. Since there is less blood flowing in the more distal artery, the velocity of blood flow decreases despite a reduction in the caliber of the artery.

**PROCESS USING
FOURIER TRANSFORMER** **SPECTRUM OF INSTANTANEOUS
FREQUENCIES (VELOCITIES)**

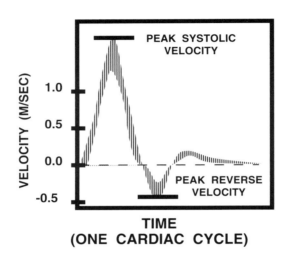

	PEAK SYSTOLIC VELOCITY	PEAK REVERSE VELOCITY
COMMON FEMORAL ARTERY	0.9-1.4 M/SEC	0.3-0.5 M/SEC
SUPERFICIAL FEMORAL ARTERY	0.7-1.1 M/SEC	0.25-0.45 M/SEC
POPLITEAL ARTERY	0.5-0.8 M/SEC	0.2-0.4 M/SEC

Figure 7.11. B.

within both the pseudoaneurysm and the feeding communication to the artery. In the pseudoaneurysm itself, a swirling pattern of blood flow is set up. This motion of blood flow resembles a colorized version of the "yin-yang" sign. Some sonographers have noted a similarity of this continuous motion of blood to what is seen in the window of a washing machine, hence the expression color "Maytag" sign. This motion persists during the full duration of a cardiac cycle (Fig. 7.12A). During systole, blood flows into the collection (Fig. 7.12B). The higher systemic arterial pressure drives blood into the collection. During diastole, blood flows back out from the collection through the communicating channel into the artery. The energy stored in the soft tissues is such that the pressure in the collection is higher than the pressure in the artery during diastole. Flow is therefore directed outward from the collec-

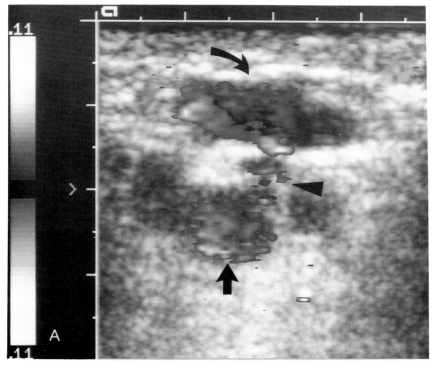

Figure 7.12. **A** (see color plate V), The typical appearance of iatrogenic injury to the femoral artery with subsequent pseudoaneurysm formation is shown here. The native femoral artery is identified lying more deeply (*arrow*). The actual communication from the rupture in the arterial wall is shown by color Doppler signals (*arrowhead*). The pseudoaneurysm is located more superficially (*curved arrow*). **B,** The compliant nature of the soft tissues surrounding and containing a pseudoaneurysm explains the persistent flow pattern that is established within it and at its communication with the native artery. During systole, blood flows into the collection due to the relatively higher pressure in the artery lumen. Energy is stored in the collection as the surrounding soft tissues are compressed. During diastole, the stored energy is released as the pressure within the artery becomes less than that generated by the elastic recoil of the soft tissues. This promotes flow into the artery. The swirling pattern of blood flow normally persists during the full cardiac cycle. A longer communicating channel will increase resistance to flow and disrupt the steady state responsible for setting up this constant motion.

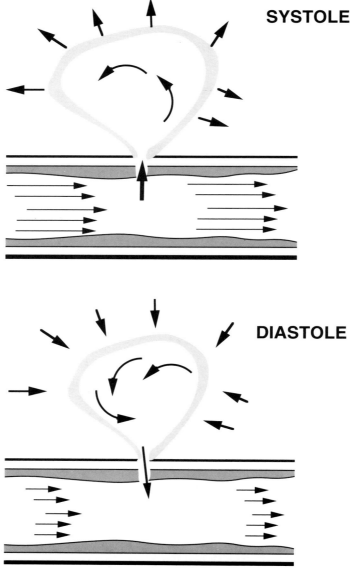

SYSTOLE

DIASTOLE

Figure 7.12. B.

tion. This motion will start to disappear as the pseudoaneurysm becomes partly thrombosed. It is also less apparent when the collection is connected by a long, tortuous channel to the native artery. The energy of the incoming blood is dissipated by the resistance within the smaller-caliber communication. The pattern of blood flow in the channel can be shown when a Doppler gate is positioned over it. This typically shows a to-and-fro motion of blood entering and exiting the collection (Fig. 7.13). Although this sign was originally described by duplex sonography alone, color Doppler mapping has made it possible to quickly identify this communication and to help place the sample gate over it (Fig. 7.14). Besides the to-and-fro pattern in the communication itself, duplex sonography does not show any typical pattern of blood flow within the main portion of the pseudoaneurysm. This is partly due to the fact that the pattern of blood flow varies as the jet of blood enters the collection, with some areas within the jet sharing strong systolic signals and others, at the periphery, having smaller-amplitude signals, which may or may not reverse during the cardiac cycle. These patterns will vary as a function of the size of the feeding artery, the size of the collection, the length of the communicating channel, the amount of surrounding tissue, and the elasticity of these tissues as they accommodate the collection.

The availability of Doppler imaging techniques has made it possible to follow the natural history of these pseudoaneurysms. Thrombosis has been observed in non-surgically treated collections when examinations are sequentially performed over intervals of up to 3 months. This approach is somewhat difficult to adopt, since there is still the risk of rupture or continued growth during the observation period, and bed rest or limited ambulation is required. A more recent approach to the problem is the use of compression ultra-

sound to help thrombose the pseudoaneurysm. This is a potential alternative to the surgical approach. The transducer is held over the neck of the pseudoaneurysm and pressure is applied until flow ceases into the pseudoaneurysm. However, the applied pressure should never cause flow within the native artery to cease. A preliminary report has shown a high rate of success if recently formed pseudoaneurysms that present 2 to 3 days following catheterization are treated with this approach. If there is a longer interval, the likelihood that the channel will become partly endothelialized increases and the effectiveness of this type of intervention decreases. Surgery should then be considered the logical alternative.

A thrombosed pseudoaneurysm should not necessarily be thought of as being "safe" (Fig. 7.15). If it is associated with a synthetic graft, the possibility of coexistent infection should be considered. Aspiration biopsy and culture should then be performed.

AV Fistulas

The presence of an arteriovenous fistula is normally suspected by clinical palpation of a "thrill." This physical sign is due to the transmission of the high-velocity signals hitting the wall of the vein as vibrations into the surrounding soft tissues. Duplex sonography will normally show a distended vein, most commonly the common femoral, and artery-like Doppler flow signals within the vein lumen. These high-velocity signals are very different from the normal low-amplitude venous signals. This can be quickly verified by comparison with the signals obtained in the vein of the opposite limb.

This must be also be distinguished from another source of high-velocity signals in the vein due to the presence of an extrinsic process compressing the vein, narrowing its lumen, and causing high-velocity flow

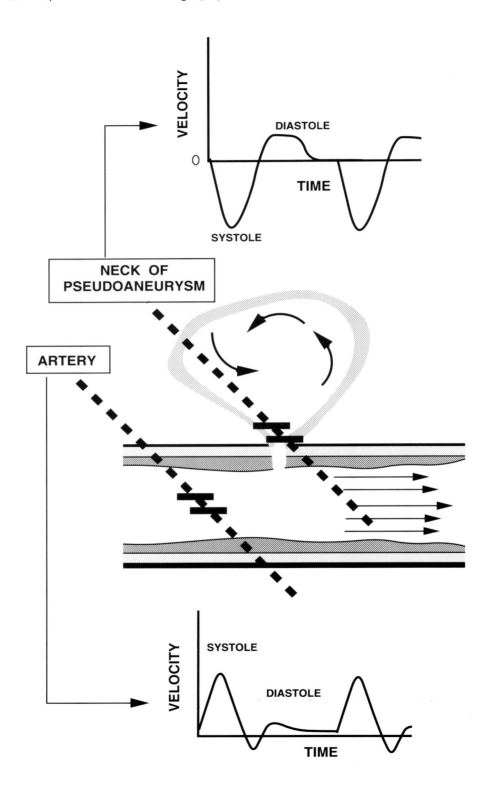

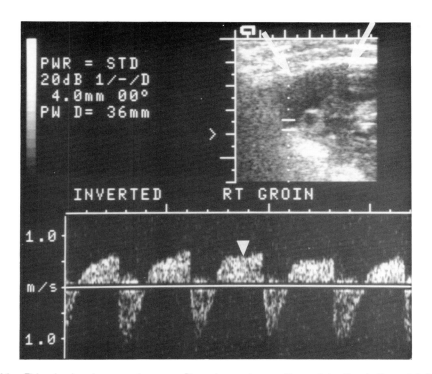

Figure 7.14. This duplex image shows a Doppler gate positioned to the left and inferior to a heterogeneous collection (*arrows*). The corresponding Doppler waveform clearly shows a typical "to-and-fro" pattern associated with a pseudoaneurysm. The diastolic flow (*arrowhead*) is of lower amplitude and is caused by the elasticity of the soft tissues, which forces blood back into the artery during diastole when arterial pressure is low. The systolic flow is caused by the arterial impulse driving blood out from the artery during systole, through the channel, and into the collection. This collection is in fact partly thrombosed, thereby explaining its heterogeneous appearance. The site where the Doppler gate was placed was determined using color Doppler mapping. This greatly facilitated the identification of the communicating channel, which could not be seen on the gray-scale image.

Figure 7.13. Confirmation of the presence of a pseudoaneurysm is normally acheived by color Doppler sonography alone. The color Doppler image also permits the exact identification of the channel communicating with the collection. The Doppler waveform measured in the channel will show the typical to-and-fro pattern. The sharp peak corresponds to the inflow during systole, while the broader, lower-amplitude flow takes place as the collection empties into the artery.

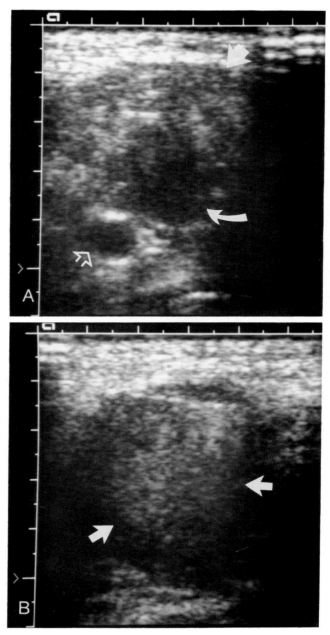

Figure 7.15. The natural history of pseudoaneurysms is becoming better understood with the help of sonography. **A,** This enlarging collection at the site of a previous carotid endarterectomy consists of a central sonolucent area (*curved arrow*) surrounded by a more echogenic mass (*arrow*). The carotid artery is located more deeply and to the left (*open arrow*). The sonolucent area corresponds to blood that is still communicating with the arterial rupture. The echogenic rim is early thrombus forming at the periphery of the pseudoaneurysm. **B,** An image taken slightly higher shows that the majority of the pseudoaneurysm is in fact thrombosing. The collection is mostly echogenic (*arrows*) and consists of freshly aggregated blood.

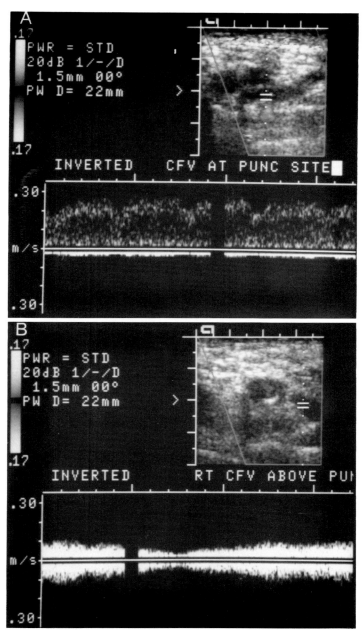

Figure 7.16. The differential diagnosis of an iatrogenic AV fistula includes the possibility of an extrinsically compressing mass causing increased venous signals due to the relative narrowing of the vein. **A,** Following catheterization, a clinically heard bruit instigated a sonography study. A first Doppler gate was positioned over the site of abnormal velocity signals. A high-velocity signal was detected. The color lumen of the vein was seen to be narrowed because of a surrounding hematoma. **B,** Doppler waveforms obtained above the site of extrinsic compression showed a venous pattern with normal respiratory phasicity.

signals. These can be readily distinguished from any "significant" AV fistula by having the patient perform a Valsalva maneuver. The flow signals in a "normal" or extrinsically compressed vein will cease (Fig. 7.16). The signals due to a large AV communication will persist even during the Valsalva maneuver. These are likely to require surgical repair (Fig. 7.17). Color Doppler mapping is often the only means of

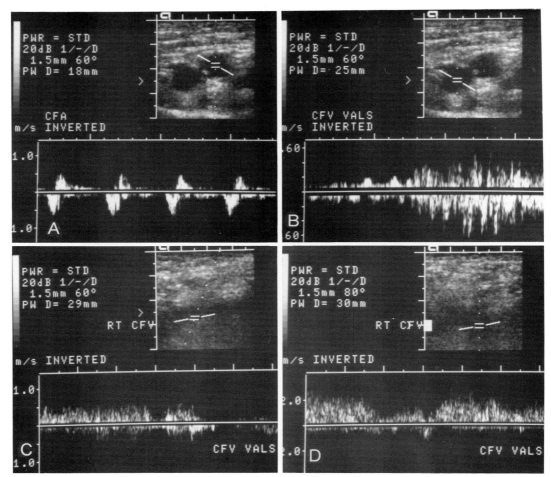

Figure 7.17. The incidence of AV communication between the femoral artery and vein following arterial catheterization is estimated at 0.5%. **A,** This first study was performed on a patient 1 day following cardiac catheterization. A transverse image of the common femoral artery and vein shows a Doppler sample within the artery and a typical arterial waveform. **B,** The Doppler gate was then moved into the adjacent vein and an abnormal waveform with high-intensity signals was obtained. This appearance is quite distinct from the normal venous waveform, which consists of constant flow with a slow respiratory phasicity superimposed. **C,** The flow signals could be completely extinguished during a Valsalva maneuver. Because of the latter, the patient was discharged but with a follow-up examination scheduled 2 weeks later. **D,** The follow-up sonogram shows that the abnormal flow signals from within the vein could not be stopped by the Valsalva maneuver. This suggested that the AV communication had increased in size and was not likely to close on its own. The fistula was repaired under local anaesthesia. **E** (see color plate V), The color Doppler image shows the physical communication between the superficial femoral artery and the superficial femoral vein (*arrow*).

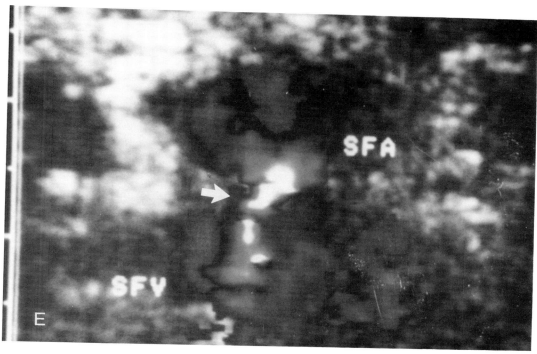

Figure 7.17. C to E.

identifying the site of the communication. Imaging is best performed transversely to better identify the actual communication. Searching for the communication with duplex sonography alone can be quite time consuming and unrewarding. Operative intervention does not normally require a preprocedure angiogram once the communicating channel has been located and confirmed by sonography.

Smaller AV fistulas can be restudied at 2-week intervals. These will typically lose the artery-like signals during the Valsalva maneuver. They are likely to close spontaneously by the first visit. If they persist at 1 month, surgical ligation is normally performed.

A perivascular artifact with color signals extending beyond the vessel walls is often observed. This is believed to represent the soft tissue vibrations due to the jet of the AV fistula as it impacts the wall of the vein. These vibrations are picked up and encoded as color signals on the color Doppler map (see Fig. 1.45**B**). They can also be shown on the Doppler spectra sampled at the same location in the soft tissues. Larger AV fistulas can affect the flow pattern in the artery proximal to the communication (Fig. 7.18). This is more likely to occur in a congenital AV fistula (Fig. 7.19).

Miscellaneous Masses

There are a variety of masses that are likely to be identified when imaging the lower extremities. The popliteal cyst normally lies posterior to the knee. It shows a large variation in the amount of echogenic structure. It is easily distinguished from a pseudoaneurysm since it does not contain any flow signals and is distant from the artery. However, it may be difficult to differentiate from a hematoma, a seroma, or an abscess.

The region of the groin will often con-

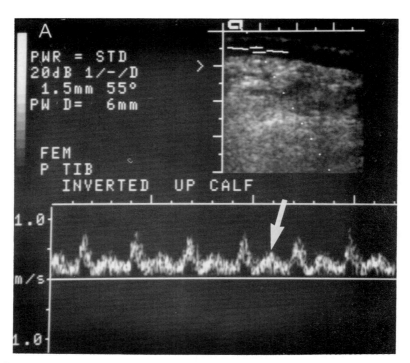

Figure 7.18. The presence of an arteriovenous fistula normally affects the flow profile of the artery proximal to the fistula and the flow pattern within the recipient vein. This can be more easily demonstrated by the effects of an open fistula following in situ arterial bypass surgery. **A,** The Doppler waveform taken in the proximal graft shows a low-resistance pattern with a significant amount of diastolic flow present (*arrow*). **B,** The Doppler waveform taken distal to the AV communication now shows a normal triphasic pattern. The *small arrow* indicates the site of the fistula, which was identified by color Doppler mapping. **C,** A Doppler waveform obtained at the fistula shows the high-velocity signals due to rapid flow through the small communication.

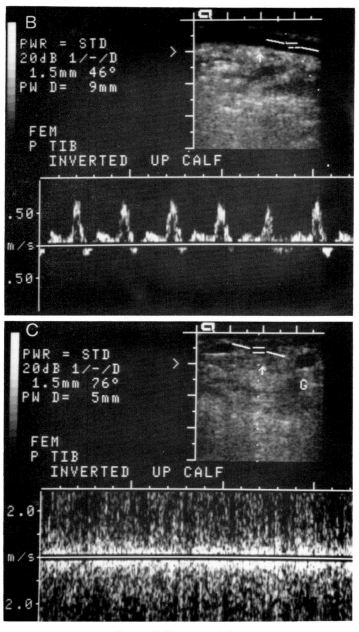

Figure 7.18. **B** and **C.**

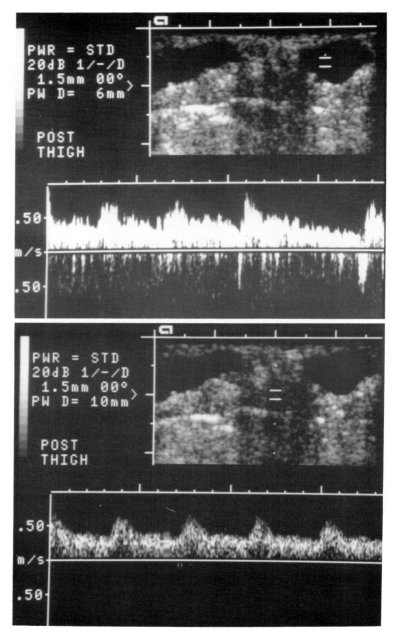

Figure 7.19. Persistent arteriovenous malformations are normally quite evident clinically. The presence of superficial skin changes, including discoloration and palpable vascular channels, are common findings. The malformation has dilated vascular channels that resemble varicosities on gray-scale imaging. **A,** The Doppler spectrum sampled from within the dilated channel shows an arterial waveform of a low-resistance pattern with relatively high diastolic velocity. This is very different from the low-velocity signals seen in a varix. **B,** Aided by color Doppler mapping, a small feeding artery was identified. The Doppler gate was then positioned at the corresponding site, and a low-amplitude, low-resistance waveform was obtained. This feeding arterial branch is but one of many that normally feed such malformations.

tain soft tissue masses. These are often enlarged lymph nodes. Benign inflammatory lymph nodes are often hyperplastic and retain the typical shape; they show both color Doppler signals and a mixed pattern of arterial and venous signals (Fig. 7.20). These signals extend from the hilum toward the periphery of the lymph node. A more irregular and rounded shape change in the lymph node should suggest the possibility of involvement by a neoplastic tumor. Flow signals are also occasionally seen in these masses. Malignant and hyperplastic lymph nodes have been confused with AV fistulas.

Aneurysms

Aneurysms develop as the structural integrity of the arterial wall weakens. Focal enlargement of the artery is most likely to occur at the level of the popliteal or distal superficial femoral artery. They are often bilateral (50%) and can remain asympto-

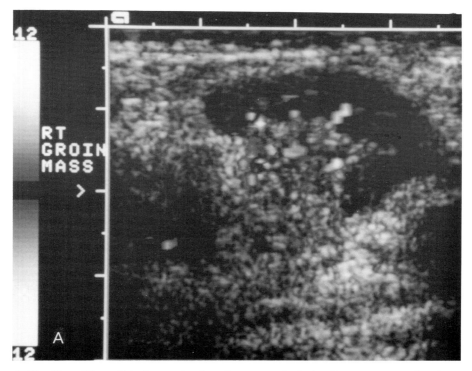

Figure 7.20. The differential diagnosis of groin masses includes the presence of enlarged lymph nodes. Those associated with malignancies tend to be large and rounded and show varying degrees of hypervascularity. The benign hyperplastic lymph node is often seen with an inflammatory process such as cellulitis. Its appearance has been confused with either an AV fistula or a pseudoaneurysm. **A** (see color plate V), An entity that has on occasion been confused with a pseudoaneurysm is the hypervascular lymph node. More careful interrogation of the suspected mass shows color Doppler signals radiating in a branching pattern from the hilum of the lymph node. **B,** On gray-scale imaging, the node has an iso- or hypoechoic outer core (*arrows*) surrounding the hilum, which is hyperechoic (*curved arrow*). The vascular channels—afferent artery and efferent vein—enter the lymph node at the base of the hilum. **C,** The Doppler gate was positioned in the hilum. Because of the small size of the vessels, the gate simultaneously received signals from both artery and vein. The Doppler waveform shows the arterial afferent signals above the baseline (*arrow*) and signals from returning venous blood below the baseline (*curved arrow*).

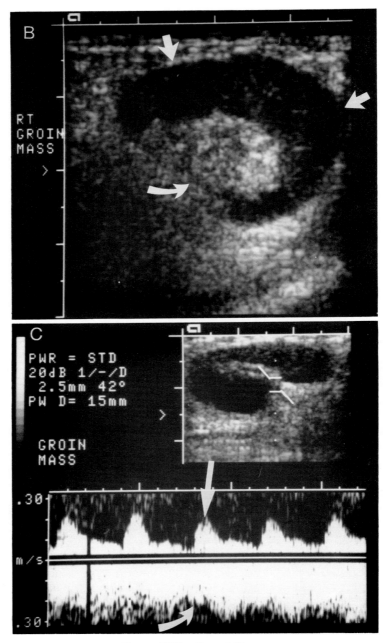

Figure 7.20. B and **C.**

matic for long periods of time. Coexistence of an abdominal aortic aneurysm is also quite likely (25 to 30%). Ultrasound imaging has become the gold standard for confirming this suspected diagnosis and has replaced arteriography. The diagnostic superiority of ultrasound is due to the fact that it can detect the progressive thrombus that fills in the aneurysm from the periphery. This gives an almost normal appearance to the lumen of the artery at the level of the aneurysm during angiography despite the fact that quite a large aneurysm may be present.

Doppler sonography is useful in the preoperative and postoperative evaluation of aneurysms. It often confirms that a thrombosing aneurysm is responsible for evidence of peripheral embolization. It is also useful in confirming occlusion following bypass surgery. A bulge or focal enlargement of greater than 20% of the expected vessel diameter constitutes a simple functional definition of an aneurysm (Fig. 7.21). Serial monitoring of asymptomatic aneurysms is now becoming an option in most noninvasive laboratories. Sonography offers a means of monitoring for possible aneurysm growth and the development of mural thrombus likely to embolize. A commonly quoted diameter of 2 cm is considered a threshold value above which the aneurysm is likely to cause symptoms and acute arterial thrombosis (Fig. 7.22).

Direct pathological verification of ultrasound diagnosed aneurysms has shown the technique to be quite sensitive and specific. It is in fact superior to angiography because of the tendency for mural thrombus to deposit along the wall. The accuracy of Doppler techniques for confirming patency or for the diagnosis of occlusion has yet to be reported.

STENOSIS AND OCCLUSIONS

The spectrum of lesions present in the leg arteries of patients with claudication is quite varied. It is not uncommon for long segmental arterial occlusions to coexist with almost normal arterial segments. The most common sites of disease are the distal superficial femoral and proximal popliteal artery segments. Diabetics tend to have preferential involvement of the tibial and peroneal arteries.

The diagnosis of peripheral disease is often made by noting a change in the flow pattern on the Doppler spectrum sampled distal to the site of an arterial lesion (Fig. 7.23). Arterial lesions of hemodynamic significance cause the period of early diastolic flow reversal to decrease and ultimately disappear as the lesion becomes more severe. The late diastolic component of forward flow increases in magnitude as the severity of the proximal lesions worsens. With the more severe lesions, a monophasic pattern showing low-amplitude forward flow velocities persists during the cardiac cycle, with the diastolic velocities reaching 30 to 50% of the peak systolic values. This pattern is thought to represent a combination of factors such as progressive dilatation and recruitment of the peripheral arterioles within the distal vascular bed of the leg as well as the development of many small collateral branches. In combination, these changes diminish the effective resistance of the artery distal to obstructing lesions.

These patterns may not be seen on selective sampling within conduit vessels proximal to high-grade focal lesions. Under such circumstances, the high resistance caused by the distal lesion and the absence of collaterals can cause an absence of any significant diastolic flow. The Doppler waveform appearance is then one of mainly forward flow during systole with or without a significant diastolic flow component (Fig. 7.24). If large collaterals are present, the diastolic component of blood flow may not be lost. Overall, the peak systolic velocity component of the Doppler velocity spectrum is less affected by the presence or absence of collaterals or by

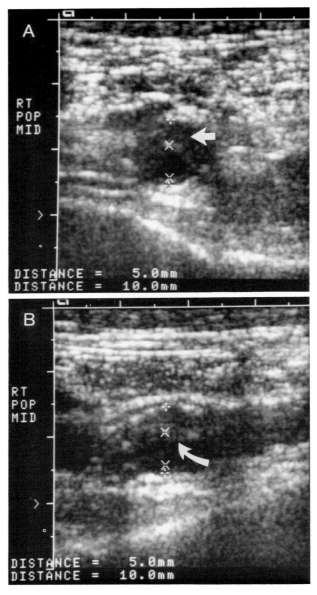

Figure 7.21. Sonography has emerged as a diagnostic gold standard for the diagnosis of arterial aneurysms. This small popliteal artery aneurysm is asymptomatic and constitutes an incidental finding. A clinically palpable aneurysm was present in the opposite extremity. **A,** On transverse imaging, the AP diameter of the aneurysm was measured at 1.0 cm. The wall of the aneurysm is lined with mildly echogenic material (*arrow*) representing laminar thrombus. The presence of this laminar thrombus creates an effective lumen of 0.5 cm (between X markers). This apparently normal lumen was seen on arteriography, which missed the presence of the aneurysm. **B,** The extent of the aneurysm is better seen on longitudinal imaging. The thrombus is more clearly delineated (*curved arrow*) and located more posteriorly.

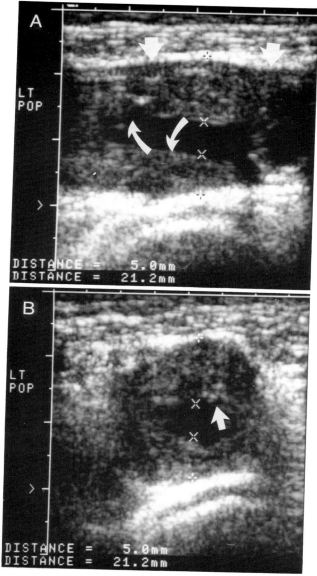

Figure 7.22. This patient developed acute discoloration of the toes suspicious for an episode of peripheral embolization. A mass was palpated behind the knee. The arteriogram showed a mildly ectatic popliteal artery. **A,** On longitudinal imaging, a large mass (*arrows*) was found contiguous to and surrounding the popliteal artery. This represents a large popliteal artery aneurysm. The arterial lumen measures 0.5 cm between the X markers. The enlarged artery measures 2.1 cm. Most of the wall of the aneurysm is made up of mildly echogenic thrombus (*curved arrows*). **B,** The eccentric nature of the aneurysm is better appreciated on this transverse image. Thrombus accounts for almost 1.5 cm of the total diameter of the aneurysm, which is 2.1 cm. Most of the thrombus is located posteriorly (*arrow*). This lining of thrombus is more than likely the source of the acute episode of peripheral arterial embolization. Aneurysms of this type will often continue to enlarge. They can completely thrombose and will often block with thrombus the smaller peripheral arteries located downstream. They can also rarely rupture. In both cases, acute loss of limb is a common complication.

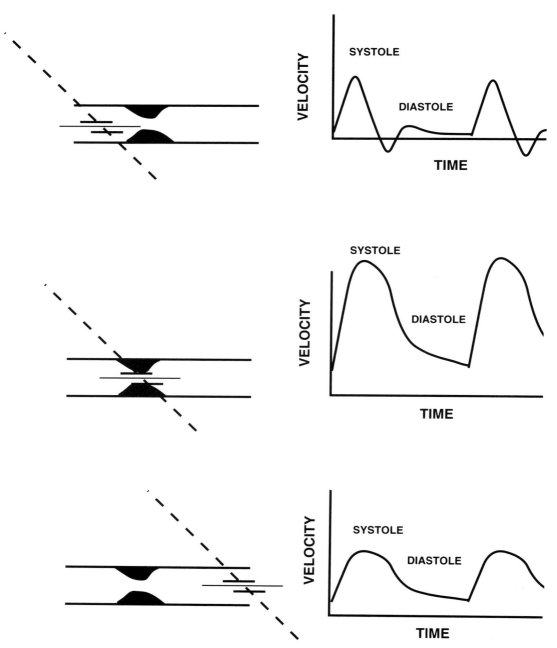

Figure 7.23. The use of the peak systolic velocity ratio to grade stenosis severity requires that the velocity be sampled proximal to the stenosis (*top row*). This is normally done 4 cm proximally. The peak systolic velocity is then measured at the point of maximal velocity or color shift on the Doppler map (*middle row*). The diastolic portion of the waveform will often show marked variability, being alternatively absent or quite pronounced for the same grade of stenosis severity in different individuals. Velocities distal to the stenosis (*lower row*) may remain perturbed for a few centimeters, depending on the grade and shape of the stenosis. In general, however, the diastolic component of the waveform will stay elevated.

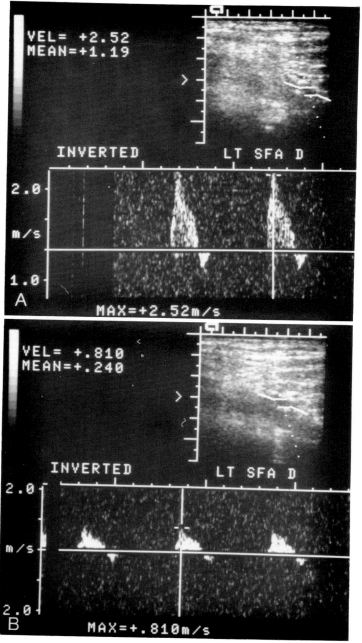

Figure 7.24. The presence of a significant stenosis (>50% diameter narrowing) of the superficial femoral artery normally causes at least a doubling of the peak systolic velocity at the site of the stenosis. **A,** Once a site of abnormal color Doppler signals is detected, a Doppler gate is used to sample the peak systolic velocity. In this case, the peak systolic velocity reaches 2.5 m/sec and the triphasic arterial waveform is preserved. **B,** The peak systolic velocity is then sampled at a point located 2 to 4 cm proximal. The peak velocity is measured at 0.8 m/sec. The calculated peak systolic velocity ratio is 3.1, suggesting the presence of a focal 75% narrowing of the artery lumen despite preservation of the typical waveform.

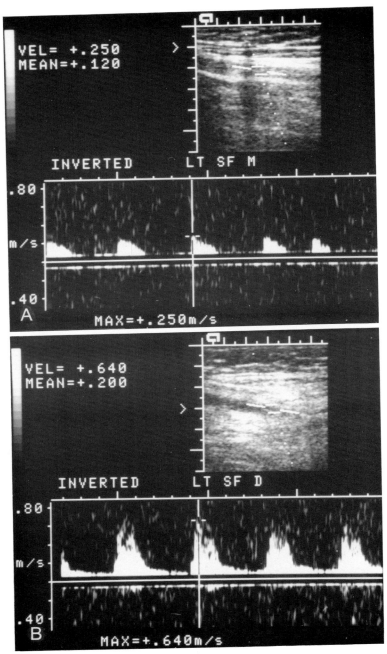

Figure 7.25. Poor inflow into a lower-extremity arterial segment due to the presence of an iliac occlusion normally causes decreased flow into the more distal arteries. **A,** The Doppler waveform sampled in the mid superficial femoral artery distal to an iliac occlusion shows a very low velocity of 0.25 m/sec. The diastolic component of blood flow is depressed and is barely at the level of the wall filter. The presence of a significant stenosis can nevertheless be detected during color Doppler mapping. A survey of the superficial femoral artery showed a focal zone of slightly increased color signals. **B,** The Doppler waveform sampled at this site shows a peak systolic velocity of 0.64 m/sec. This value is considered to be within normal limits. However, when the peak systolic velocity ratio is calculated, a value of 2.6 suggests the presence of a hemodynamically significant stenosis.

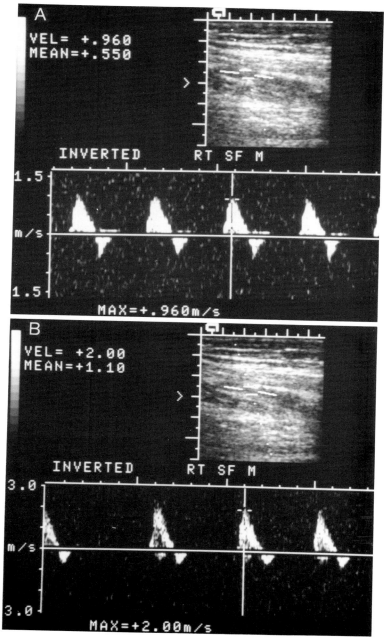

Figure 7.26. Moderately severe stenoses of 40 to 60% narrowing are less likely to perturb the normal triphasic arterial waveform. **A,** This longitudinal image of the superficial femoral artery shows a normal peak systolic velocity of 0.96 m/sec and a normal contour of the Doppler waveform. **B,** A focal lesion of approximately 50% is nevertheless seen 1 cm distal to this point. The waveform at the stenosis does not show a low-resistance pattern.

proximal as well as distal occlusions (Fig. 7.25). It is therefore considered a more useful index for grading stenoses in the leg arteries.

Peak systolic velocity decreases as one progresses down the leg arteries. It is 1.1 m/sec at the level of the common femoral, 0.9 m/sec in the superficial femoral, 0.7 m/sec in the popliteal, and 0.4 to 0.5 m/sec in the tibioperoneal branches. This normal decrease in the peak systolic velocity occurs despite a gradual decrease in the diameter of the arteries from 0.6 to 0.8 cm in the femoral to 0.2 to 0.3 cm in the tibioperoneal branches. This decrease appears paradoxical, since the reduced diameter of an arterial conduit normally causes the velocity to increase. In the case of the leg arteries, major branches that arise along their course are responsible for a decrease in the amount of blood reaching the more distal artery. This is responsible for the progressive decrease in velocity.

Focal areas of doubling of the measured peak systolic velocity have been shown to correspond to hemodynamically significant lesions of greater than 50% narrowing in the lumen diameter of the artery. For the reasons discussed above, there are no reliable parameters for grading stenosis severity based on the diastolic component of the velocity spectrum (Fig. 7.26).

A diagnostic sensitivity above 80% and a specificity above 90% can be achieved for detecting segmental arterial lesions with duplex sonography of the femoropopliteal arteries. The Doppler gate must be moved sequentially along the full length of the femoral and popliteal arteries. Since these arteries are over 30 to 40 cm in length, a survey of Doppler velocities takes 1 to 2 hours. Any site where the peak systolic velocity at least doubles is considered to have a significant lesion. The velocity at the site of a suspected stenosis is normally compared to that at a point 2 to 4 cm proximal to it. Occlusions are considered present whenever there is a failure to detect any flow signals within the segment in question (Fig. 7.27). A simple way of ensuring that the Doppler gain is properly set is to sample flow in the adjacent venous segment. The comparative efficacy of this technique with respect to angiography has been mostly done by comparison of the findings of Doppler sonography for segments of femoral or popliteal artery 7 to 15 cm in length. Depending on the author, the femoral artery is separated into two or three segments, while the popliteal artery is treated as either one or two segments. The common femoral and profunda femoral arteries are treated as separate segments. No systematic studies have included an evaluation of the three tibioperoneal branches. The iliac arteries can be surveyed with a lower-frequency transducer. It is part of our protocol to sample the spectrum at the common femoral artery and to infer the presence of any significant iliac lesions by the resultant effect on the shape of the velocity spectrum. A lower-amplitude signal (<0.6 m/sec) or the appearance of a strong forward diastolic flow component without flow reversal is considered evidence of significant aortoiliac pathology (>75% stenosis) (Fig. 7.28).

Color Doppler sonography has recently been shown to decrease by 40% the time needed to examine the carotid artery for sites of suspected stenosis. A similar advantage emerges when color flow mapping is used to detect focal lesions in the femoropopliteal artery. The diagnostic accuracy of this type of examination is slightly better than for non–color assisted duplex sonography. The criteria used to perform the examination include the presence of a typical decrease in the color saturation at the site of stenosis and the absence of color signals at the site of an occlusion. The perceived size of the flow lumen may also be used. This approach is more likely to underestimate or overestimate the extent of lumen diameter narrow-

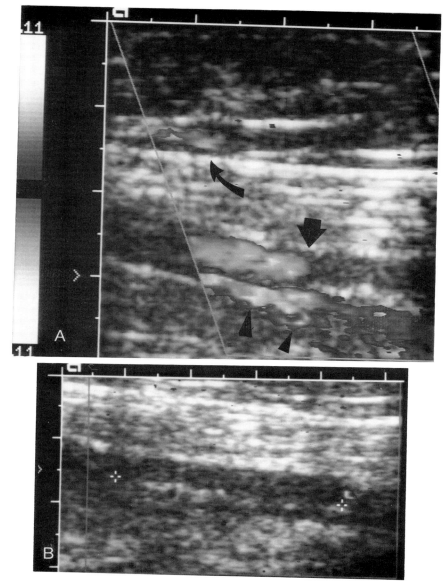

Figure 7.27. **A** (see color plate V), Total occlusion of the superficial femoral artery is shown in this color Doppler image. The color Doppler signals within the superficial femoral artery terminate abruptly (*arrow*). The superficial femoral vein is deep to the artery (*arrowheads*). A proximal arterial collateral is also present (*curved arrow*). **B,** The presence of a totally occluded portion of the femoral artery is clearly shown in this longitudinal image. The cross-hairs span the length of the occluded segment—approximately 4.0 cm. **C,** The absence of flow is confirmed by sampling the Doppler spectrum in this arterial segment. **D,** Proximal to the occlusion, flow velocities are markedly depressed at 0.23 m/sec peak systolic velocity. **E,** The presence of a large collateral detected on the color Doppler map is confirmed by the Doppler spectrum, which shows a peak systolic velocity of 0.25 m/sec. The collateral cannot be followed on the same longitudinal image because of its markedly tortuous course.

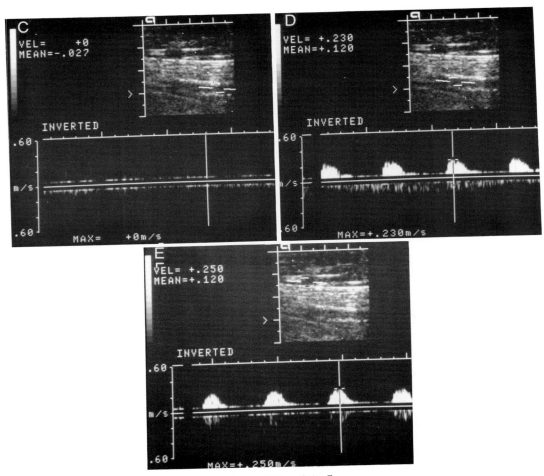

Figure 7.27.   C to **E.**

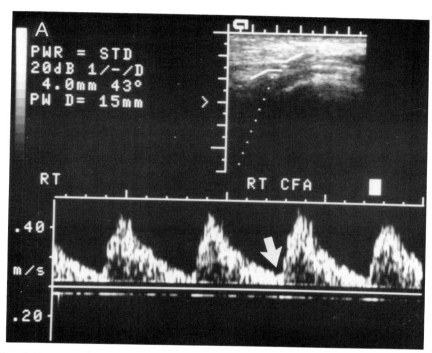

Figure 7.28. **A,** The presence of either occlusion or high-grade stenosis of the aorta or iliac artery can be suspected whenever the Doppler waveform sampled at the common femoral artery shows low amplitude—peak systolic velocity of 0.45 m/sec—and a low-resistance pattern with elevated diastolic velocities (*arrow*). The effect of this aortoiliac lesion is to depress blood flow and therefore the measurable peak systolic velocities in the more distal arterial segments. **B,** This is shown on the Doppler waveform obtained in the superficial femoral artery of this same extremity. The peak systolic velocity is 0.5 and the diastolic velocity is 0.3 m/sec. **C,** The Doppler waveform taken at a site of increased velocities on a color Doppler map shows a peak systolic velocity of 1.2 m/sec. The calculated velocity ratio is 4.0 and therefore is consistent with a stenosis of greater than 75%.

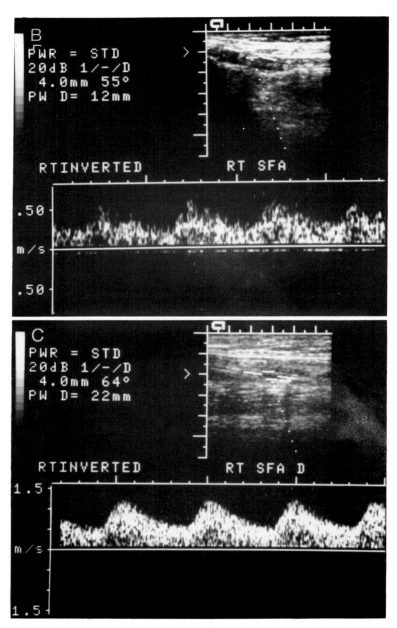

Figure 7.28. **B** and **C.**

ing depending on the actual blood flow velocities. It will underestimate the lumen size when the velocities are elevated due to color overflow beyond the boundaries of the artery. Blood flow velocities are actually decreased in long segmental stenoses (greater than 7 to 10 cm). The color flow lumen appreciated on transverse images rather than longitudinal images may then be used to subjectively grade the extent of lumen diameter narrowing. This may in fact overestimate the severity of a focal stenosis, since the velocity at the periphery of the arterial lumen may drop below the velocity sensitivity of the color Doppler velocity scale and be encoded as black. This situation is likely to occur whenever there is a high-grade lesion or a totally occluded segment located more proximally.

Lower-Extremity Examination Protocol

The survey is normally performed by moving the transducer from the common femoral to the low popliteal artery. A Doppler spectrum is first sampled over the junction of the external iliac and common femoral arteries. Velocities less than 0.6 m/sec or a loss of the normal early diastolic reversal of blood flow is considered to be evidence of aortoiliac pathology. This will normally correspond to stenoses above 75% in lumen diameter narrowing.

The transducer is held longitudinally, parallel to the proximal superficial femoral artery. The color window is steered forward and the color scale is set to a maximum of 0.4 to 0.6 m/sec. The transducer is held fixed for one to two cardiac cycles to perceive flow in the arterial segment. Once flow signals have been perceived along the length of this segment, the transducer is then slid a distance equal to its length. Doppler signals are then observed in this more distal segment. This is repeated until the vessel lumen cannot be further visualized due to the increased depth at the level of the adductor canal. The transducer is then placed behind the knee. The proximal popliteal artery is sampled upward until the site where the signals were previously lost is reached. If imaging from the anterior or posterior aspect of the thigh cannot fully show the arterial lumen, the examination is incomplete. The velocity window is normally decreased to the 0.2 to 0.4 m/sec range at the level of the popliteal artery. The popliteal artery is also followed downward until the anterior tibial artery origin is identified and then the tibioperoneal branches.

It normally takes a series of 10 to 12 sliding motions to survey the length of the femoropopliteal arteries using a transducer with a 4-cm-wide footprint. A larger transducer with a 5- to 6-cm footprint can reduce the time needed for the examination further, since the number of stations necessary to cover the arterial segments is reduced by 25 to 50% (i.e., to a minimum of 5 to 9 stations).

Areas of abnormal flow velocities are subjected to Doppler spectral analysis (Fig. 7.29). A point 2 to 4 cm proximal to sites of abnormal velocity is sampled to obtain a velocity ratio. At least one velocity spectrum is acquired for each of the common femoral, superficial femoral and popliteal arteries. The presence of collateral branches is noted whenever possible. They are indirect evidence of significant lesions located downstream. Transverse imaging is used as needed. The area with color flow signals is compared to the cross-section area of the artery. This gives an approximate estimate of the degree of stenosis.

Lesions develop in the femoropopliteal arteries and progress in severity until they cause an occlusion. The segment involved by the occlusion will then thrombose proximally and distal to the lesion until a major collateral branch is reached. These collateral branches, as they develop, take on a greater proportion of the blood flow (Fig.

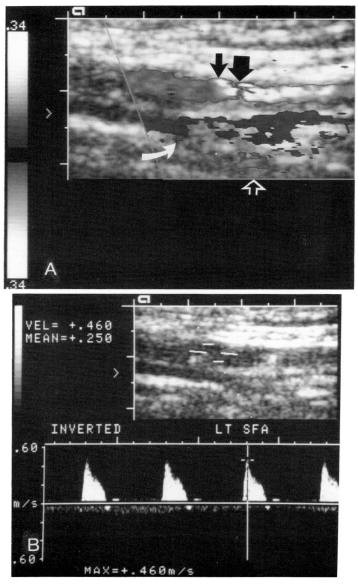

Figure 7.29.   The presence of a high-grade stenosis in the superficial femoral or popliteal artery will affect blood flow and the peak systolic velocities measured proximal to the lesion. **A** (see color plate V), The presence of a focal high-grade stenosis in the native superficial femoral artery is shown here. This corresponds to the site of a previous endarterectomy. The actual stenosis is identified as a zone of aliasing with transition in the color Doppler signal from red to white (*small arrow*) and then aliasing into blue (*large arrow*). The partly compressed superficial femoral vein is shown lying deep to the artery (*curved arrow*). An arterial collateral is also present (*open arrow*). **B,** A velocity spectrum taken proximal to the superficial femoral lesion shows a depressed peak systolic velocity of 0.46 m/sec. **C,** The Doppler gate was positioned at the stenosis, giving a peak systolic velocity of 2.38 m/sec. The calculated velocity ratio is 5.2, consistent with a greater than 75% lumen diameter stenosis. **D,** A final longitudinal image shows the Doppler spectrum distal to the stenosis. The peak systolic velocity is still elevated due to the length of the stenosis. The shape of the Doppler waveform

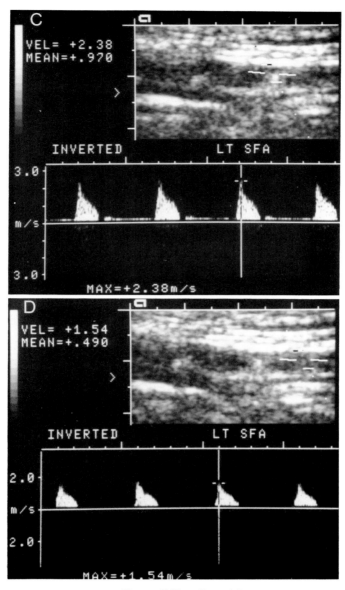

Figure 7.29. C and D.

remains relatively unaffected. There is no elevation of the diastolic velocities so typical of stenoses of similar severity affecting the carotid arteries. Waveforms such as this are the main reason for using the peak systolic velocity and the derived ratio as a means of gauging lesion severity in the peripheral arteries.

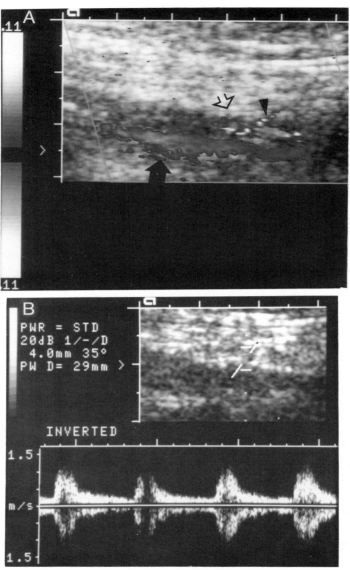

Figure 7.30. Arterial collateral branches will tend to preserve blood flow distal to segmental arterial occlusions. This reconstitution of blood flow to the artery distal to the occlusion can be shown with the aid of color Doppler imaging. **A** (see color plate V), This superficial femoral vein (*arrow*) lies deep to a superficial femoral artery containing low-amplitude color Doppler signals (*open arrow*). A small arterial collateral channel (*arrowhead*) feeds the superficial femoral artery distal to an occlusion. It contains signals showing increased velocities. This is a common finding. It is caused by the smaller caliber of the collateral with respect to the native artery. **B,** This collateral branch was identified on the color Doppler map. The Doppler waveform shows that the collateral delivers antegrade flow delivered into this segment of the superficial femoral artery. **C,** The superficial femoral artery distal to this point now has antegrade blood flow with a peak systolic velocity of 0.4 m/sec. **D,** The superficial femoral artery is also patent for a few millimeters proximal to the collateral. Flow within this blind segment of the artery is mostly reversed (*arrow*) and of low amplitude.

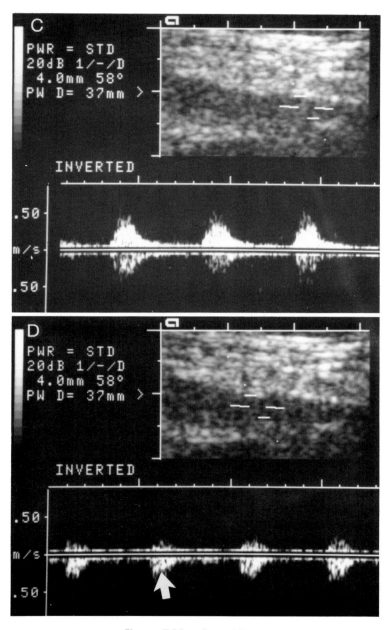

Figure 7.30. **C** and **D.**

7.30). There is therefore a point of transition where flow through the occluding segment is equal to if not less than that within the collateral (Fig. 7.31). A high-grade lesion might therefore be undetected, since a velocity ratio might be taken between the lesion in the segment with depressed velocities compared to the segment just proximal to the developing collateral (Fig. 7.32). A simple strategy adopted to compensate for this effect is to construct the velocity ratio with a point distal to the stenosis. However, this might not be effective. The lesion might therefore only be inferred by the presence of a low-velocity profile without a diastolic component proximal to the stenosis. The actual stenosis might not be detectable. A similar situation can arise when calcifications are present. The lesion is then suspected only due to the presence of low-flow signals proximal and distal to the lesion. The severity and length of the lesion might not be accurately determined. Conversely, occluded segments may be inadvertently considered stenotic because Doppler signals are inadvertently obtained in the developing collateral (Fig. 7.33). With color-assisted Doppler sonography, the examination takes approximately 30 minutes to cover both lower extremities. The diagnostic accuracy of this approach is the same if not better than with traditional duplex sonography.

Rare cases of suspected popliteal artery entrapment require a modification to the

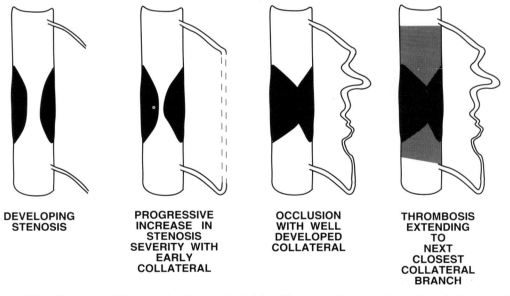

| DEVELOPING STENOSIS | PROGRESSIVE INCREASE IN STENOSIS SEVERITY WITH EARLY COLLATERAL | OCCLUSION WITH WELL DEVELOPED COLLATERAL | THROMBOSIS EXTENDING TO NEXT CLOSEST COLLATERAL BRANCH |

Figure 7.31. The natural history of a stenosis is slightly different in the leg arteries than in the carotid arteries. The leg arteries do not feed a critical organ like the brain, and the progression of significant stenoses and occlusions is much better tolerated. As a stenosis develops and becomes more severe, potential collateral pathways develop. These form through muscular feeding arteries or through other unnamed branches. At the time the arterial segment occludes, the collateral pathways are normally well enough developed to prevent the appearance of more severe symptoms such as rest pain. The underlying stenosis may be quite small, whereas the length of the occlusion tends to be much longer. There is a normal tendency for thrombus to deposit in the artery lumen both proximal and distal to the occlusion. The occluded lumen normally extends from the origin of the first large collateral branch proximal to the occlusion. The distal end of the occlusion normally corresponds to the site where a collateral branch feeds into the main arterial lumen.

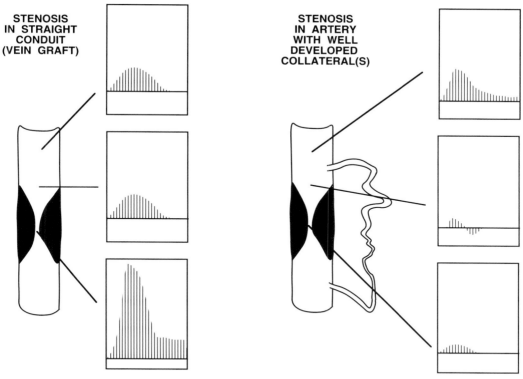

Figure 7.32. On the left side of the diagram is the ideal situation where Doppler sonography is best used to grade a stenosis by the increase in blood flow velocities. The velocity of blood just proximal to the stenosis and at a point a few centimeters above is essentially the same. The artery behaves as a simple conduit. This situation is typical of most peripheral arterial stenoses, all bypass graft stenoses, and all internal carotid stenoses. On the right of the diagram is the situation that can occasionally cause inaccurate grading of the stenosis severity. The presence of a large collateral branch shunts blood flow away from the main artery segment with the high-grade stenosis. The peak velocities measured 2 to 4 cm above the stenosis, when compared to the velocity at the stenosis, suggest that there is no stenosis present. The velocities sampled immediately distal to the origin of the collateral branch correctly suggest that we are dealing with a subtotal occlusion.

imaging protocol. High-resolution imaging is first performed to exclude the presence of the portion of the gastrocnemius muscle or tendon that is abnormally located between the popliteal vein and artery (Fig. 7.34). In addition, color Doppler or duplex sonography is performed longitudinally over the popliteal artery as the patient performs provocative maneuvers such as dorsiflexion and plantarflexion of the foot. A greater than doubling of the peak systolic velocity is considered evidence of significant entrapment.

Upper Extremity

NORMAL ANATOMY AND FLOW PATTERNS

The arterial system of the upper extremity parallels the deep venous branches (Fig. 7.35).

The subclavian artery originates from the innominate artery on the right and from the aorta on the left. Both junctions can be identified using a sonographic window just superior to the sternoclavicular joint. The location of this bifurcation can

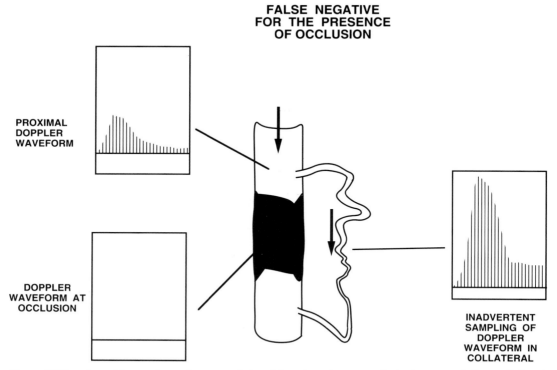

FALSE NEGATIVE FOR THE PRESENCE OF OCCLUSION

PROXIMAL DOPPLER WAVEFORM

DOPPLER WAVEFORM AT OCCLUSION

INADVERTENT SAMPLING OF DOPPLER WAVEFORM IN COLLATERAL

Figure 7.33. A problem arises when a collateral lies close to an occluded segment. The collateral branch itself may inadvertently be sampled. The Doppler signal is then inappropriately ascribed to a patent arterial segment and the occlusion is missed.

be easily determined using the following maneuver. The transducer is held transverse to the carotid artery and the more superficially located internal jugular vein. It is then slowly slid downward toward the clavicle and the transduceer is pointed slowly toward the feet. The carotid artery is kept in the image as the subclavian and brachiocephalic arteries appear. The subclavian artery will lie superficial to the vein while the transducer is kept in the supraclavicular fossa. The junction of the mid and proximal third of the clavicle is often a blind spot for direct sonographic imaging. The lack of space in the more lateral aspect of the supraclavicular fossa often makes it necessary to place the transducer below the clavicle. The artery now appears to lie deep to the subclavian vein.

The axillary artery originates near the junction of the cephalic and the axillary veins (Fig. 7.36) at the proximal aspect of the pectoralis minor muscle. The axillary artery can be followed as it courses medially over the humeral head to become the brachial artery. This artery can be followed to the antecubital fossa, where it trifurcates into the radial, ulnar, and interosseous branches. The ulnar and radial branches can be followed downward toward the wrist. From the level of the brachial artery downward there are two veins accompanying every artery.

The Doppler waveform of these arterial branches is one of high resistance and is similar to that of the leg arteries. With careful technique, it is possible to visualize the smaller digital branches.

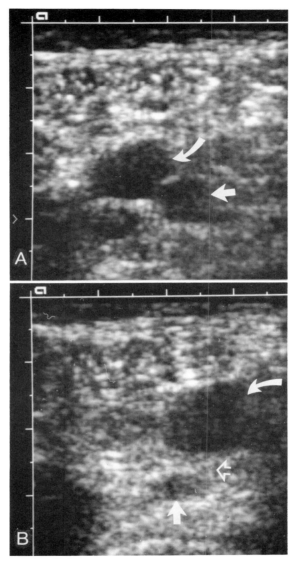

Figure 7.34. Popliteal artery entrapment is caused by the presence of either a muscular or tendinous portion of the medial head of the gastrocnemius muscle that is abnormally located between the popliteal artery and vein. **A,** Normally, there should not be any separation between the artery (*arrow*) and the vein (*curved arrow*). **B,** On the opposite side, however, this patient shows an abnormal separation (*open arrow*) between the popliteal artery (*arrow*) and vein (*curved arrow*). The diagnosis of entrapment, however, requires that the popliteal artery be extrinsically compressed and that a flow disturbance be present at the site of entrapment whenever the patient performs maneuvers such as plantarflexion or dorsiflexion of the foot.

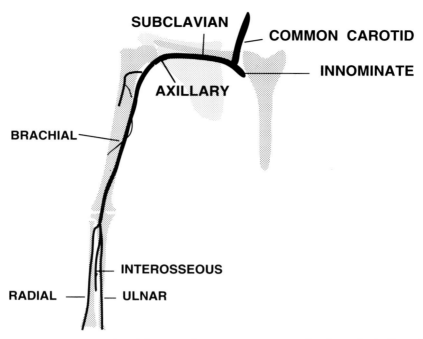

Figure 7.35. The arterial supply of the arm has many more anatomic variants than the arteries supplying the legs. These occur mostly in the forearm. Significant stenoses or atherosclerotic occlusions are quite uncommon in the subclavian and more distal arteries. The lesions commonly seen include iatrogenic injuries and peripheral embolizations.

PATHOPHYSIOLOGY AND DIAGNOSTIC ACCURACY

The noninvasive evaluation of the upper-extremity arterial branches is directed to diagnosing atherosclerotic occlusions, detecting focal stenosis due to thoracic outlet syndrome, confirming native arterial occlusion secondary to emboli or trauma, determining the presence of vasculitis, detecting complications following cardiac catheterization, and evaluating dialysis shunts. The upper-extremity arteries are normally spared the same type of severe atherosclerotic lesions that affect the legs. The most likely site of stenotic lesion is the proximal subclavian artery. Progressive stenosis of the proximal artery causes an important collateral to develop using the vertebral artery. Except for this type of proximal lesion, atherosclerotic occlusion of the more distally located branches is quite uncommon. The same diagnostic criteria used in the leg arteries are applied to the arm arteries. Doubling of the peak systolic velocity is considered diagnostic for significant stenosis above 50% narrowing of the artery diameter. Absence of Doppler signals is suggestive of occlusion.

There are increasing reports on the use of Doppler imaging for making the diagnosis of thoracic outlet syndrome (Fig. 7.37). To induce arterial stenosis, the arm is positioned in the orientation that normally elicits symptoms. This is most often in abduction with the head rotated away from the arm. The entrapment of the artery can occur at one of three sites in the subclavian artery. The first is at the level of an additional first cervical rib, the second is at the level of the scalene muscle, and the third is

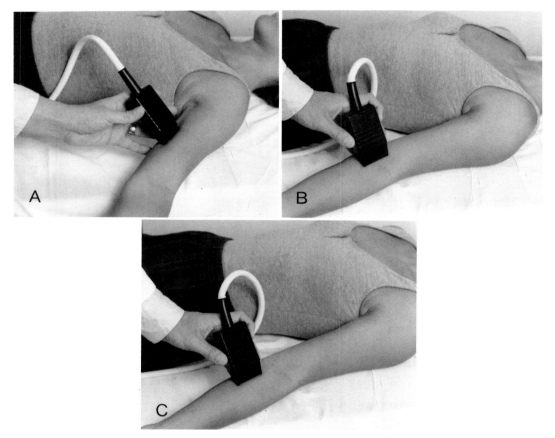

Figure 7.36. Evaluation of the peripheral arteries of the upper extremity can be quickly performed. **A,** The transducer is normally positioned longitudinal from the junction of the axillary and brachial arteries. **B,** The transducer is kept medial as it is displaced more inferiorly to the level of the elbow. **C,** The three separate branches of the interosseous, radial, and ulnar arteries can be visualized by displacing the transducer from a more medial to a lateral position.

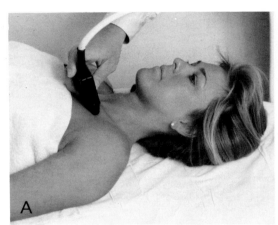
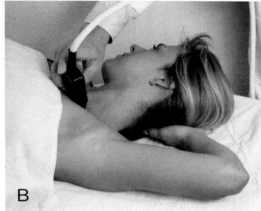

Figure 7.37. The thoracic outlet syndrome will normally cause a decrease in the blood velocity measured in the axillary and more peripherally located arteries of the arm when certain ancillary maneuvers are performed. **A,** The artery is first imaged in a neutral position. **B,** The arm is then placed in abduction behind the head and the head is rotated to the side opposite that being imaged. **C,** The site of stenosis is often located at a point accessible to the transducer. In the neutral position corresponding to **A,** a gray-scale image shows the subclavian artery (*arrow*) just as it passes underneath the clavicle (*curved arrow*). **D,** With the arm in abduction **B,** the lumen of the subclavian artery appears constricted (*curved arrow*). **E,** The Doppler waveform of the artery with the arm in the neutral position does not show any abnormality. **F,** This situation quickly changes in the abducted position. Peak systolic velocities have now more than doubled compared to baseline, suggesting a greater than 50% stenosis in the subclavian artery.

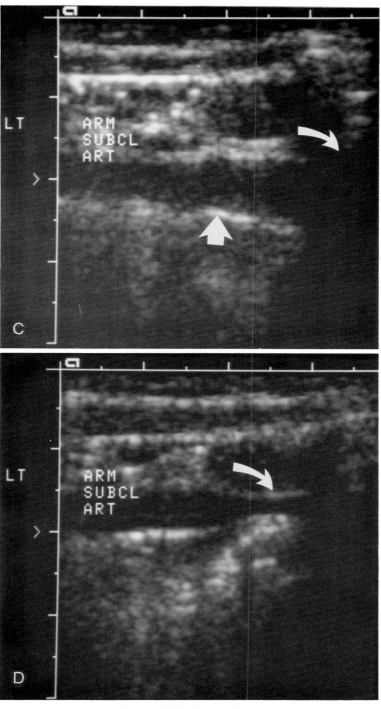

Figure 7.37. **C** and **D.**

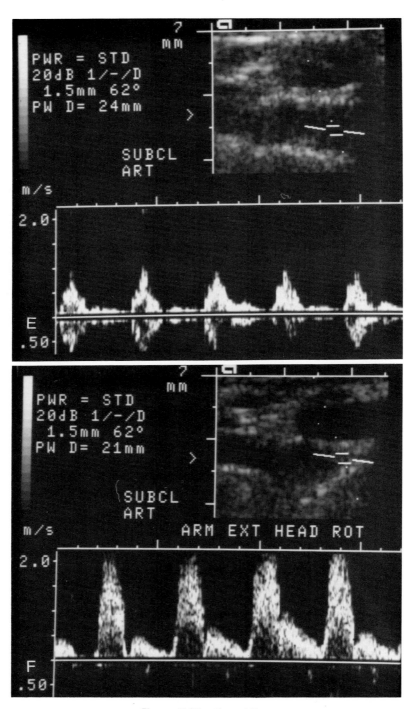

Figure 7.37. E and F.

at the crossing of the subclavian artery above the first rib at the level of the mid clavicle. There is a frequent association between thoracic outlet syndrome and distal arterial embolization. These occur because of thrombus deposition in an aneurysmal segment of the artery downstream from the stenosis. The extent of any acute or chronic occlusions can be mapped out and can help assess the feasibility of bypass surgery or thrombolysis before angiography. The type of information obtained with sonography is useful in helping to clarify patients with upper-extremity arterial symptoms. The most common physical finding of the thoracic outlet syndrome is the presence of paresthesia (altered sensation) in up to 80% of patients, with the ulnar nerve distribution most often being the site of symptoms. Surprisingly, venous compression is much less likely to coexist in these patients.

The first site of possible compression is at the level where the proximal subclavian artery passes between the anterior scalene muscle and the first rib. The vein normally passes anterior to the anterior scalene muscle and is therefore not affected by the compression of the artery within a triangle formed by the anterior scalene muscle anteriorly, the middle scalene muscle posteriorly, and the first rib inferiorly. A second site of compression is the space between the first rib and the clavicle. Finally, more laterally, the *axillary artery* can be compressed between the tendon of the pectoralis minor and the attachment at the coracoid process. To these likely sites of extrinsic compression is added the possibility of an anomalous rib arising at the level of the cervical vertebrae. Compression of the subclavian artery occurs more proximally and is often due to an abnormal ligamentous structure connecting the cervical rib to the first (thoracic) rib. We image the subject supine, with the arm in the neutral position (palm upward). Two additional positions are always taken: with the

arm in abduction and the head in neutral position, and with the arm held in abduction but with the head rotated away and the chin held upward. The more traditional maneuvers are difficult to implement when performing simultaneous Doppler imaging.

In cases of vasculitis, the length of the subclavian and axillary arteries are imaged. The extent of arterial involvement can normally be determined. The flow patterns, however, are quite variable. Velocities can be either decreased or increased as a function of the location, length, and severity of the stenoses. Since the process tends to be diffuse, the cumulative resistance of the pathologically narrowed arteries can blunt the expected increase in peak systolic velocities. Instead, a decrease in peak systolic velocities is often seen in long, diffusely narrowed arterial segments. As in the lower limb, transverse imaging of a narrowed flow lumen is useful to confirm that this is in fact the pathological process responsible for the patient's symptoms. Patients with Raynaud's syndrome can be screened for the presence of a more proximal process responsible for their symptoms.

Preprocedure evaluation of the arm arteries is normally done in patients with known severe peripheral arterial disease. This is mostly useful before performing arterial catheterization.

Following cardiac catheterization, suspected arterial occlusions can be rapidly confirmed and acted on. Large hematomas can be readily evaluated. Any suspected pseudoaneurysms can be confirmed and readily acted on. Supplemental arteriography is often not needed.

Dialysis fistulas can be readily evaluated by Doppler sonography. These are discussed in greater detail in Chapter 8. They do, however, tend to show a variety of pathologies typical of peripheral vascular diseases. Since heparin is utilized during dialysis, the incidence of small pseudoaneurysms is quite high. Similarly, the multiple punctures to which the shunts are subjected encourage the development of arterial thickening due to thrombus deposition and myointimal proliferation. Progressive stenosis leads to the development of a poor result during dialysis due to the large pressure differences that hamper the exchange of dialysates. Ultimately, these lesions progress and cause failure of the shunt. The accuracy for the detection of stenoses and small pseudoaneurysms is above 90%. Detection of stenoses is somewhat more reliable in dialysis shunts that have straight interposition segments.

SUGGESTED READINGS

Altin RS, Flicker S, Naidech HJ. Pseudoaneurysm and arteriovenous fistula after femoral artery catheterization: association with low femoral punctures. AJR 1989;152:629–631.

Cossman DV, Ellison JE, Wagner WH, et al. Comparison of contrast arteriography to arterial mapping with color-flow duplex imaging in the lower extremities. J Vasc Surg 1989;10:522–529.

Coughlin BF, Paushter DM. Peripheral pseudoaneurysms: evaluation with duplex US. Radiology 1988;168:339–342.

Cronenwett JL, Warner KG, Zelenock GB, et al. Intermittent claudication. Current results of nonoperative management. Arch Surg 1984;119:430–436.

Gooding GA, Effeney DJ. Ultrasound of femoral artery aneurysms. AJR 1980;134:477–480.

Helvie MA, Rubin JM, Silver TM, Kresowik TF. The distinction between femoral artery pseudoaneurysms and other causes of groin masses: value of duplex Doppler sonography. AJR 1988;150:1177–1180.

Kohler TR, Nance DR, Cramer MM, Vandenburghe N, Strandness DE Jr. Duplex scanning for diagnosis of aortoiliac and femoropopliteal disease: a prospective study. Circulation 1987;76:1074–1080.

Lynch TG, Hobson RW 2d, Wright CB, et al. Interpretation of Doppler segmental pressures in peripheral vascular occlusive disease. Arch Surg 1984;119:465–467.

MacGowan SW, Saif MF, O'Neill G, Fitzsimons P, Bouchier-Hayes D. Ultrasound examination in the diagnosis of popliteal artery aneurysms. Br J Surg 1985;72:528–529.

Moneta GL, Strandness ED Jr. Peripheral arterial duplex scanning. JCU 1987;15:645–651.

CHAPTER EIGHT

Postoperative Imaging

Doppler sonography has become an important addition to standard real-time two-dimensional sonography since it adds the ability to determine the presence and character of blood flow within masses located in close proximity to vascular prostheses, to confirm patency of an artery or graft following bypass surgery or endarterectomy, and to evaluate an arterial site for possible complications that may ultimately cause an intervention to fail. Although the presence of blood flow within a perivascular mass can be diagnostic of a pseudoaneurysm, the absence of blood flow makes it easier to justify a more conservative approach. In the case of a suspected hematoma, serial follow-up examinations can be used to document resolution of the process. In the case of a suspected abscess, a biopsy can be performed without fear of uncontrolled hemorrhage. This is, however, only a small portion of what Doppler sonography now offers in terms of monitoring the results of surgical and percutaneous interventional procedures. The detection of small AV fistulas in in situ grafts is an example of the use of intraoperative color Doppler mapping. Early postoperative surveys can document the patency of a graft despite the technical inability to perform ankle-brachial pressure measure-

ments. The color Doppler ultrasound device is also finding an increased number of applications in the operative suite, the interventional suite, and in the follow-up examinations performed in the noninvasive laboratory. These studies rely on all three components of sonographic imaging: high-resolution imaging to detect surgical defects, duplex sonography to quantitate flow abnormalities, and color Doppler sonography to rapidly survey and identify abnormal blood flow patterns at the site of arterial interventions.

Carotid Endarterectomy
INTRAOPERATIVE SURVEY

Duplex sonography is increasingly used to document patency and confirm a technically normal appearance of the carotid branches following endarterectomy (Figs. 8.1 and 8.2). The two most important changes are the presence of intimal flaps and stenoses formed secondary to positioning of clamps both proximal and distal to the arteriotomy site (Fig. 8.2). Less common are evidence of retained plaque or thrombus formation (Fig. 8.3).

The examination is performed on completion of the procedure, before skin clo-

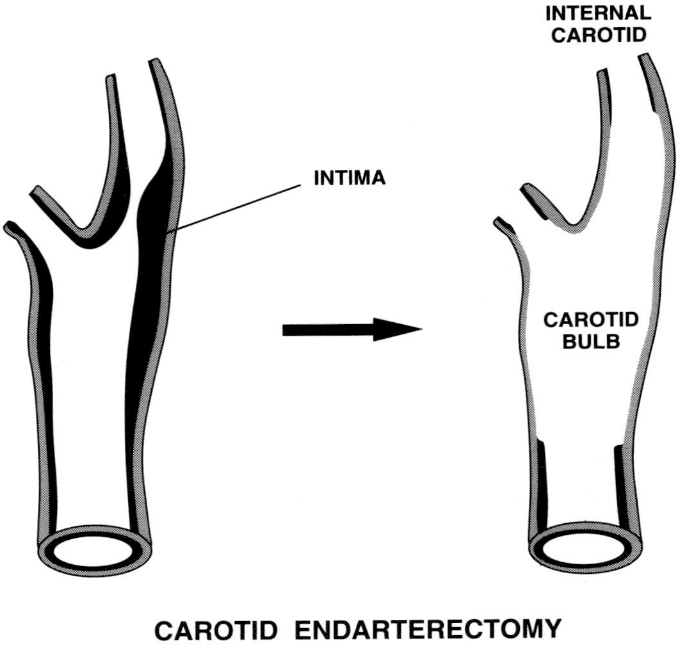

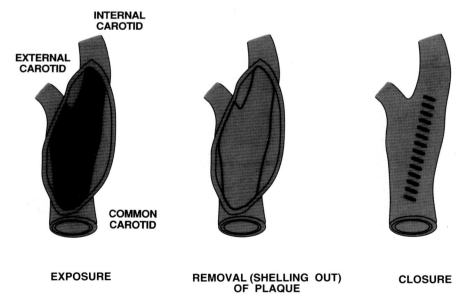

CAROTID ENDARTERECTOMY

Figure 8.1. Carotid endarterectomy consists of the removal of most of the diseased intima of the carotid bulb and proximal internal carotid artery. Some of the diseased media is also often removed.

Figure 8.2. The different steps of the endarterectomy are summarized here. The diseased intima is exposed following incision into the arterial wall. The plaque is then "shelled" out. Finally, the artery wall is closed. The same basic steps are also followed when the procedure is performed in the peripheral arteries.

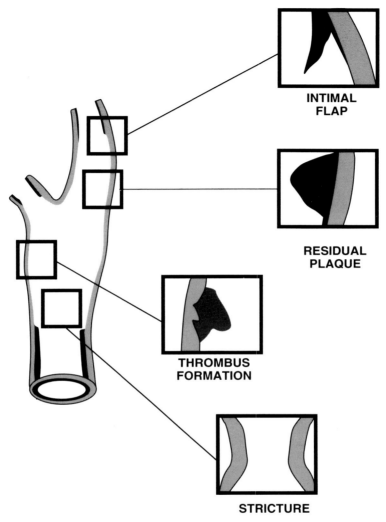

**INTIMAL
FLAP**

**RESIDUAL
PLAQUE**

**THROMBUS
FORMATION**

STRICTURE

Figure 8.3. The mechanisms responsible for poor surgical success of a carotid—or any—endarterectomy are summarized here. These can be visualized on high-resolution gray-scale imaging. Doppler sonography will identify the defects that cause a significant flow abnormality. The latter are more likely to be corrected.

sure. The transducer, kept in a sterile glove, is placed against the exposed artery. High-resolution imaging is performed and flow signals are also sampled along the length of the artery. Intimal flaps are normally detected during high-resolution imaging. Intimal flaps or strictures that do not cause any blood flow abnormality remain a diagnostic problem. No criteria are currently available except for experimental data, which suggest that intimal flaps greater than 3 mm in size are likely to progress and affect vessel patency. In general, sites showing increased velocities above a baseline of 1.2 m/sec are suspect and warrant re-examination. In the majority of cases these are caused by an intimal flap or stricture. The abnormal flow pattern

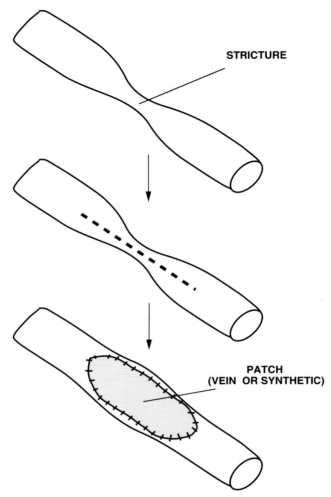

Figure 8.4. The patch plasty is often used to enlarge a site of stenotic narrowing in an artery following endarterectomy or in a vein graft stenosis. It is used to enlarge the residual lumen and to compensate for the fibrointimal thickening that almost always develops (*top*). Either a small piece of vein or synthetic material is used. The vessel is incised over the stenosis (*middle*). The patch is then sutured at the level of this incision (*bottom*).

seems to be more discriminative in identifying lesions that are likely to cause early postoperative failures.

Color Doppler facilitates this portion of the examination by helping to quickly localize any sites of abnormal blood flow. This decreases the need to perform too many manipulations on the machine console. Consecutive sampling of the artery by duplex ultrasound alone is complicated by the intraoperative environment.

POSTOPERATIVE SURVEY

Although it is uncommon, a stroke or transient ischemic attack (TIA) following surgery warrants immediate noninvasive evaluation to exclude acute occlusion of the operated vessel.

Early postoperative evaluation of carotids that have had patches can be made difficult by the synthetic material (polytetrafluoroethylene, or PTFE) (Fig. 8.4). The ultrasound beam often will not penetrate the material until 1 or 2 days postoperatively. Until the gas present in the interstices of the synthetic material has been resorbed it is necessary to evaluate the portion of the artery proximal and distal to the patch.

The normal postendarterectomy carotid shows flow signals that return to a normal baseline (Fig. 8.5) or a harsher pattern with more turbulence and filling in of the spectral window. This is believed to be due to the exposure of a rougher subintimal layer without endothelial lining. Over the ensu-

ing months, flow abnormalities suggestive of 50% diameter stenosis are seen in 20% of patients (Fig. 8.6).

Longer-term follow-up examinations are performed at 6 months and 12 months due to the concern that these fibrointimal hyperplastic lesions will continue to progress. This thickening of the arterial wall is less likely to cause any problem when the native vessel has a large diameter. However, in up to 10% of patients, it causes a relative narrowing of the artery of 50% or more at 12 months. There is also a high incidence (up to 30%) of apparent stenosis

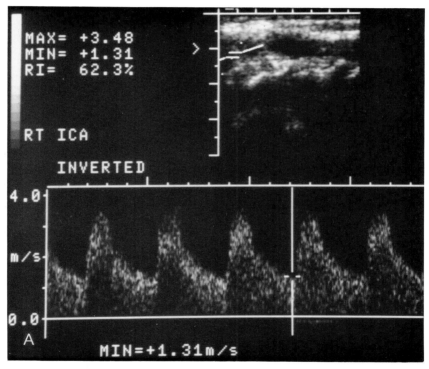

Figure 8.5. **A,** The presence of a high-grade stenosis of the right internal carotid artery is documented by a high-grade flow abnormality with a peak systolic velocity of 3.48 m/sec. **B,** The corresponding gray-scale image shows loss of definition of the lumen and echogenic signal within the course of the proximal internal carotid artery (*arrows*). **C,** The postoperative image of the carotid bifurcation following endarterectomy shows good definition of the proximal internal carotid artery (*arrow*). The Doppler spectral waveform shows a pattern resembling the common carotid artery with increased pulsatility of the waveform in systole. The appearance of the Doppler spectral waveform of the internal carotid artery following endarterectomy often resembles that of either the common or the external carotid artery. Similarly, in a good proportion of patients, the peak systolic velocity will show a mild increase to the velocity range of 1.2 to 1.5 m/sec. The presence of turbulence manifested as spectral broadening in the Doppler window is also a common finding.

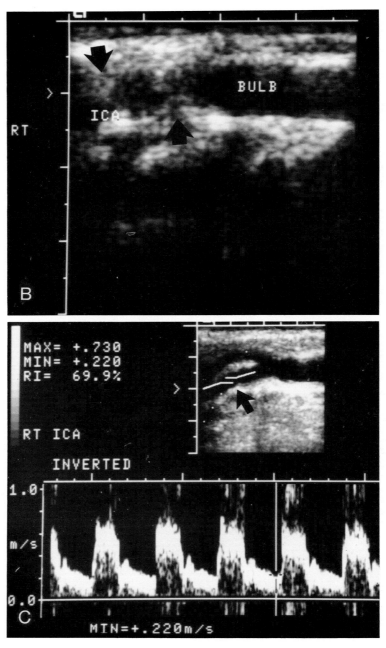

Figure 8.5. **B** and **C.**

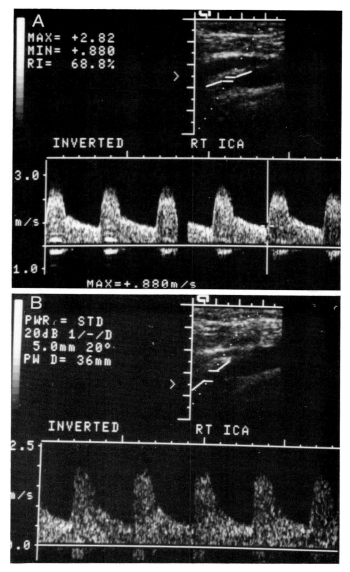

Figure 8.6. **A,** Preoperative evaluation of an asymptomatic patient revealed high-grade stenosis of the right internal carotid artery with a corresponding peak systolic velocity of 2.82 m/sec. **B,** Three months following surgery, a follow-up Doppler examination was performed as part of a normal surveillance program. A moderate flow abnormality was detected with a peak systolic velocity of 2.0 m/sec. This finding, suggestive of a 50 to 75% narrowing, is not uncommon in the early postoperative period following carotid endarterectomy. Most of these flow abnormalities resolve within 6 months to a year. A very small percentage, estimated at less than 10%, will persist and actually progress secondary to the development of fibrointimal hyperplasia. Stenosis greater than 75% warrants more careful examination. There is currently a mild controversy as to whether or not these asymptomatic recurrences should be treated.

at 6 months. This decreases to 16% by 1 year. Stenoses in the 50 to 75% category are more likely to revert to a normal Doppler waveform by 1 year. The strategy is then to perform serial noninvasive examinations with the understanding that progression to velocities equivalent to 75% lumen diameter narrowing or above (>2.25 m/sec peak systolic velocity or >1.4 m/sec peak end-diastolic velocity) will more than likely require operative intervention. The reproducibility of peak systolic velocity values is such that changes of more than 30% from a previous examination are considered significant. These correspond to stenosis progression of approximately 20% lumen diameter narrowing.

The postoperative Doppler waveform of the internal carotid will often have an "externalized" waveform similar to the appearance of the external carotid. The use of the temporal tap maneuver is often necessary to differentiate the external from the internal carotid. This is more important in patients who have only one open carotid branch, thereby helping to differentiate an occluded internal carotid from an occluded external carotid.

Peripheral Bypass Surgery

The patency of a peripheral bypass graft is normally confirmed by either the pres-

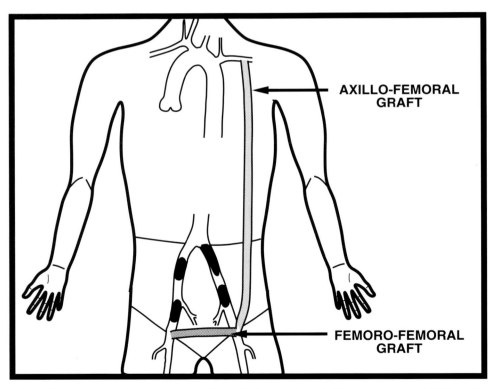

Figure 8.7. The longest arterial bypass is the axillofemoral graft. It is composed of PTFE or Dacron. The proximal anastomosis is made at the junction of the subclavian and axillary arteries. The graft conduit is placed subcutaneously and is tunneled down to the level of the common femoral artery. The clinical situations that prompt the use of such an elaborate graft are few. When they are placed, however, an accompanying femoral-to-femoral bypass graft is almost always needed to supply blood to the opposite leg.

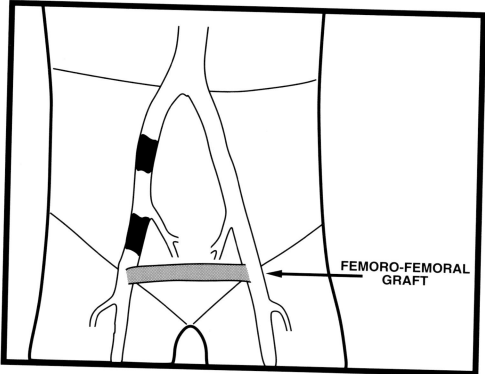

Figure 8.8. The femoral-to-femoral artery bypass graft connects the two common femoral arteries together. It permits the bypassing of an iliac artery system that is severely diseased on only one side.

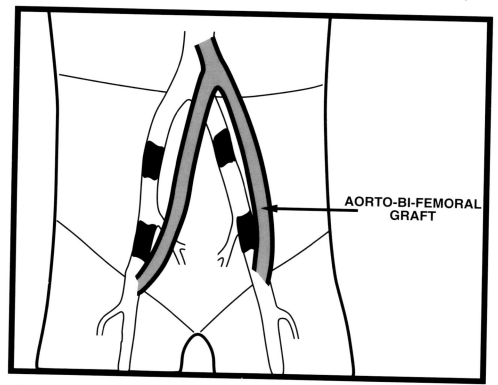

Figure 8.9. The aortobifemoral bypass graft is most often made of Dacron. It connects the distal abdominal aorta to both common femoral arteries, bypassing bilateral severely diseased iliac arteries.

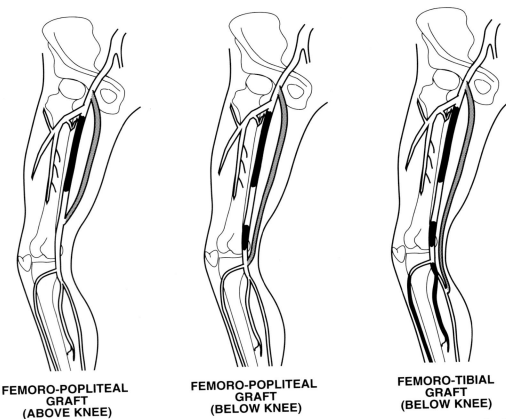

**FEMORO-POPLITEAL
GRAFT
(ABOVE KNEE)**

**FEMORO-POPLITEAL
GRAFT
(BELOW KNEE)**

**FEMORO-TIBIAL
GRAFT
(BELOW KNEE)**

Figure 8.10. The peripheral arterial bypass grafts are identified by their composition—synthetic or autologous vein—as well as the location of their proximal and distal anatomosis. The increasing trend is not to use synthetic materials such as PTFE but rather vein. The principal types of grafts are shown here. The autologous vein is increasingly used for above-the-knee grafts. Synthetic material is still used on occasion. Autologous vein is normally used for the below-the-knee graft. The first type is to the popliteal artery proper. The second type is to the more peripheral arterial branches in the calf. In situ vein grafts are slightly favored for the more distal bypass grafts. Variations on these three types are common. The proximal anastomosis need not be from the common femoral artery but can be placed in the superficial femoral artery or even in another graft. Multiple segments of vein can also be added together to form composite vein grafts.

ence of a palpable pulse or a persistently improved postoperative ankle-brachial pressure index (Figs. 8.7 to 8.10). This is normally referred to as the primary rate if no other intervention is performed on the graft. If the graft shows evidence of failure and the problem is then corrected, the continued patency of the graft is then quoted as being the secondary patency rate. Confusion still exists as to how to define patency rate when more sophisticated composite grafts are sequentially performed in response to the progression of atherosclerotic lesions in the native arteries or in response to recurrent lesions within the bypass graft.

SYNTHETIC VASCULAR BYPASS GRAFTS

The complications likely to affect the function of synthetic lower-extremity bypass grafts are varied. They are a function of the location of bypass graft insertion, its material, and the time since operative placement.

In the first and second years following operation, graft failure can occur secondary to technical errors or to the development of fibrointimal lesions at the anastomoses. Later failures are more often due to the progression of atherosclerotic lesions in the native vessels proximal and distal to the graft (Fig. 8.11). The late complication of an anastomotic pseudoaneurysm occurs an average of 5 to 10 years following graft placement and preferentially affects the femoral anastomosis of aortofemoral grafts.

Infections can occur at any time following graft placement and can be associated with the development of an anastomotic pseudoaneurysm. With time, atherosclerotic changes and fibrointimal hyperplastic lesions mixed with areas of chronic thrombus deposition will develop in the synthetic graft conduit. The two types of synthetic material used have distinct appearances on sonography. These are best appreciated on longitudinal imaging. Dacron, often used for aortobifemoral grafts, has a corrugated or saw-blade appearance (Fig. 8.12), while PTFE grafts typically show two parallel echogenic lines (Fig. 8.13).

Masses (Hematoma versus Pseudoaneurysm)

The diagnostic accuracy of duplex sonography is above 95% for making the diagnosis of pseudoaneurysms. However, there are no specific waveform patterns that can be used to make this diagnosis.

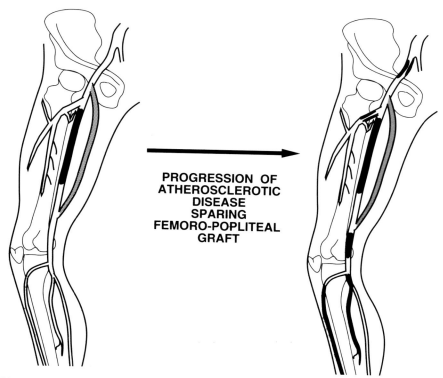

PROGRESSION OF
ATHEROSCLEROTIC
DISEASE
SPARING
FEMORO-POPLITEAL
GRAFT

Figure 8.11. A problem that will ultimately plague the success of a well-functioning bypass graft is the progression of atherosclerotic disease in the arteries proximal or distal to the graft. This problem starts to gain in importance 2 to 3 years following surgery.

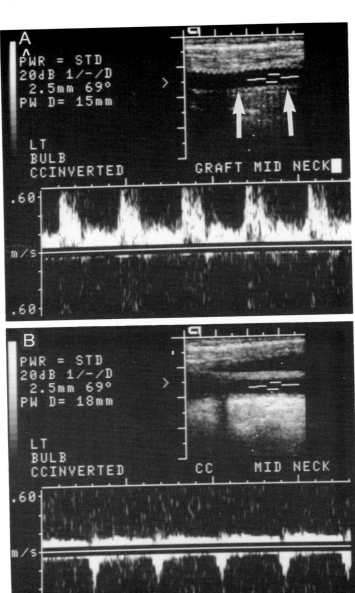

Figure 8.12. **A,** This image shows antegrade flow in a subclavian artery to common carotid artery bypass graft. The material utilized is Dacron, as witnessed by the "sawtooth" appearance at the interface between the conduit and blood (*arrows*). **B,** The second image shows evidence of a technical error at the time of the surgery. The common carotid artery, whose origin had a high-grade stenosis, was not ligated. The vessel remained patent and, because of the relatively slow flow and stagnation, served as a source for thrombus formation and repeat episodes of transient ischemic attacks. Following this diagnostic Doppler sonographic study, the common carotid was explored and ligated.

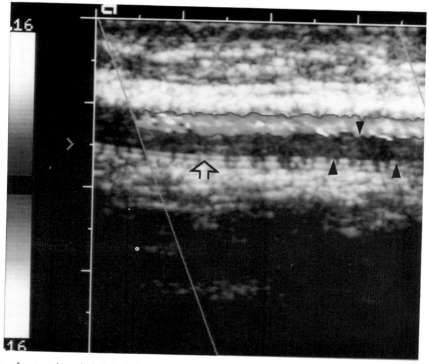

Figure 8.13. (see color plate VI). Diffuse deposition of thrombus within a PTFE bypass graft is clearly shown as a zone of absent color Doppler signal (*arrowheads*). Flow is restricted to a portion of this graft. The PTFE material typically causes a double line on high-resolution imaging (*open arrow*).

The waveforms within the pseudoaneurysm have varied appearances depending on the location of the Doppler gate. Color Doppler imaging reveals an almost classic appearance of swirling motion of blood in the perivascular mass (Fig. 8.14). This sign is not specific to a pseudoaneurysm, since saccular aneurysms share similar flow patterns. The differential diagnosis is normally made when careful real-time imaging confirms that the mass communicates with the normal lumen of the vessel or with the bypass graft contiguous to the anastomosis. On occasion, a patulous anastomosis may mimic the appearance of a pseudoaneurysm (Fig. 8.15). The flow signals, however, are more discordant and tend to lose the swirling motion during a portion of the cardiac cycle.

The Doppler spectral "to-and-fro" sign is seen in the flow channel between the perivascular collection and the native vessel. This is often not seen in perianastomotic pseudoaneurysms because these tend to have a broader communicating neck between the extravascular collection and the graft or artery. The pseudoaneurysm will tend to have some thrombus deposition within it.

As in the case of simple iatrogenic pseudoaneurysms, care must be taken to differentiate perivascular pulsations transmitted into a hematoma from those due to flowing blood. The flow sensitivity of the color Doppler is adjusted to minimize this artifact. This is accomplished by decreasing the sensitivity of the color Doppler display so that no abnormal color signals are detected over the graft or native artery at a

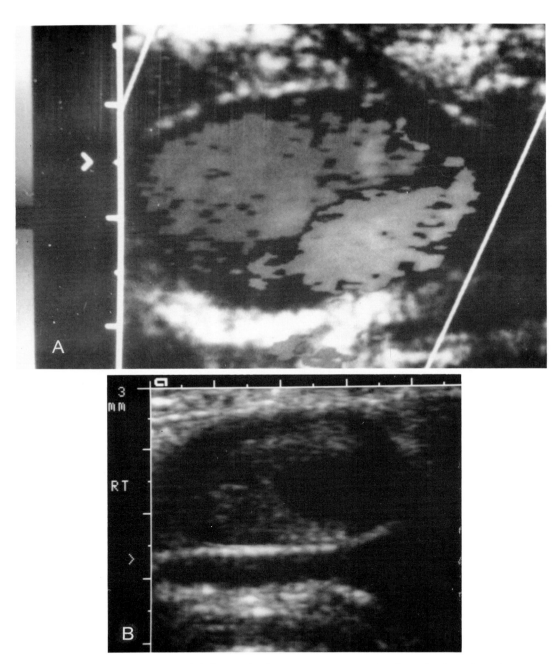

Figure 8.14. **A** (see color plate VI), The typical appearance on color Doppler imaging of a pseu-doaneurysm associated with a bypass graft is shown here. There is a mixture of antegrade and forward flow, commonly referred to as the color "yin-yang" sign or the "color washing machine" sign. This swirling motion of blood is accentuated by the large diameter of the communication between the pseudoaneurysm and the bypass graft anastomosis. **B,** A longitudinal image shows a hypoechoic collection above the bypass graft. **C,** The transverse image taken at this level shows the large collection (*arrows*) and a more central area devoid of signal (*curved arrows*). This lies superior to the actual bypass graft, which is partly compressed (*arrowheads*). The echogenic material lying

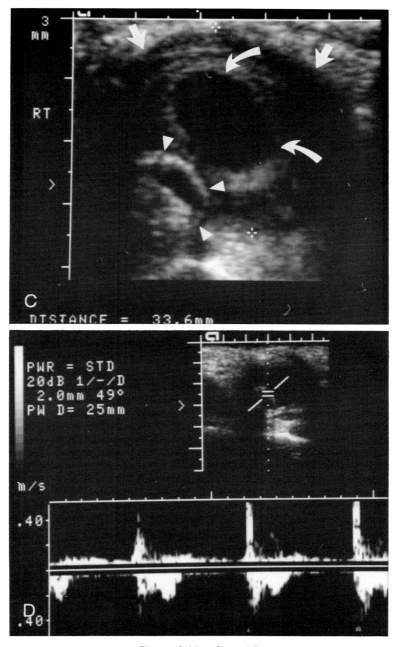

Figure 8.14. C and D.

between the physical confines of the collection and the central sonolucent area corresponds to thrombus deposition. **D,** The Doppler spectral waveform is acquired at the communication between the bypass graft and the collection. In distinction to the flow pattern seen in many of the pseudoaneurysms caused following catheterization, pseudoaneurysms occurring at the anastomotic sites tend to have wider communications and often do not show the typical to-and-fro pattern of flow at the site of the communication.

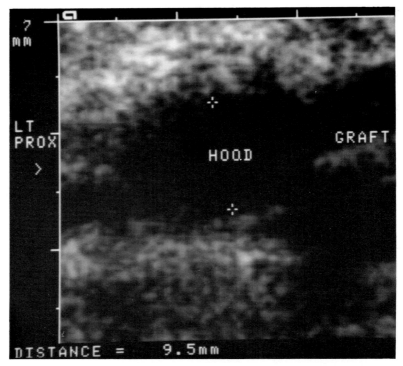

Figure 8.15. The differential diagnosis of pulsatile masses includes a patulous anastomotic site at the origin of the bypass graft. In this figure, the hood or proximal anastomosis of this vein bypass graft shows moderately severe dilatation secondary to the reconstructive surgery performed and the use of a patch angioplasty. Continuity in the conduit between graft and artery as well as the lack of thrombus deposition is consistent with the diagnosis of a patulous anastomosis.

site distant from the suspected pseudoaneurysm. A heterogeneous perigraft collection with absent flow signals should suggest the possibility of hematoma, seroma, or abscess (Fig. 8.16).

Occlusions and Perianastomotic Stenoses

A Doppler sonographic examination is useful for differentiating total from subtotal graft occlusions. The absence of Doppler signals within a graft is diagnostic of an occlusion. The color Doppler must be set to a high sensitivity level and at the lowest velocity scale possible, since subtotally occluded grafts will still maintain very slow flow within them despite the absence of a palpable pulse.

An anastomotic stenosis can be detected and graded using the peak systolic velocity ratio described in the previous section. However, there is a normal tendency for perturbed flow patterns to develop at the anastomosis. At the proximal anastomosis, a hood is occasionally created when a patch angioplasty enlarges the site of insertion of a graft into the native artery. When present, these cause a zone of altered flow signals with mixtures of low-velocity forward and reversed flow signals. The best way to ensure that no stenosis is present is to set the Doppler gate 2 cm proximal to the anastomosis and to follow the course of the flow channel into the proximal 2 cm of the graft. If the flow signals remain less than twice the velocity in the proximal artery, a stenosis is unlikely. If the velocity increases, this should be compared to the proximal velocity in the graft. A well-matched graft conduit should not contain velocity signals more than twice those in the native artery. On occasion, a small-diameter graft will carry higher-velocity signals than expected.

Increases in peak systolic velocities are quite common at the distal anastomosis of bypass grafts. These increases are often due to the geometry of the anastomotic construction, which often causes increases of 50% in the peak systolic velocities. This effect is more pronounced in below-knee popliteal and tibioperoneal grafts. There

are few studies addressing the actual distribution of velocities at the anastomosis and the significance of this finding. Serial monitoring of these sites of disturbed flow must therefore be used with the premise that an increase in peak systolic velocity or peak systolic velocity ratio over the next few months is indicative of a developing stenosis. Rather than rely on doubling of the peak systolic velocity as a diagnostic threshold, we now favor using tripling of the ratio (>75% stenosis) as a sign of a significant stenosis. This eliminates the high number of false-positive examinations that would be found when doubling of the peak systolic velocity is used as a threshold.

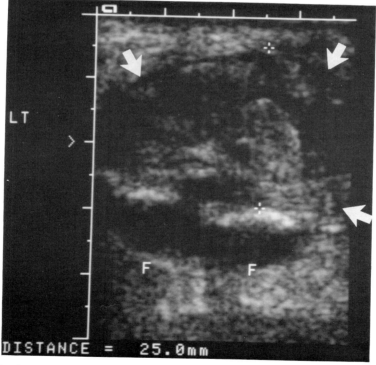

Figure 8.16. The large heterogeneous collection (*arrows*) lies superficial to a synthetic femoral-to-femoral bypass graft. The differential diagnosis is of a large hematoma or thrombosing pseudoaneurysm. Aspiration biopsy of the collection shows it to be infected. The aspiration procedure was performed on the basis of absent color Doppler and duplex waveform signals within this collection.

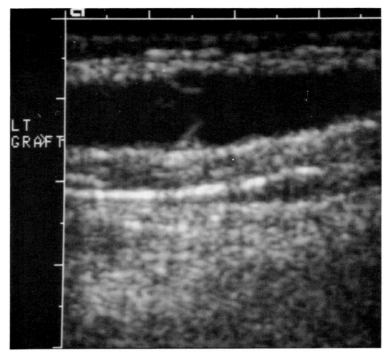

Figure 8.17. The presence of persistent venous valves is normally appreciated as in this case of a reversed vein bypass graft. The use of in situ vein bypass graft requires complete lysis in disruption of the valves so that retrograde flow can be established in the vein before it is connected to the arterial circuit.

AUTOLOGOUS VEIN GRAFTS

Two types of venous bypass grafts are currently used for arterial revascularization: the reversed vein and the "in situ" vein grafts. The reversed vein is a segment of a native superficial vein that has been harvested from its normal anatomic location, reversed, and then anastomosed to the native artery segments proximal and distal to the diseased segments. Segments of the greater saphenous, lesser saphenous, cephalic, and basilic veins can be harvested and used (Fig. 8.17).

The in situ technique uses the closest superficial vein, leaving it in its native bed. The valves are lysed and the side branches that are normally anastomosed to the deep venous system are ligated (Fig. 8.18). The proximal and distal portions are then mobilized and anastomosed to the selected proximal and distal arterial segments. When the greater saphenous vein is used, the distal anastomosis is often to the tibioperoneal arteries. There is an ongoing argument as to which of the two techniques performs best with respect to patency rates for below-the-knee bypass surgery. Patency rates up to 80% (secondary) are reported with both techniques. The reversed bypass graft normally causes a patulous distal anastomosis since the caliber of the reversed vein is largest at the distal anastomosis. The in situ approach requires that the valves be lysed, since arterial blood flow is in the reverse direction to venous flow. There is a better match between vein diameter and diameter of the recipient artery.

Composite grafts are normally achieved by anastomosing a segment of vein to another segment. Segments of different lengths and from different anatomic locations are often spliced together to reach the target artery.

Preoperative Assessment

The postoperative appearance of the bypass graft and its hemodynamics are the main focus of Doppler sonographic imaging. Preoperative evaluation of the superficial veins, while it plays an important role, is not necessary in all patients presenting for bypass procedures. The preoperative survey is indicated in those with a previous history of vein stripping, deep vein thrombosis, and harvesting of veins for coronary or peripheral bypass surgery.

The major importance of the technique is in documenting a vein caliber above 2.5 mm. These can be used for both in situ and reversed vein bypass procedures. Survey of the superficial vein should include localizing the site of major branches and documenting that the vein course is not serpiginous or tortuous. These findings suggest either that the vein is varicose or that collaterals are present. These vein segments are normally not suitable for harvesting. The survey is performed with the transducer held transverse to the vein. The

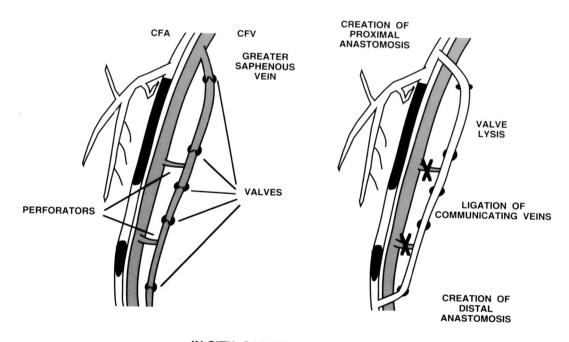

**IN-SITU SAPHENOUS
FEMORO-POPLITEAL
GRAFT
(BELOW KNEE)**

Figure 8.18.   The reversed vein bypass grafts are placed in two steps. The vein is surgically removed and reversed. It is then anastomosed to the artery. The in situ bypass graft is left in its normal anatomic bed. The valves must by lysed, however, since they normally prevent blood flow down the leg. The perforator veins must also be ligated so as not to create an AV fistula when the vein is connected to the arterial circuit. The anastomoses are created by mobilizing the ends of the vein. This may entail moving the distal portion of the vein over longer distances than the few centimeters necessary for the proximal anastomosis.

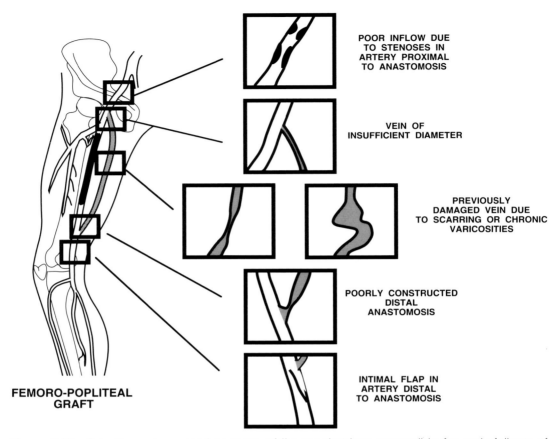

Figure 8.19. This diagram summarizes some of the mechanisms responsible for early failures of reversed vein bypass graft. These will all manifest abnormal Doppler sonographic findings. They either will be noticeable during surgery or will cause problems within the first 1 or 2 months following placement of the graft.

hand holding the transducer is normally stabilized by using one or two fingers to help keep the same distance from the skin surface and to minimize the amount of pressure transmitted from the transducer to the vein located beneath. Surveys of the greater saphenous and lesser saphenous veins are normally conducted with the patient standing. The transducer is moved down the leg as a slight amount of pressure is intermittently applied to the skin. This confirms the patency of the vein lumen. The diameter of the vein is measured every 10 cm and the largest conduit is followed downward along the medial aspect

of the thigh, past the knee, and down the medial aspect of the calf. Major branches are noted on the skin and as centimeters of distance from the groin crease.

For the lesser saphenous, the origin of the vein is identified in the popliteal fossa. It is then followed as it traverses the fascia and slowly migrates to lie anterior to the lateral malleolus. Additional surveys of the upper extremity veins, both basilic and cephalic, are occasionally needed when the greater and lesser saphenous are not sufficiently long for the contemplated surgery. The patient is imaged supine, again with the transducer held transverse.

The basilic vein is identified in the mid proximal arm at its junction with the brachial vein and is followed downward along the medial aspect of the arm. The cephalic vein is more superficial and courses along the lateral aspect of the arm. It is more easily identified at the level of the antecubital fossa and can then be followed upward.

The sonographic estimates of vein diameter correlate well with the findings at venography or surgery.

Intraoperative Assessment

The intraoperative survey is performed when the vein has been anastomosed to the proximal and distal arterial segments.

The more traditional procedure is performed with the vein exposed along its full length. The intraoperative graft is scanned with Doppler imaging looking for either focal regions of abnormal flow or patent veins to the deep system. This type of survey is also easily performed with a hand-held Doppler probe. Real-time imaging is used to assess the anastomosis for the presence of intimal flaps, strictures, or early thrombus deposition.

Newer surgical approaches that combine angioscopy and limited sites of exposure along the vein to ligate side branches require a more comprehensive intraoperative duplex or color Doppler sonographic examination. The length of the vein can

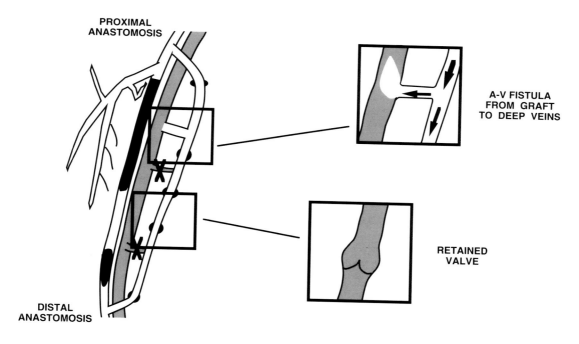

PROXIMAL ANASTOMOSIS

A-V FISTULA FROM GRAFT TO DEEP VEINS

RETAINED VALVE

DISTAL ANASTOMOSIS

IN-SITU SAPHENOUS FEMORO-POPLITEAL GRAFT (BELOW KNEE)

Figure 8.20. The in situ vein graft is subject to the same failure mechanisms that plague the reversed vein grafts. Two additional modes of dysfunction are shown here: the presence of an AV fistula shunting blood away from the distal graft and the presence of retained valves, which create obstructions to blood flow.

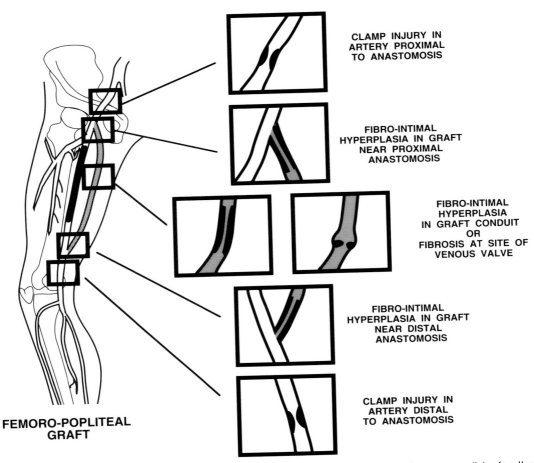

CLAMP INJURY IN
ARTERY PROXIMAL
TO ANASTOMOSIS

FIBRO-INTIMAL
HYPERPLASIA IN GRAFT
NEAR PROXIMAL
ANASTOMOSIS

FIBRO-INTIMAL
HYPERPLASIA
IN GRAFT CONDUIT
OR
FIBROSIS AT SITE OF
VENOUS VALVE

FIBRO-INTIMAL
HYPERPLASIA IN GRAFT
NEAR DISTAL
ANASTOMOSIS

CLAMP INJURY IN
ARTERY DISTAL
TO ANASTOMOSIS

**FEMORO-POPLITEAL
GRAFT**

Figure 8.21. This diagram summarizes the many mechanisms that may be responsible for the development of a stenosis and graft failure in a reversed vein bypass graft. These typically start to be seen 1 to 2 months after the surgical placement of the graft. All of these lesions will manifest themselves as a site of abnormal blood flow with increased peak systolic flow velocities measurable by Doppler ultrasound.

then be followed more quickly and efficiently, and potential AV fistula focal stenoses can be quickly detected. Absolute Doppler velocity measurements should be a standard part of the examination. Velocities below 0.4 m/sec should suggest a significant problem and pending occlusions. This rule is broken only when a large discordance in size is observed between graft and artery, the graft being much wider than the artery.

Postoperative Assessment

Three different failure mechanisms come into play. Early failures are normally ascribed to technical errors likely to cause graft occlusion within the first 2 months following surgery (Fig. 8.19). These include poor suture line placement, the opening of unsuspected venous channels in the in situ grafts, poor selection of anastomotic sites, and poorly lysed vein valves (Fig. 8.20). During the first 2 years following surgery, fibrointimal or fibrotic lesions can develop either at the anastomosis or within the graft conduit, most often at the site of a vein valve (Fig. 8.21). Late failures beyond this 2-year period are thought to be secondary to continued progression of the atherosclerotic process in the native vessels proximal and distal to the anastomoses.

Early Suspected Occlusion

In the early days following surgery, it is often very difficult to clinically verify graft patency or occlusion. This is especially true when large hematomas are present or when short-segment vein bypass grafts have been used.

Short-segment bypass grafts are often placed in patients who have had previous peripheral or coronary bypass surgery and who have a shortage of usable vein. They are often placed deep near the bed of the artery, whereas the more traditional grafts are superficial and easily evaluated by clinical palpation. This approach is also more likely to be used for a salvage procedure or to help promote healing of a wound.

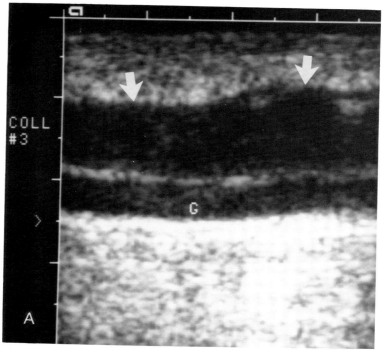

Figure 8.22. The standard noninvasive evaluation of the postoperative bypass graft is often aided by color Doppler and duplex sonography. **A,** In this patient, the ankle-brachial index failed to increase following bypass surgery. Imaging of the proximal graft shows a large sonolucent collection (*arrows*) lying superficial to a vein bypass graft (G). **B,** The corresponding transverse image shows the collection partly pressing on the graft. **C,** Imaging more distally on the thigh reveals yet another collection (*arrows*) lying deep to a bypass graft. The graft velocities are normal and there is no evidence of stenosis. The presence of these multiple hematomas made it difficult to adequately compress the lower extremity while performing the segmental pressure measurements. Evaluation with the Doppler approach revealed normal graft velocity and no evidence of focal lesions. On serial follow-ups, these hematomas slowly resolved and the ankle-brachial index improved.

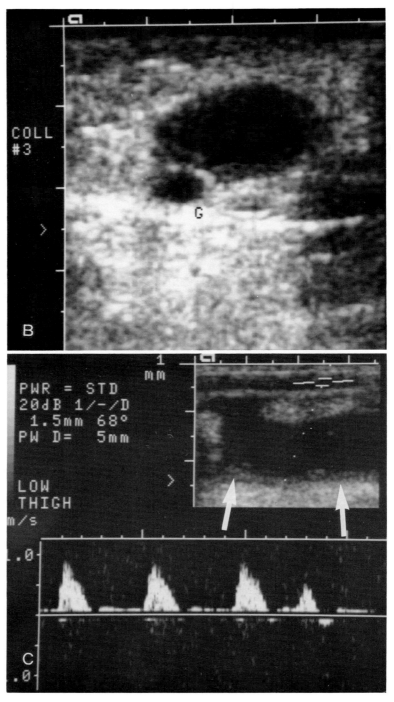

Figure 8.22. B and C.

Patency of the graft is normally confirmed by the detection of flow signals within it. On occasion, we have seen poor ankle-brachial ratios despite a normal flow pattern in the bypass graft. These have subsequently gone on to do well, with improvement of the ankle-brachial ratio to normal within 2 to 3 months. This apparent loss in pressure is thought to be due to local compression and obstruction of the graft inflow and proximal conduit by hematoma (Fig. 8.22). As these slowly resolve, the extrinsic compression improves and perfusion pressure also improves.

AV Fistula

This complication is apt to occur with the "in situ" technique. AV fistulas can easily be missed at operation or immediately postoperatively, since a good percentage open in the few weeks following surgery. Color Doppler assisted sonography is a simple and elegant means of documenting their presence. Our current protocol identifies sites of AV communication between the in situ superficial veins and the deeper native veins. These are then operated on and ligated directly, without the need for angiography.

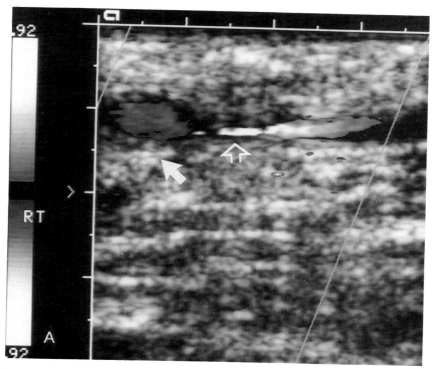

Figure 8.23. **A** (see color plate VI), The site of relative constriction in this venous bypass graft was identified by color Doppler imaging. The proximal high-grade stenosis at the anastomosis of a bypass graft shows up as a zone of narrowing of the color Doppler lumen as well as high color velocity signals (*open arrow*). Flow reversal is occurring in the hood proximal to the stenosis (*arrow*). **B,** The corresponding duplex sonogram shows marked increase in peak systolic velocity consistent with a high-grade stenosis (2.6 m/sec). **C,** Imaging more distally in this bypass graft the peak systolic velocity is significantly decreased to 0.13 m/sec. This is below the reported threshold of 0.45 m/sec often used as a discriminant value to predict a high likelihood of occlusion. The relative peak systolic velocity ratio was estimated at 20.

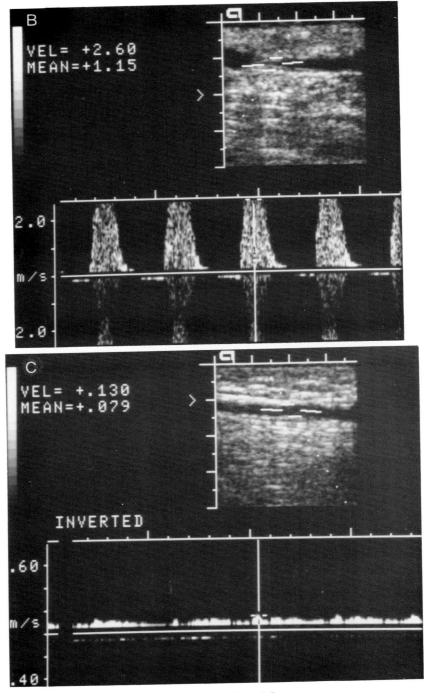

Figure 8.23.   B and **C.**

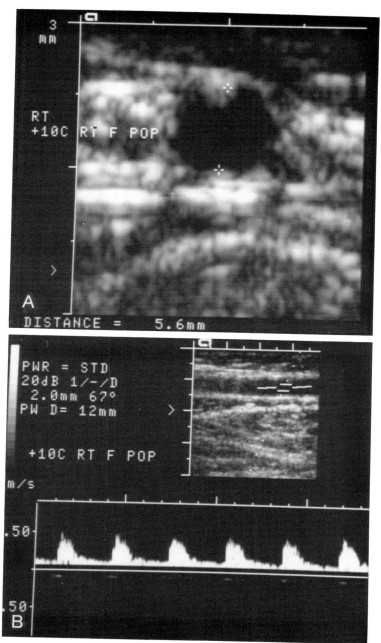

Figure 8.24. **A,** This femoral-popliteal bypass graft imaged transversely measures 5.6 mm in diameter. **B,** The corresponding velocity profile shows a diastolic antegrade flow but, more importantly, a peak systolic velocity of 0.45 m/sec. Such a low velocity is artificially created due to the larger than normal diameter of the bypass graft utilized. A first evaluation of the Doppler velocity waveforms within the vein graft should take into consideration the relative size of the graft. This diameter normally varies between 3 and 4 mm.

Stenosis

The measurement of graft velocity in either the early or late postoperative period can be used to detect grafts with a high likelihood of incipient failure. Bandyk et al. have suggested that a peak systolic velocity below 0.4 or 0.45 m/sec can be used to identify such grafts (Fig. 8.23). This measurement can be made in the distal graft, approximately 5 to 10 cm from the anastomosis. This criterion can identify only the more severely diseased grafts. It does not identify grafts with less significant stenoses and causes false positives when the graft is of large diameter (Fig. 8.24). The early stenoses that are missed are likely to continue to progress over the ensuing months until they become flow re-strictive, cause a drop in flow velocity, and finally result in graft thrombosis. These lesions are commonly the result of fibrointimal hyperplasia. Once they are located, they can then be monitored for evidence of progression. Color Doppler sonography has been used to survey the length of these bypass grafts, whose lengths vary from 30 to 75 cm. The site of a suspected stenosis is quickly identified by the telltale color shift of a high-grade stenosis. Doppler spectral analysis is then used to grade the severity of the stenosis by measurement of the peak systolic velocity ratio.

Color Doppler Extremity Protocol

The examination is performed as follows. The transducer is first held trans-

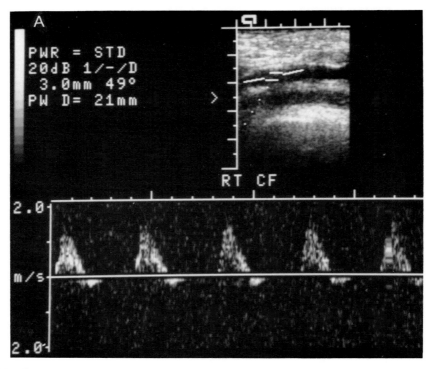

Figure 8.25. The flow patterns established at the anastomotic connections between native arteries and bypass grafts are often complex. **A,** The first step in the evaluation of the anastomosis proper consists of a sampling of the native artery proximal to the anastomosis. This evaluation typically starts 4 cm proximally and is confirmed on longitudinal imaging. In this example, a normal velocity profile is noted in the common femoral artery. **B,** A search is made for evidence of any high-velocity jet. **C,** This is repeated in the different portions of the anastomosis. Areas of flow reversal are quite common.

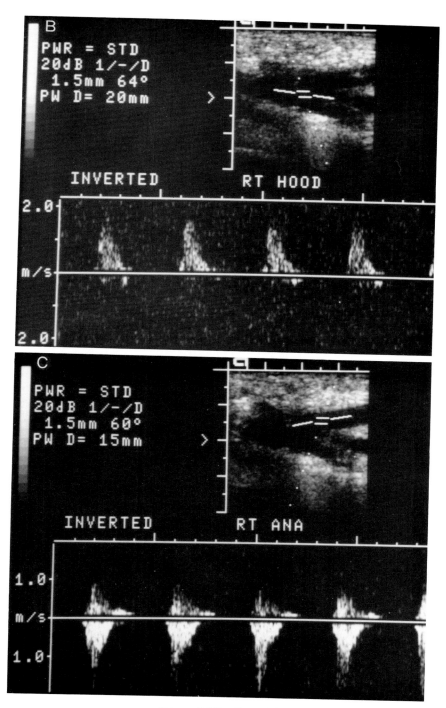

Figure 8.25. **B** and **C**.

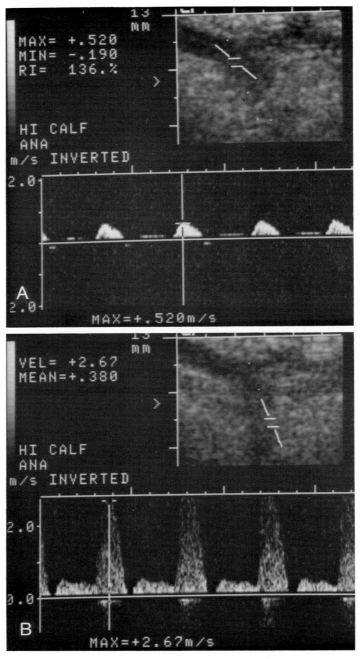

Figure 8.26. A, Imaging of the distal portion of this femoral-popliteal bypass graft shows peak systolic velocities at the lower limits of normal (0.52 m/sec). **B,** The graft distal to this point is poorly visualized on the gray-scale image. The color Doppler image was used to position the Doppler gate and to perform angle correction. Sampling at the site of velocity disturbance under the color image shows a peak systolic velocity of 2.67 m/sec, consistent with a greater than 75% stenosis when the velocity ratio is calculated. Because of the lower Doppler frequency used, the color Doppler image will often reveal flow abnormalities while the gray-scale image acquired at the higher frequency will not penetrate as well. This is most likely to occur when the vessel wall interfaces are not parallel to the imaging plane, as is the case in this example.

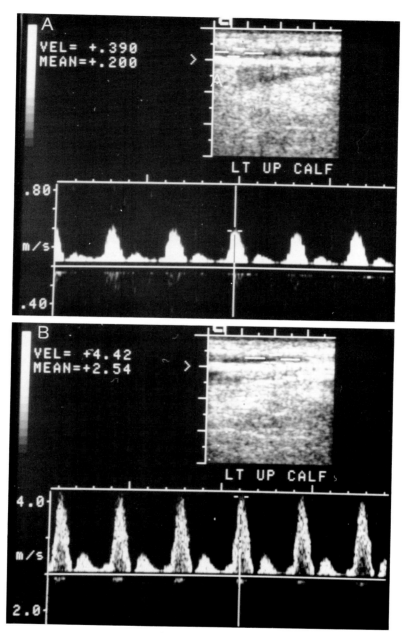

Figure 8.27. A, A more typical Doppler waveform is present in this bypass graft. Proximally, peak systolic velocities are depressed to 0.39 m/sec. There is a short component of early diastolic retrograde flow and a more prolonged antegrade diastolic flow. **B,** This triphasic pattern is preserved at the stenosis proper where the peak systolic velocity reaches 4.4 m/sec.

verse and is used to identify the location and course of the bypass graft from the proximal to the distal anastomosis. Acoustic coupling gel is generously laid along this course.

The transducer is then placed parallel to the graft. The proximal anastomosis is identified and Doppler spectra are examined from the artery 2 cm proximal to the graft anastomosis to the proximal 2 cm of the graft. Flow patterns are often quite complex in this region and it is more efficient to move the Doppler gate along these few centimeters (Fig. 8.24). Color Doppler imaging will normally detect any abnormal flow jets present in this region (Fig. 8.25). These tend to blend in with generally disorganized flow pattern within the anastomosis proper.

The conduit of the graft is then scanned by moving the longitudinally oriented transducer down the graft in increments equal to the length of the transducer. The color window is angled forward or backward, depending on the course of the graft. The transducer is held in the same position for one to three cardiac cycles, long enough to have visualized flow signals in the lumen. The scale of the color map is set to a maximum of 0.4 to 0.6 m/sec in most cases. Any areas of abnormal flow are sampled and the peak systolic velocity is measured. The Doppler spectrum is then sampled in the region 2 to 4 cm proximal to the site of flow abnormality. The peak systolic velocity ratio is calculated by dividing the peak systolic velocity measured at the site of suspected stenosis on

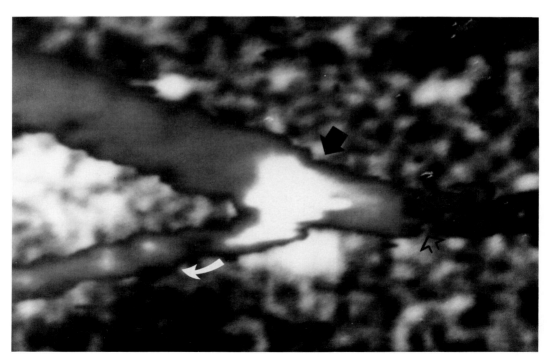

Figure 8.28. (see color plate VI). This distal anastomosis of a femoral-tibial bypass graft shows a mild increase in velocity at the anastomosis proper (*arrow*). This is often seen and suggests an estimated 50% narrowing. There is flow directed more proximally in the posterior tibial artery (*curved arrow*). Antegrade flow into the more distal posterior tibial artery (*open arrow*) is compromised by more distal arterial disease.

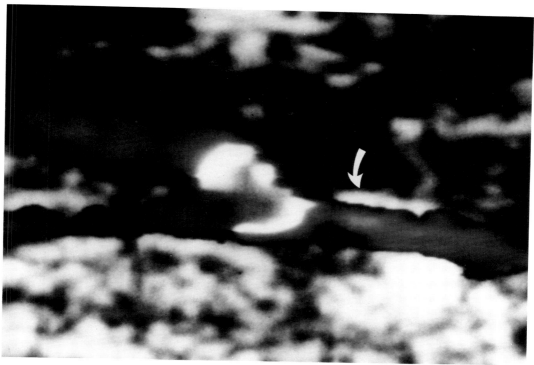

Figure 8.29. (see color plate VI). This distal anastomosis shows a more even tapered zone of increased peak systolic blood flow velocities. This corresponds to an estimated 50 to 75% stenosis. There is antegrade flow in the anterior tibial artery (*curved arrow*).

the color Doppler image (Fig. 8.26) by that measured in the portion of the graft 2 to 4 cm proximal (Fig. 8.27). The only exception to this rule is in the case of a stenosis at the proximal anastomosis. A peak systolic velocity must then be measured in the proximal graft 4 to 6 cm downstream from the stenosis, in the portion of the graft with a normal color Doppler flow pattern. If no sites of abnormal flow are detected, velocities are sampled at the anastomoses and at every 10-cm increment along the graft conduit. The distal anastomosis almost always shows some slight elevation in the peak systolic velocity (Figs. 8.28 and 8.29). Although doubling of the peak systolic velocity ratio is considered significant everywhere else in the graft, tripling of this ratio is considered significant at the distal anastomosis (Fig. 8.30).

This type of survey works best with a transducer with a 4-cm footprint. The longer transducers tend to slip more easily and need to be repeatedly positioned over the same graft segment.

DIALYSIS FISTULA

There is a large amount of interest in the evaluation of dialysis AV fistulas (Fig. 8.31). These are typically inserted in the forearm and are either synthetic or made of autologous vein. Problems common to these include the development of microaneurysms, larger aneurysms, or stenoses. Duplex sonography can be used to detect stenoses; the accuracy of the technique is close to 90%. A loss of accuracy may be due to the turbulent flow patterns that are caused by a quite tortuous course

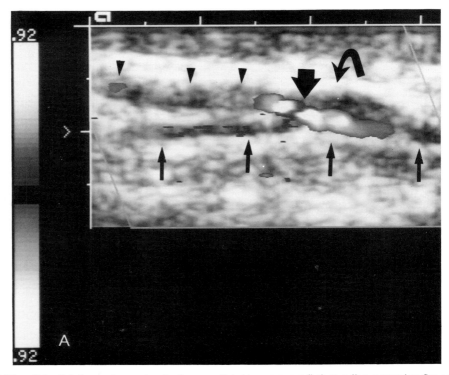

Figure 8.30. This distal anastomosis of a femorotibial bypass graft shows the complex flow patterns that often coexist. **A** (see color plate VI), The distal anastomosis of the femoral-tibial bypass graft is involved by a high-grade stenosis. Color Doppler signals are displayed on a high-velocity scale. They have aliased from red to white to blue (*arrow*) at the anastomosis proper. The distal graft is outlined by the *arrowheads;* the color Doppler signals within are too low to show up on this color Doppler map. The native artery is identified by the *small arrows.* The actual anastomotic hood is indicated by the *curved arrow.* **B,** Graft velocities proximal to the anastomosis show a peak systolic velocity of 0.45 m/sec. **C,** There is a high-grade stenosis at the anastomosis proper. Peak systolic velocities are greater than 5.0 m/sec. This finding suggests a high-grade 90% narrowing at the anastomosis. **D,** Distal to the anastomosis proper there is reestablishment of antegrade flow and evidence of turbulence as shown by the irregular contour of the Doppler waveform (*arrows*). **E,** The posterior tibial artery proximal to the anastomosis shows retrograde flow. This confirms the importance of this bypass graft, since blood supply to the proximal calf is dependent on the retrograde flow in the posterior tibial artery.

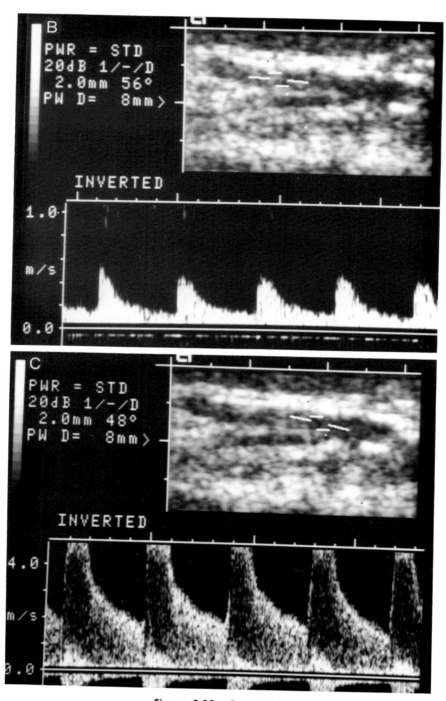

Figure 8.30.   B and C.

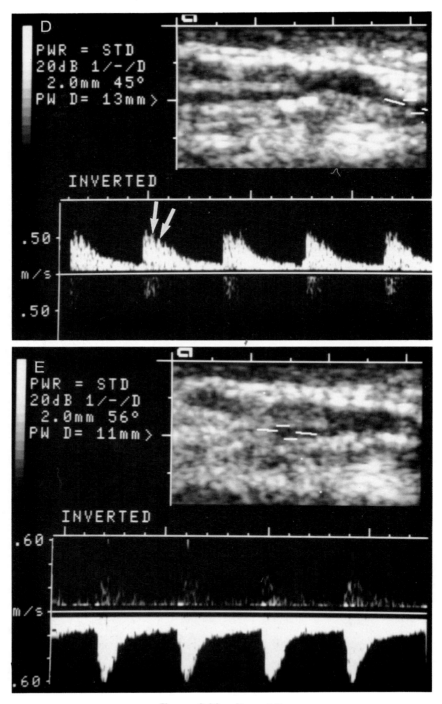

Figure 8.30. D and E.

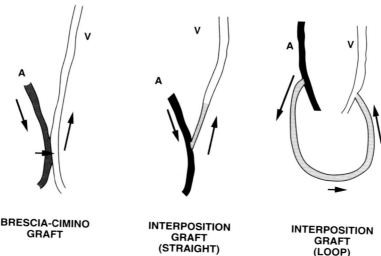

BRESCIA-CIMINO GRAFT   **INTERPOSITION GRAFT (STRAIGHT)**   **INTERPOSITION GRAFT (LOOP)**

Figure 8.31. Dialysis grafts often develop areas of stenosis and small pseudoaneurysms. There are three types of dialysis shunts placed subcutaneously in the forearm and in the upper arm. The first type is a side-to-side connection of artery to vein (*left*). The second has a straight segment interposed between artery and vein (*middle*). The last (*right*) has a longer loop interposed between artery and vein. The diagnostic accuracy of Doppler sonography for detecting pseudoaneurysms is roughly the same in the different types of dialysis shunts. The accuracy for detecting stenoses is slightly better in the straight interposition graft than in the loop type. This is due to the fact that the flow dynamics of curved channels are more complex and difficult to analyze using Doppler sonography. A common site for a stenosis to develop in all of these grafts is the efferent vein downstream from the anastomosis. This site should be included in the evaluation of the shunt, as should the flow profiles in the proximal artery. The etiology of these stenoses is thought to be secondary to previous catheter insertions, which cause a fibrointimal reaction at the site of a damaged valve.

and sharp bends in these arteriovenous shunts. In the straight segment of the efferent veins, the sensitivity for detecting stenosis is closer to 95%. The addition of color Doppler does not seem to improve diagnostic accuracy, nor is it always needed. However, it does facilitate the examination. Detection of smaller pseudoaneurysms is facilitated by the color flow mapping. Surgical revision of the graft for only a few smaller aneurysms is unlikely unless dialysis is compromised.

FOLLOWING INTERVENTIONAL PROCEDURES

Doppler ultrasound lends itself well to the evaluation of sites of percutaneous interventions. These include a broad family of interventions ranging from thrombolysis to percutaneous balloon angioplasty

(Fig. 8.32), atherectomy (Fig. 8.33), laser angioplasty (Fig. 8.34), and stent placement (Fig. 8.35).

Thrombolysis

Sonography can be used to identify the site for percutaneous access, monitor the delivery of the lytic agent, and evaluate the results of therapy.

Percutaneous Access

On occasion, direct access is needed into thrombosed synthetic grafts such as axillofemoral, aortobifemoral, or femorofemoral grafts. Direct puncture into these grafts is greatly facilitated by previous or concurrent sonographic imaging. Thrombolysis can then be accomplished with the assurance that the catheter lies in the appropriate vascular structure.

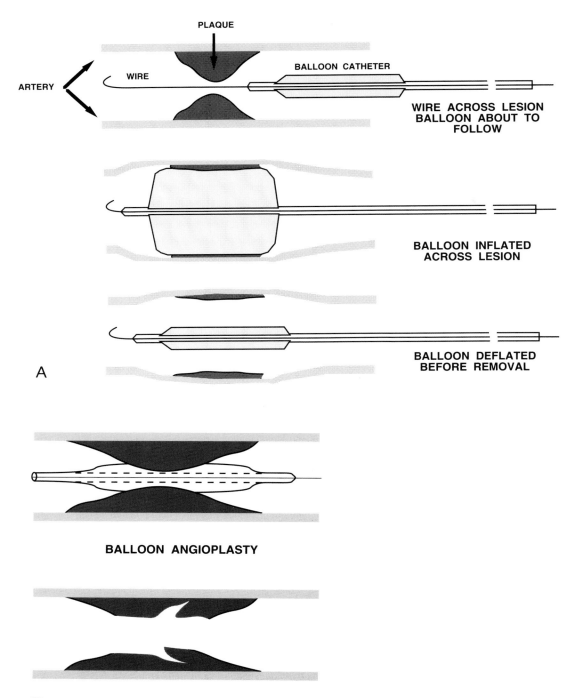

Figure 8.32. **A,** Angioplasty is performed in three steps. First, the lesion to be treated is crossed and a wire is left across the lesion. A balloon is then introduced over the wire. The balloon is then inflated and the lesion is treated. **B,** The mechanism of action of percutaneous angioplasty is of a controlled fracture and dissection of the plaque. This is also accompanied by an outward expansion of the artery at this level. The size of the dissection must be large enough to relieve the stenosis yet not large enough to cause occlusion of the artery.

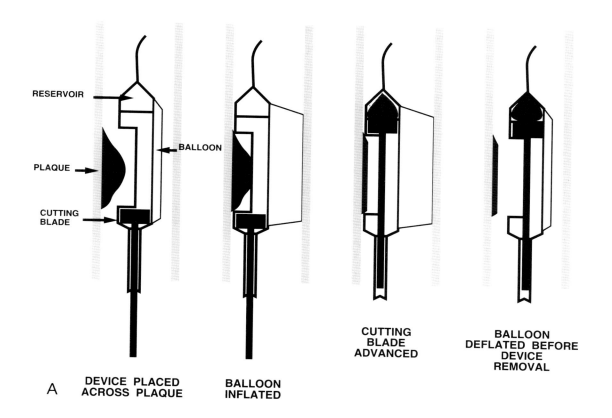

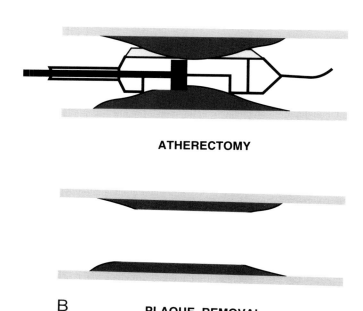

Figure 8.33. **A,** Percutaneous atherectomy is performed in four steps. The lesion is first crossed. The device is then positioned over the plaque to be removed. A stabilizing balloon is then inflated, pressing the device against the plaque. A cutting blade is then advanced over the lesion and the plaque material removed and pressed into a retrieval reservoir at the tip of the device. **B,** The mechanism of action of percutaneous atherectomy is removal of the plaque material. It will normally leave a smooth surface of the artery at the site of treatment.

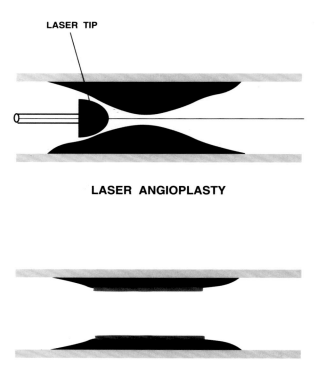

LASER TIP

LASER ANGIOPLASTY

**THERMAL EFFECTS
OR SUBLIMATION**

Figure 8.34. Laser angioplasty has mostly been performed using the laser energy to heat and "cook" the stenotic lesion. Another approach uses the photoenergy of the beam to directly vaporize the plaque material. The lumen of the artery is left smooth following the procedure. The size of this new lumen is, unfortunately, roughly the size of the laser device itself.

An antegrade arterial puncture is often the most efficient way of entering a femoropopliteal or infrapopliteal graft. Identification of the proximal anastomosis is accomplished by imaging the artery proximal to the location of the graft. This helps to confirm that there is enough room for the catheter to be inserted and helps orient the catheter for a more efficient and rapid entry into the occluded graft.

Percutaneous entry into arteries distal to occlusions is also facilitated by sonographic imaging. In the groin, a patent femoral artery distal to an iliac occlusion can be cannulated much more rapidly once it has been localized by sonography. Entry into the popliteal artery using a retrograde approach can be performed from the back of the knee. This approach is useful when attempting recanalization of occluded superficial femoral segments. Ultrasound has shown that this is more safely performed from the posteromedial aspect of the knee since the veins rarely overlie this portion of the artery. A rapid sonographic survey confirms this fact and helps guide the needle used for arterial access.

Monitoring

Current strategies for monitoring intraarterial thrombolysis require that repeat angiography be performed and that decisions on catheter position then be made accordingly. With the availability of color Doppler sonography, it has become possible to perform some of these manipulations using information obtained from the Doppler spectra. For example, when normal flow patterns are seen in the graft, the catheter can be incrementally pulled back without the need for repeat angiography. An obstructive flow pattern suggests worsening and the need for continued lysis and repeat angiographic evaluation.

Postprocedure

Following successful thrombolysis, it is often necessary to determine the source of the acute occlusion. The Doppler sonogram can then survey the length of the graft to detect sites of flow abnormality. Most angiograms are performed on one projection. Instances of apparently normal angiograms have been shown, following abnormal Doppler surveys, to have high-grade stenosis visualized by angiography with additional oblique views. The Doppler sonogram can also help to identify sites of dissection. These are more likely in grafts affected by diffuse fibrointimal hyperplasia. This information is useful in determining the need for further intervention in a graft that might appear almost normal by angiography.

Angioplasty and Atherectomy

In the following paragraphs, the percutaneous interventions are discussed as a group with occasional mention given to the strength or weakness of a specific intervention.

Preprocedure

Doppler sonographic arterial mapping adds important information not available

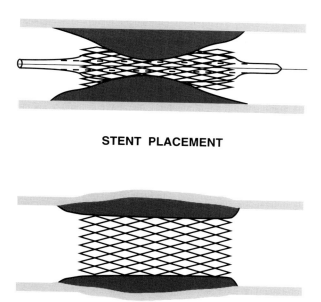

STENT PLACEMENT

CONTROLLED EXPANSION

Figure 8.35. The mechanism of action of stent placement is of a controlled expansion of the treated arterial segment. The stent can be placed at first attempt or following angioplasty. The latter approach offers the advantages of angioplasty while preventing possible complications such as elastic recoil or extension of the dissection.

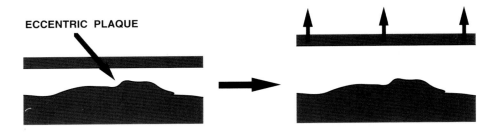

ELASTIC RECOIL

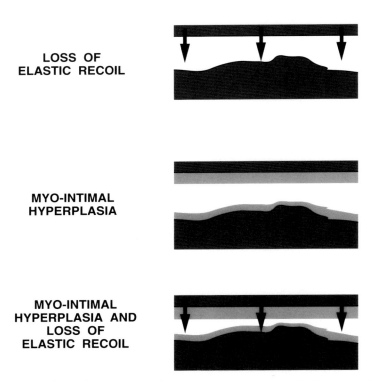

LOSS OF ELASTIC RECOIL

MYO-INTIMAL HYPERPLASIA

MYO-INTIMAL HYPERPLASIA AND LOSS OF ELASTIC RECOIL

Figure 8.36. The reason that atherectomy is favored over angioplasty for the percutaneous treatment of eccentric plaques and nonatherosclerotic lesions is shown here. The application of angioplasty may only cause an apparent increase in lumen size without affecting the plaque itself (*top*). Following the apparent success of the intervention, elastic recoil may cause a return of the stenosis. Local trauma during the intervention may incite fibrointimal proliferation, which will also narrow the lumen. Finally, both effects may combine so that the lesion may return and be more severe than it was originally.

by other noninvasive means. Even before any intervention is attempted, the presence of occluded segments can be readily determined. If these occlusions are treated by surgical approaches, then the patient can be triaged toward surgery. If, however, focal lesions amenable to angioplasty are detected, the likelihood of surgery decreases and the possibility of percutaneous intervention is recommended to the patient. The survey performed is the same as that described in Chapter 7. Doppler sonography is very accurate for detecting segmental occlusions. It will detect most focal stenoses and, in fact, will tend to overestimate lesion severity. This may cause a dilemma when patient symptoms are minimal or absent in the limb being studied.

During the Procedure

Once the suspected stenosis is identified and a is decision made to perform angioplasty, it can be located, the flow velocity can be measured at the stenosis and a peak systolic velocity ratio can be determined. The only significant limitation to

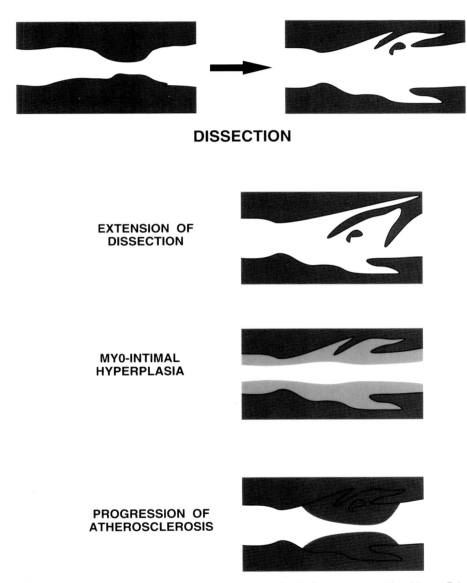

DISSECTION

**EXTENSION OF
DISSECTION**

**MYO-INTIMAL
HYPERPLASIA**

**PROGRESSION OF
ATHEROSCLEROSIS**

Figure 8.37. The different modes of failure of an angioplasty site are summarized here. Extension of the dissection is a problem related to the mode of action of angioplasty. It is seen semi-acutely following the intervention. Fibrointimal hyperplasia plagues almost all of the percutaneous interventions within a few months of the procedure. Progression of atherosclerosis comes into play a few years following the intervention.

this approach is for high-grade lesions having large collaterals just proximal to them. Under these circumstances, sampling in the channel with the stenoses can give falsely low velocity signals since the segment that contains the lesion is in fact subtotally occluded and has decreased blood flow and flow velocities compared to the collateral.

The success of the intervention is nor-mally evaluated by repeat angiography. There are two additional ways of assessing the results of the intervention.

The first is intraluminal sonography. This is performed at a frequency of 10 to 20 MHz using a transducer mounted on a catheter. This catheter transducer is used to image the lesion while slowly moving up and down the arterial segment in question. The results of the intervention are

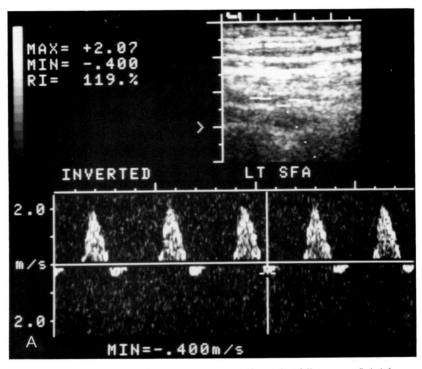

Figure 8.38. **A,** The presence of a moderately severe stenosis of the superficial femoral artery is documented by the presence of a flow abnormality with a peak systolic velocity of 2.07 m/sec. **B,** Sampling of the velocities more proximally shows a peak systolic velocity of 1.03 m/sec. **C,** The waveform of the distal superficial femoral artery does not show evidence of a low-resistance pattern. The peak systolic velocities are also within normal limits at 1.0 msec. **D,** Following percutaneous artherectomy, the peak systolic velocity at the site of artherectomy has decreased to 1.61 m/sec. **E,** The comparative velocity proximal to the site of endarterectomy is also slightly increased to 1.39 m/sec. **F,** The peak systolic velocity distal in the superficial femoral artery is also slightly increased compared to before the procedure with a peak systolic velocity of 1.26 m/sec. Both preceding and following the percutaneous intervention, this approximately 50% stenosis of the superficial femoral artery did not cause any significant resting flow abnormalities demonstrable by the shape of the Doppler waveform. Following atherectomy, the peak systolic velocity ratio at the site of the procedure showed improvement from a preprocedure ratio of 2 to a postprocedure ratio of 1.2. A mild improvement or increase in the peak systolic velocities in the artery proximal and distal to the percutaneous intervention is often seen following the procedure.

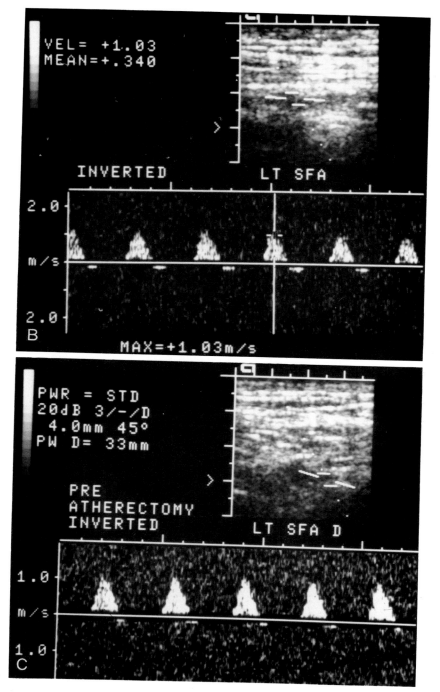

Figure 8.38. B and **C.**

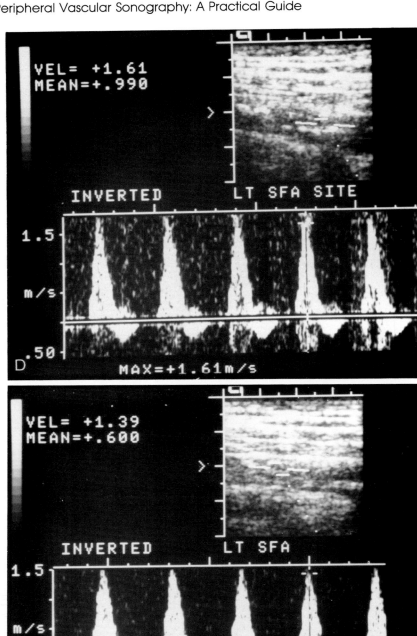

Figure 8.38. D and **E.**

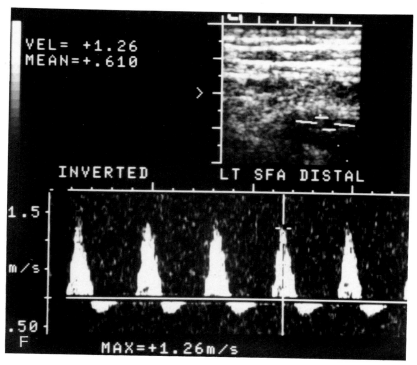

VEL= +1.26
MEAN=+.610

INVERTED   LT SFA DISTAL

1.5

m/s

.50
F

MAX=+1.26m/s

Figure 8.38.   F.

evaluated from the real-time two-dimensional images. Such surveys have shown that 10 to 20% of cases thought to show satisfactory results on angiography have persistent significant reductions in the residual lumen—persistent stenosis—or large dissections within the atherosclerotic plaques that warrant repeat angioplasty or atherectomy. For example, cases of elastic recoil during attempted angioplasty of asymmetric plaques are recognized and the procedure is changed to atherectomy. Repeat intervention is then performed until the postprocedure abnormality has been corrected.

The second approach is color Doppler mapping. Since most of the interventions are likely to be performed in native arteries, deep in the soft tissues, the resolution of gray-scale imaging is insufficient to accurately visualize and characterize most arterial lesions. The Doppler velocity parameters are easily obtained, however.

The same strategy as described for arterial or graft mapping is adopted. The peak systolic velocities are measured both proximal and distal to the stenosis. This type of approach has shown that the peak systolic velocity proximal to the stenosis often improves, while velocities at the stenosis decrease, thereby causing a reduction in the peak systolic velocity. This decrease parallels the improvement in lesion severity following the intervention. This approach can be expanded to using serial noninvasive measurements of artery velocities as a means of following the results of percutaneous interventions. Differences seen early when examining the results of angioplasty (Figs. 8.36 and 8.37) and atherectomy (Fig. 8.38) might be predictive of long-term success of the intervention.

Following the Procedure

The evaluation of the results of percutaneous intervention is an interesting challenge. How does one compare the results of procedure A to the results of procedure B in patients with peripheral vascular disease?

The first question is what should we evaluate?

The obvious answer is symptoms. The patient who undergoes percutaneous intervention is likely to have symptoms of claudication or rest pain. Resolution of the symptom is a clinical endpoint. This, however, may be confused by the presence of symptoms caused by another arterial lesion or by a pathological process unrelated to arterial disease. This is often the case in patients with spinal stenosis or degenerative disk disease. Finally, the arterial symptomatology in nonoperated patients may show a dramatic response to an exercise program alone. It is then difficult to determine which caused the improvement in symptoms, the percutaneous intervention or the adoption of an exercise program following the intervention.

The second set of parameters that is followed is that of ankle-brachial pressures supplemented by pulse-volume recordings or segmental pressure measurements. At the outset, many diabetics cannot be followed since their noncompliant vessels are difficult to compress, making pressure measurements inaccurate. Among patients who have serial monitoring of their pressures, three scenarios are likely. In the first, early lesions that develop within the first 2 years following the intervention manifest themselves by a drop in pressure on any one of the serial follow-up examinations made at 6 weeks, 3 months, 6 months, 12 months, and then yearly. These measurable pressure drops occur despite the absence of symptoms in up to two-thirds of patients and relate to the development of a significant stenosis in the graft. In the second scenario, the earlier lesions are not detected on a given visit. The lesion progresses to total occlusion in the interval of time before a return visit to the noninvasive laboratory. Finally, a third scenario sees a persistent improvement in ankle-brachial index despite graft occlusion. This is likely because of the better care undergone by the patient who has now adopted an exercise program and stopped smoking. The distinction between these three outcomes is normally made by angiography. Doppler sonography is also very useful since graft peak systolic velocities decrease in response to a developing stenosis before there is any evidence of a pressure drop detectable by ankle-brachial index measurements.

Color Doppler imaging can be further used to localize the site of the stenosis and to estimate its severity. The issue of what constitutes a significant change between repeat visits has yet to be determined. In the carotid, a change of 30% in the Doppler velocity is considered significant and corresponds to a 20% change in lesion severity. These changes can be seen in a peripheral graft or artery even before the proximal velocity has dropped below the critical value of 0.45 m/sec. Zones showing more than a tripling of the peak systolic velocity ratio should be considered to represent significant stenosis of greater than 75% lumen diameter narrowing.

There are no other noninvasive approaches currently available that permit this type of serial monitoring. A developing technology is magnetic resonance (MR) angiography. Focal lesions can manifest themselves as areas of signal loss on the MR angiograms. A current limitation of this technology is its inability to grade stenosis above 50% with any accuracy.

Invasive evaluations should be put in two broad categories. The first is sonography, the second angiography.

Intravascular sonography is a procedure requiring entry into the artery and physical manipulation across the area of narrowing. This type of approach is hard to justify since the stenosed segment is often likely to be smaller than the imaging catheter. The risk of complications related to the manipulation are not negligible.

Quantitative angiography is the most objective method available for quantitating the severity of arterial stenosis. It is normally done with two projections to better define the lesion and requires high-resolution cut-film angiography and not digital approaches. The reproducibility for lumen diameter changes has been reported to be better than 5%. This approach does require catheterization.

Summary

The early role of Doppler sonography in evaluating perigraft masses and confirming graft occlusions has broadened. It replaces angiography in selected cases when localized lesions—AV fistulas, pseudoaneurysms, or focal stenoses—are detected. Doppler sonography is also a flexible and cost-effective means of detecting perioperative failures and is becoming critical for the serial monitoring of arterial bypass graft function. This application is broadening to include a more prominent role in the serial monitoring of the results of percutaneous interventions.

SUGGESTED READINGS

Aldoori MI, Baird RN. Prospective assessment of carotid endarterectomy by clinical and ultrasonic methods. Br J Surg 1987;74:926–929.

Altin RS, Flicker S, Naidech HJ. Pseudoaneurysm and arteriovenous fistula after femoral artery catheterization: association with low femoral punctures. AJR 1989;152:629–631.

Atnip RG, Wengrovitz M, Gifford RR, Neumyer MM, Thiele BL. A rational approach to recurrent carotid stenosis. J Vasc Surg 1990;11:511–516.

Bandyk DF, Cato RF, Towne JB. A low flow velocity predicts failure of femoropopliteal and femorotibial bypass grafts. Surgery 1985;98:799–807.

Bandyk DF, Jorgensen RA, Towne JB. Intraoperative assessment of in situ saphenous vein arterial grafts using pulsed Doppler spectral analysis. Arch Surg 1986;121:292–299.

Bandyk DF, Kaebnick HW, Adams MB, Towne JB. Turbulence occurring after carotid bifurcation endarterectomy: a harbinger of residual and recurrent carotid stenosis. J Vasc Surg 1988;7:261–274.

Bandyk DF, Moldenhauer P, Lipchik E, Schreiber E, Pohl L, Cato R, Towne JB. Accuracy of duplex scanning in the detection of stenosis after carotid endarterectomy. J Vasc Surg 1988;8:696–702.

Bandyk DF, Seabrook GR, Moldenhauer P, et al. Hemodynamics of vein graft stenosis. J Vasc Surg 1988;8:688–695.

Cook JM, Thompson BW, Barnes RW. Is routine duplex examination after carotid endarterectomy justified? J Vasc Surg 1990;12:334–340.

Grigg MJ, Nicolaides AN, Wolfe JH. Detection and grading of femorodistal vein graft stenoses: duplex velocity measurements compared with angiography. J Vasc Surg 1988;8:661–666.

Hedgcock MW, Eisenberg RL, Gooding GA. Complications relating to vascular prosthetic grafts. J Can Assoc Radiol 1980;31:137–142.

Leahy AL, McCollum PT, Feeley TM, et al. Duplex ultrasonography and selection of patients for carotid endarterectomy: plaque morphology or luminal narrowing? J Vasc Surg 1988;8:558–562.

Middleton WD, Picus DD, Marx MV, Melson GL. Color Doppler sonography of hemodialysis vascular access: comparison with angiography. AJR 1989;152:633–639.

Polak JF, Donaldson MC, Whittemore AD, Mannick JA, O'Leary DH. Pulsatile masses surrounding vascular prostheses: real-time US color flow imaging. Radiology 1989;170:363–366.

Scheible W, Skram C, Leopold GR. High resolution real-time sonography of hemodialysis vascular access complications. AJR 1980;134:1173–1176.

Schwartz RA, Peterson GJ, Noland KA, Hower JF Jr, Naunheim KS. Intraoperative duplex scanning after carotid artery reconstruction: a valuable tool. J Vasc Surg 1988;7:620–624.

Tordoir JH, de Bruin HG, Hoeneveld H, Eikelboom BC, Kitslaar PJ. Duplex ultrasound scanning in the assessment of arteriovenous fistulas created for hemodialysis access: comparison with digital subtraction angiography. J Vasc Surg 1989;10:122–128.

Wilson SE, Wolf GL, Cross AP. Percutaneous transluminal angioplasty versus operation for peripheral arteriosclerosis. Report of a prospective randomized trial in a selected group of patients. J Vasc Surg 1989;9:1–9.

APPENDIX

Vascular Evaluation Forms

BRIGHAM AND WOMEN'S HOSPITAL
NON-INVASIVE VASCULAR LABORATORY

CAROTID ARTERY EVALUATION

PRESENTING SYMPTOMS : _____

_____

_____

_____

_____

DATE : ___ / ___ / _____ . _____

PHYSICIAN : _____

TIA _____ AMA. FUG. _____ CVA _____ BRUITS _____

ENDARTERECTOMIES _____ PRE-OPERATIVE SCREENING _____ FOLLOW-UP _____ .

REAL TIME IMAGING

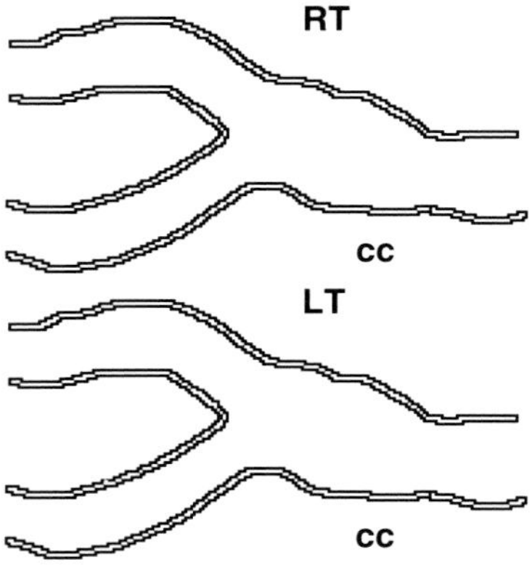

C - W DOPPLER (HZ)

RIGHT	LEFT	
_____	_____	CCA
_____	_____	ECA
_____	_____	ICA

PULSE DOPPLER (M / SEC)

RIGHT	LEFT	
___/___	___/___	CCA
___/___	___/___	ECA
___/___	___/___	ICA

RT
ic
ec
cc
LT
ic
ec
cc

PERIORBITAL DOPPLER

RIGHT	LEFT
SO_____	SO_____
ST_____	ST_____

_____

_____

_____

PRELIMINARY:

RT_____ LT_____

BRIGHAM AND WOMEN'S HOSPITAL

NON-INVASIVE VASCULAR LABORATORY

LOWER EXTREMITY VENOUS EVALUATION

PRESENTING SYMPTOMS : _____

_____

_____

_____

DATE : ___ / ___ / ___

PHYSICIAN : _____

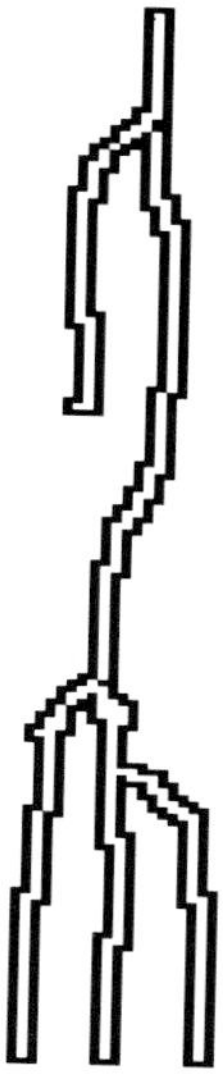

RIGHT   **LEFT**

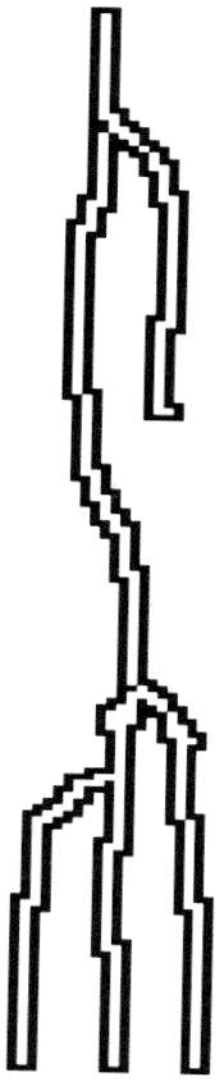

	AUGMENTATION		PHASICITY		VALSALVA	
	RIGHT	LEFT	RIGHT	LEFT	RIGHT	LEFT
CFV						
SFV						
PFV						
POP						
P T						
PER						

VENOUS RESPONSE
0 = absent,
1 = decreased
2 = normal

IMPRESSION: _____

_____

_____

_____

_____

BRIGHAM AND WOMEN'S HOSPITAL

NON-INVASIVE VASCULAR LABORATORY

UPPER EXTREMITY VENOUS EVALUATION

PRESENTING SYMPTOMS : _____

_____

_____

_____

DATE : ___ / ___ / ___

PHYSICIAN : _____

_____

_____

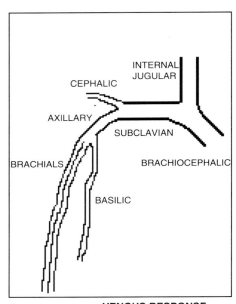

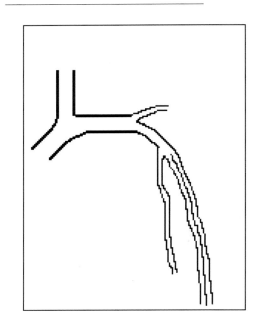

VENOUS RESPONSE
o=absent, 1=decreased, 2=normal

	R	L	R	L
	DOPPLER SIGNALS		**DIAMETER CHANGE**	
BCEPH				
PROX SUB				
DIST SUB				
AXIL				

_____

_____

_____

FINAL   IMPRESSION: _____

_____

_____

_____

BRIGHAM AND WOMEN'S HOSPITAL
NON-INVASIVE VASCULAR LABORATORY

LOWER EXTREMITY GRAFT EVALUATION

PRESENTING SYMPTOMS : _____

_____

_____

_____

DATE :   /   /   .____

PHYSICIAN : _____

VELOCITIES

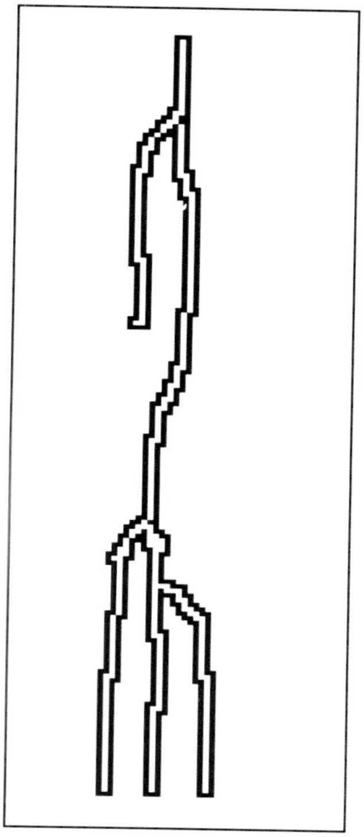

RIGHT   LEFT

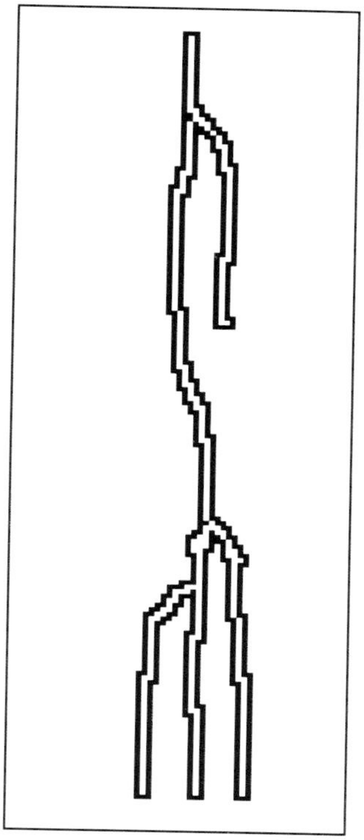

FINAL   IMPRESSION: _____

_____

_____

_____

INDEX